16⁰⁰

Quantitative Techniques
for Hospital Planning
and Control

Quantitative Techniques for Hospital Planning and Control

John R. Griffith
University of Michigan

Lexington Books
D.C. Heath and Company
Lexington, Massachusetts
Toronto   London

Copyright © 1972 by D.C. Heath and Company.

All rights reserved. No part of this publication may be reproduced or transmitted in any form or by any means, electronic or mechanical, including photocopy, recording, or any information storage or retrieval system, without permission in writing from the publisher.

Second printing September, 1973.

Published simultaneously in Canada.

Printed in the United States of America.

International Standard Book Number: 0-669-84087-4.

Library of Congress Catalog Card Number: 72-3550.

To Helen

Contents

	List of Figures	xi
	List of Tables	xv
	Preface	xvii
Chapter 1	**Introduction**	1
	The Feedback Loop: Meaning of Planning and Control	1
	Demand in Hospital Planning and Control	4
	The Role of the Hospital	13
Part I	*Forecasting Demand*	15
Chapter 2	**The Forecasting Problem and Simple Time Series Analysis**	17
	The Logic of Demand Analysis and Forecasting	17
	A Procedure for Forecasting	22
	Forecasting Expected Values of a Stochastic Process from Historic Data on the Same Process	23
	Appendix	31
Chapter 3	**Forecasting by Multivariate Analysis and Techniques for Forecasting Variation**	37
	Multivariate Analysis	38
	Examples of Multivariate Analysis of Demand for Inpatient Care	46
	Short-Term Forecasting Techniques	50
	Analysis of Randomness	55

Chapter 4	**Determining Population Service Areas and Calculating Use Rates**	65
	The Concept of a Service Population	65
	Equal Likelihood Service Areas–The Poland-Lembcke Procedure	68
	Relevance and Commitment Indices for Service Area Definition	75
	Data Collection for Service Area Population Estimates	78
	Birth and Death Rates as Service Area Indicators	79
	Use Rates	81
	Application to the Urban Setting	82
	Forecasting from Use Rate and Service Area Population	85
	Appendix–Data Collection Aids for Service Area Definition	87
Chapter 5	**Demand Forecasts in Specialized Situations**	93
	Demand Rates	93
	Demand Rates on Bases Other than Population	96
	Analysis of Variance to Evaluate Demand Rates	96
	Forecasting Demand for Nonexistent Services	99
	Summary	110
Part II	*Models for Resource Allocation*	111
Chapter 6	**Total Value Analysis**	113
	Nature of Resource Allocation Problems	113
	Inventory Control Problems– Deterministic Model	121
	Other Uses of Total Value Analysis	126
	Summary	133

Chapter 7	**Queueing and Simulation Models for Resource Allocation**	135
	Resource Allocation in Stochastic Processes	135
	Queueing Theory Models	140
	Simulation as a Solution to the Facility Size Problem	146
	Use of Simulation in Scheduling Policies	154
Chapter 8	**PERT and Mathematical Programming Models**	167
	Introduction	167
	PERT and CPM	168
	Modeling for Mathematical Programming	175
	Programming Models	200
	Hospital Applications of Mathematical Programming	202
Chapter 9	**Evaluating Capital Investment Opportunities**	209
	Introduction	209
	Decisions Involving Principally Monetary Costs	210
	Cost-Benefit Analysis	225
	Capital Budgeting Decisions	238
Part III	*Control Systems*	245
Chapter 10	**Nature and Application of Control Systems in Hospitals**	247
	Concept of Control Systems	247
	General Considerations in Control Systems	251
	Statistical Quality Control Techniques	259
	Meaning of Statistical Deviation	276

| Chapter 11 | Examples of Hospital Control Systems | 279 |

Introduction 279
Resource Control Systems 280
Quality Control Systems in Other than
   Medical Systems 303
CASH-Type Nursing Quality Instrument 323

| Chapter 12 | Measuring the Quality of the Medical Care Process | 331 |

Introduction 331
Manual Information-Gathering Systems 334
The Professional Activity Study—A
   Partially Computerized Procedural-
   Outcome Measurement System 337

| Chapter 13 | Advanced Information Systems for Hospital Planning and Control | 367 |

Characteristics of a Comprehensive
   Information System 367
The CUPIS Data Base 371
BURP—A Sophisticated Quality and
   Utilization Monitor System 364
Towards A Working Comprehensive
   Information System 379

Notes 385

Index 397

About the Author 405

List of Figures

1-1	Basic Feedback Loop	2
1-2	Multiple Feedback Loop	3
1-3	Basic Feedback Loop Modified for Demand	5
1-4	The Citizen and Health Care	9
1-5	Simplified Model of the Medical Care Process	10
2-1	Visual Projection of Patient-Day Demand	25
2-2	Regression Line of Patient Days in ELB Hospital	28
2-3	Patient Days at the ELB Hospital on Logarithmic Scale	30
3-1	Histogram of Absenteeism	56
4-1	Hypothetical Geographic Region	69
4-2	Hypothetical Geographic Region Showing Equal Likelihood Service Area	72
4-3	Hypothetical Geographic Region Showing Relevance Index Values	77
4-4	Hypothetical Road Map	87
5-1	Form for Survey of Expected Demand	102
5-2	Patient-Condition Checklist	106
6-1	Total Costs of a Hypothetical Laboratory Service, Manual Method	115
6-2	Costs per Unit, Manual Method	115

6-3	Total Cost of a Hypothetical Laboratory Service, Auto Analyzer	116
6-4	Cost per Unit, Auto Analyzer Method	116
6-5	Cost per Unit, Auto Analyzer Method; Cost per Unit, Manual Method	117
6-6	Cost of Resources Used in Providing a Health Service	119
6-7	Cost of Illness versus Units of Service Provided	119
6-8	Total Costs versus Units of Service	119
6-9	Inventory of a Routine Supply Item over Time	121
6-10	Annual Costs of Varying Order Quantities	123
6-11	Probability Distribution of Demand for Service D	127
6-12	Total Cost of Meeting Demand	128
7-1	Simplified Obstetrical Care Flow Chart	141
7-2	Estimating Area of an Irregular Surface	148
7-3	Average Census as a Function of Decision Level	157
7-4	Average Overflow as a Function of Decision Level	158
7-5	Probability of Turning One or More Patients Away per Day versus B	161
7-6	Optimum B-Level as a Function of Cost Ratios	162

8-1	PERT Chart of a Hypothetical Program	171
8-2	PERT Chart of a Hypothetical Program Showing Critical Path	172
8-3	Graphic Solution: Hospital Production Model	180
8-4	Graphic Solution: Hospital Production Model	183
10-1	Components of MonitorProcess	248
10-2	Nursing Audit Analysis: Daily Mean Values	265
10-3	Nursing Audit Analysis: Daily Deviations	265
10-4	Control System for Nursing Quality	268
10-5	Control Limits on "Normal Tissue" Reports	275
11-1	Comparative Report: Statement of Revenues, Statement of Expenses, and Operational and Departmental Indicators	287
11-2	Internal Report: Statement of Revenues, Statement of Expenses, and Operational and Departmental Indicators	291
11-3	Internal Report: Statistical Report and Man Hours Paid	295
11-4	Quality Control Check Sheet I: Housekeeping Department	306
11-5	Quality Control Check Sheet II: Housekeeping Department	307

11-6	Quality Control Check Sheet I: Dietary Department	309
11-7	Quality Control Check Sheet II: Dietary Department	310
11-8	Quality Control Plan: Dietary Department	312
11-9	Nursing Quality Instrument: Work Sheet Number 2	324
11-10	Nursing Quality Instrument: Work Sheet Number 5	325
12-1	PAS 1971-72 MAP Case Abstract	339
12-2	1971 Birth Abstract	343
12-3	Specimen Monthly Diagnosis Listing	346
12-4	A Form—Discharge Analysis	350
12-5	B Form—Discharge Analysis	351
12-6	M1 Form—Basic Data, Findings, Investigation	355
12-7	M2 Form—Investigation Management	357
12-8	S Form—Length-of-Stay Comparison	360
12-9	Quality of Care Report	364
13-1	BURP Model	377

List of Tables

2-1		Medical and Surgical Patient Days at ELB Hospital	24
3-1		Operating Room Demand	52
3-2		Scheduled Surgery Demand	53
4-1		Usage of Area Hospitals: Central County and Environs	73
5-1		Comparative Demand for Home Care	100
7-1		Distribution of Length of Stay in Labor Rooms	142
7-2		Distribution of Length of Stay in Delivery Rooms	143
7-3		Distribution of Length of Stay in Postpartum Area	144
7-4		Predicted Usage of Delivery Rooms	144
7-5		Cumulative Probability of Discharge from Labor Rooms	150
8-1		Hospital Technology Matrix	178
8-2		Facility Constraints	179
8-3		Maximum Patient Capacity per Year	179
8-4		Nursing Care Task Values	205
9-1		Schedule of Expenses for Ambulatory Patient Facility	228
9-2		Discounted Values of Expenses for Ambulatory Patient Facility	230

9-3	Comparison of New Program Activities	237
9-4	Net Present Cost per Beneficiary at Varying Interest	238
9-5	Present Value of $1 Received at the End of the "Year"	242
9-6	Present Value of $1 Received Annually at the End of Each "Year" for N Years	243
11-1	Supplementary Sampling for Varying Percentages Acceptable	311

Preface

This work is intended for the manager of hospitals and related health care institutions, for the operations research specialist interested in hospital applications, and for students in each of these fields. It attempts to provide conceptual understanding of a variety of techniques useful in hospital decisions—particularly planning, forecasting, scheduling, cost control and quality control—and a detailed discussion of the practicalities of applying the techniques. Measurement, data collection, utility of solutions, dangers implicit in common assumptions, and examples of promising applications are discussed in depth. Technology, on the other hand, is simplified as far as reasonable conceptual accuracy will permit. Advanced mathematics, including calculus, has been strictly avoided. Graphic and elementary algebraic solutions are common. Some elementary statistical and probability concepts, principally regarding means, deviations, and hypothesis testing are required. Technical facility with these concepts is necessary only for a relatively few identifiable sections. These sections are easily within the grasp of present-day students in management; they are elementary for operations researchers and can be skipped by most practicing managers without serious loss.

In this way I hope to have constructed a book which will provide a problem-oriented common ground which will facilitate communication between the manager and the operations researcher, and speed the sound application of these valuable aids to hospital management.

The book has been nearly six years in preparation. So many people have helped me with it that I cannot possibly thank them all. For various and sundry reasons, however, these people made extraordinary contributions which were critical to the work: Professors John D. Thompson, Robert B. Fetter and Donald C. Riedel, of Yale University, Dr. Vergil Slee of the Commission on Professional and Hospital Activities, Professors William L. Dowling and Roy Penchansky of Michigan, and Lawrence A. Hill, formerly at Michigan and now at the Rhode Island Hospital. The W.K. Kellogg Foundation supported me for much of the sabbatical year during which the first draft was written. Miss Mary L. Uranga, my secretary for most of this period, did as much of the interminable typing of manuscript as anyone could be expected to do. Several dozen students, mostly at Michigan, suffered through the sometimes incomprehensible early drafts. I thank all these people most sincerely and gratefully. Hopefully the book will provide for others what they gave to me—an opportunity to learn.

John R. Griffith

Ann Arbor, Michigan
1972

1 Introduction

The Feedback Loop: Meaning of Planning and Control

One way to describe a hospital is as a collection of functional service units, each of which performs some specialized task. The departmental organizational structure—nursing, dietary, radiology, laundry, etc.—is in fact built this way. In the typical acute hospital there may be upwards of twenty functional units of this kind. The actual functions they perform vary widely, from removing waste to psychiatric counseling. However, from a management viewpoint, all of these units can be represented as a basic *feedback loop* or *cybernetic process*. In each there is a supervisor or group of supervisors whose job it is to:

1. Establish some expectations and/or goals for the operation, including both quantity and quality of performance
2. Order the arrangement of resources—men, material, and facilities—into a system designed to reach these expectations
3. Compare the actual performance with expectations and correct the system to improve achievement of expectations

This operation can be represented as shown in figure 1-1.

The notion of the feedback loop is not unique to hospitals. It occurs in a variety of other situations including biological, mechanical, and human systems. The simplest illustration is the common thermostat-furnace system. This mechanical system consists of three elements: a space to be heated, a monitor (the thermostat) which senses the amount of heat, and the furnace, which provides heat under the control of the thermostat. Feedback systems always contain similar elements, and always work by comparing actual performance against expectations. (The expectations in the thermostat-furnace system are the preset ranges of temperature on the thermostat. Without these, the system would not function.)

Most supervisors, in hospitals or elsewhere, operate roughly in the manner suggested in figure 1-1. They may not have quantitative or even objective expectations or measures of performance, but they and their workers have personal and subjective notions. They tend to operate their functional areas so that performance meets these notions. There are, however, certain noticeable limitations in relying solely upon these subjective assessments. First, different supervisors will have different expectations, and thus performance will vary

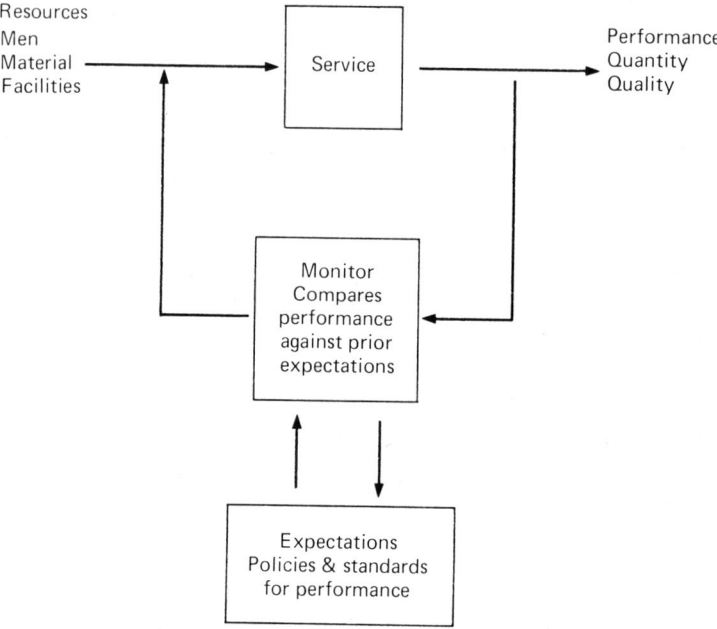

Figure 1-1. Basic Feedback Loop.

when supervisors change. Secondly, the possibility of changing these expectations is limited until they become at least partially objective and quantifiable. Third and most significant, it is extremely difficult for management to assess the performance of the supervisor if the performance and expectations of the function are not quantified.

The third disadvantage of the lack of objective and quantitative expectations and performance assessment is worthy of closer examination. Consider a functional supervisor or hospital department head who works solely on a subjective evaluation of performance. His superior, the hospital administrator or assistant administrator, is often at a loss. If the department is professional, the administrator is not familiar with the professional goals which the supervisor may have learned over years of training. Even if he were, he has little or no exposure to the information necessary to make the evaluation, because he does not see the process itself. It is quite possible that his expectations and the department head's will become widely divergent, enough so to prove very troublesome at some time. From the department head's viewpoint, there is no way good performance on his part can be recognized, let alone rewarded. He is also in a difficult position with regard to failure. Since the measure of failure is solely his perception of it, his ability to gain support in correcting it depends on his ability to present a persuasive case. He may have to make his case in competition with several other department heads. This is the situation in which most hospital department heads and administrators find themselves, because in fact the technology of measuring performance and expectations has not yet progressed far in hospitals.

If both the expectations and ways of measuring performance necessary to operate a feedback system can be made more clear, then many of these problems can be eliminated or reduced. As soon as there is a quantitative test of the function performance, there is an automatic test of the supervisor's performance. The superior who must monitor the supervisor can ask, "What is the success rate of the system of function and supervisor combined?" This in effect makes the original system a subsystem, and a new feedback loop can be constructed as shown in figure 1-2. Thus the concept of the feedback loop is expansible to any level of organization, so long as the information necessary to perform the monitor function can be communicated clearly enough. Objectivity and quantification, of course, become devices to increase clear communication.

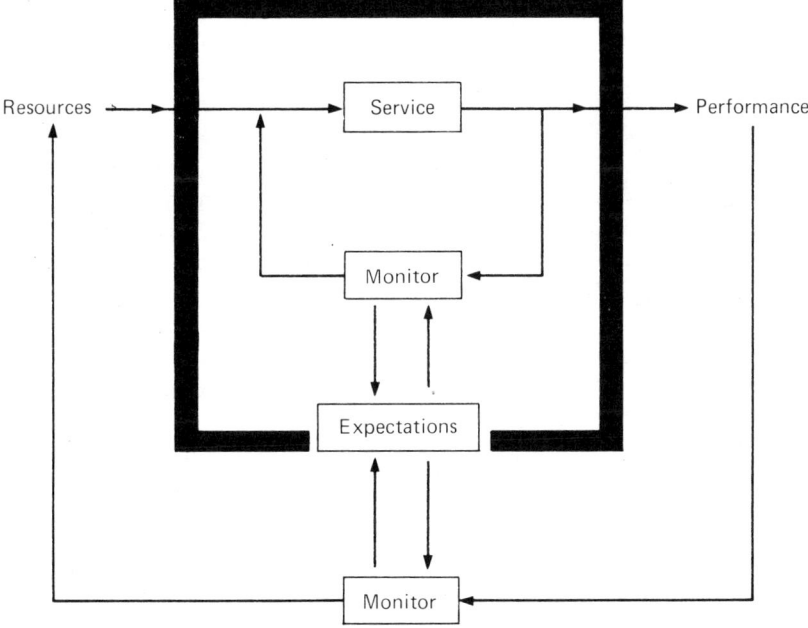

Figure 1-2. Multiple Feedback Loop.

There is another important result of reducing the information to quantitative terms. The information can then be readily stored, and it becomes accessible for management study. A variety of questions can be posed and answered by analysis of this data. For example:

— Can the arrangement of resources be altered to advantage?
— What changes will growth of the organization require?
— Should expectations be changed?
— What causes performance failure?

Although the distinction is not sharp, this sort of use of quantitative information is *planning*. The feedback loop use is *control*.

This text explores the problems of applying the concepts of planning and control to hospital organizations. The identification of what should be measured, the techniques for measurement, and the techniques for using the measurements in gaining improvement in performance are taken up within a hospital setting.

Demand in Hospital Planning and Control

In attempting to apply the concepts of figure 1-1 to hospitals, a second characteristic common to nearly all functions appears. With only trivial exceptions, *no hospital function can be effectively performed in the absence of a demand for it.* Also, demand in a hospital is generated by processes different from the functional services, and it often has a large random or unpredictable component. From the point of view of the supervisor of an individual unit, understanding, predicting, and adjusting to the variation in demand often becomes the central problem of controlling performance. The model can be adapted to show this element as in figure 1-3. The supervisor who performs as monitor has two possibilities to improve performance. The first is by operating upon the arrangement of resources. The second is by operating upon the demand. Thus in some situations part of the demand can be scheduled, or other actions can be taken which reduce the impact of variability on performance.

Modifying the basic feedback loop as shown in figure 1-3 brings the concept of demand for service into the hospital management problem at a level coequal with resources, performance, and expectations. It permits classification of all information necessary to describe a functional service into four categories:

1. *Demand*—the amount of service required
2. *Resources (inputs)*—the manpower materials and equipment available to perform the function
3. *Performance (outputs)*—the amount of service rendered

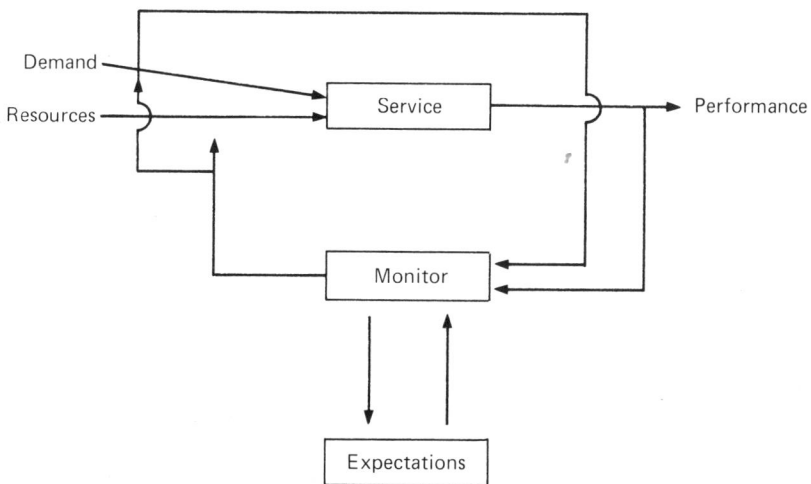

Figure 1-3. Basic Feedback Loop Modified for Demand.

4. *Expectations*—standards or policies regarding the function, including quality and efficiency of performance, resource allocation policies, scheduling rules, etc.

A number of extremely important management questions are approached by the study of demand, including the relation of demand to notions of what might be needed, the expectations for the system in terms of ability to meet demand, factors influencing demand, and the loss of performance due to unpredictable demand.

Because of its utility, the modified feedback loop shown in figure 1-3 will be the basic model of hospital operation used in this text. Any hospital can be conceived as a set of such loops, each monitored by others providing supervision of the process. Each patient service fits into the model. The job done by the doctor of analyzing the patient's needs and issuing the demands to other services can be similarly modeled, and this will be done in the following section. Certain hospital departments do not serve patients directly, but perform functions for the support of the medical services (plant maintenance, accounting, personnel, etc.). These departments usually experience demand from other departments rather than directly from doctors and patients, but the model still fits. These are the departments where exceptions to the rule about demand occur. Some of their functions could go on in the absence of demand. In any case, the level of work is independent of the level of demand. Such activities as preparing monthly statements and doing routine periodic maintenance are examples.

The generation of demand is the next question of interest: Where does demand come from, what is the underlying process which generates it, and what is important in a thorough description of the demand? For most hospital functions, demand comes from the decisions made by doctors about patients, but these decisions themselves are the result of a complex process. This process, basic to what goes on in the hospital but occurring largely outside it, is now explored.

The Demand for Medical Care

Most of the services of hospitals are not sought directly by the patient. They are demanded as a part of a larger process through which the citizen seeks the treatment or prevention of some health problem. The demand for laboratory examinations, hospital admission, x-ray, and other services is not generated by the patient but by his doctor. An understanding of the process by which demand is generated must go back to the original demand for medical care. For measurable demand to exist for medical care, three factors must be present in the attitudes of the person seeking care: (*a*) he must be convinced he has a reason to seek medical care or at least advice; (*b*) he must be able to find the care he seeks; and (*c*) he must be convinced the care will be worth the price he pays for it. Different individuals are likely to have differing viewpoints on whether to seek care in a given situation. A "persistent cough" may be reason to one man, but not to another. A two-hour bus ride and a three-hour wait may discourage some patients although it is a small matter to others. Finally, how much the patient is willing to pay, and how much a given service will cost him, depends on a number of factors which change from individual to individual. How much money the individual has, whether he has insurance coverage, or whether he is eligible for certain programs of free care will affect his demand for health care.

When the patient does decide to seek medical care, his normal course of action is to turn to a doctor. The doctor can request for the patient any of a number of services in the hospital, through the hospital, or independently of the hospital. Again, which services he actually demands depends upon a combination of factors, including his perception of what is wrong, the patient's financial and social position, and the availability of services.[1]

Considering the quantity of health care rendered to a community of people leads to the development of a long series of questions which can be shown to affect the demand upon the medical care system. Taken as a set, the answers to these questions might describe why a given group of people used more or fewer health-care resources, or received greater benefit from the resources than some other group. Many of the questions, however, are difficult in themselves, and further problems are introduced by the fact that the questions are interlocking. The following is a list of factors which might be analyzed before reaching a full understanding of demand for health services in a community. These factors provide a background to understand both the demand for care and the quality of care as rendered by a physician or in an institution in a specific situation.

1. Attitudes of the people regarding illness and death, their interest in preventing death, and their willingness to tolerate illness. These attitudes include attitudes towards such matters as birth control, abortion, suicide, and aging
2. Economic level of the community and its ability to devote resources to the prevention and cure of illness and the prolongation of life
3. Environmental health problems such as the presence of endemic infectious disease, environmental pollution, and social, economic and genetic factors predisposing to mental and physical illness
4. Morbidity, the actual incidence and prevalence of disease
5. Methods of financing health care
6. Attitudes towards the seeking of professional health care, such as the interest of the population in seeking periodic physicals for early diagnosis, prenatal care, or care of well infants. Also the attitude of the population towards the use of "quacks" and self-diagnosis and treatment
7. The availability of professional health care, including primarily doctors but also other health-care professionals
8. The attitudes of physicians regarding the extent of diagnostic services which should be rendered, particularly in regard to early diagnosis or secondary prevention
9. The attitude of physicians regarding the selection of treatment, including attitudes towards the prolongation of life in chronic disease, and attitudes towards the selection of debatable therapeutic alternatives as for example, the use of psychoanalysis versus group therapy or chemotherapy
10. Attitudes of physicians towards the use of institutional resources, that is the willingness of physicians to use hospital services on outpatient basis, as well as the tendency to admit patients to the hospital versus treating them in the home or in the office
11. The availability of institutional resources, including not only the number and variety of hospitals and related institutions available to the population, but also their convenience, attractiveness, and social, economic, or geographic restrictions which might be imposed on their use
12. The availability and adequacy of resources within the hospital or other institution for diagnosis and treatment

The process by which social institutions interact upon the patient and the doctor to influence the demand for health care is shown in figure 1-4. It should be noted that in this figure the "hospital" as a single entity is not shown, but the functional services are shown as manpower and facilities available to the physician. The upper level of the figure shows a variety of the institutions which are not primarily providers of health care, but which act on the citizen and the doctor to influence the level of demand.

A number of simplifications have been made in figure 1-4. The role of health-care professions in the social agencies and the occasional provision of care by these agencies (namely, emergency care by industrial health units) have been omitted. The interaction of the professionals and the care institutions is not shown. Quacks and cultists have not been shown. Finally and most important, the arrows on the right half of the figure do not reflect the extensive and important interaction, which occurs in both directions, between the citizen, his doctor, other professionals, and various care institutions.

The doctor has been shown in a central position as befits his importance. He alone has the legal authorization to both diagnose and prescribe for any illness. He directly controls a very large fraction of the interaction between the citizen and other professionals and completely controls the use of certain professions such as laboratory technicians. In addition, with only minor exceptions, a doctor is necessary to place the citizen in contact with any of the care institutions.

It is with these portions of the process, where the doctor draws upon the services of other professionals and the supporting facilities, that the hospital is directly concerned. In general a hospital is an organization of manpower and facilities which is brought into the process of medical care by the doctor. The extent of facilities and services included in the hospital varies with the individual institution. At the least, the hospital will include an organized medical staff relationship with the doctor, employee relationship to most of the professions in the right center section of figure 1-4, and general inpatient facilities. At the most, as exemplified by the largest teaching hospitals, the hospital includes employee relationships with nearly all the health-care professions, including doctors, and all major forms of facilities shown as care institutions. Regardless of how large the scope of activities of a given hospital, its roles are (*a*) to fill the demands for specific services made upon it by the individual doctors treating individual patients, and (*b*) to an increasing degree, to provide for the systematic review and improvement of the process by which the doctor discovers and meets the patient's needs. This process can be called the "medical care process," and it is shown in detail in figure 1-5.

The medical care process begins with the individual patient seeking the services of an individual physician. The initial decision to seek care is usually the patient's. All subsequent decisions are generally those of his physician, except that the patient may at any time terminate his relationship with his physician and break off the process. The physician makes his decisions based on his professional assessment of the total collection of patient's needs and wishes. The medical care process may involve no other individual or institution. In fact, for the great majority of the occurrences the doctor will not find it necessary to go

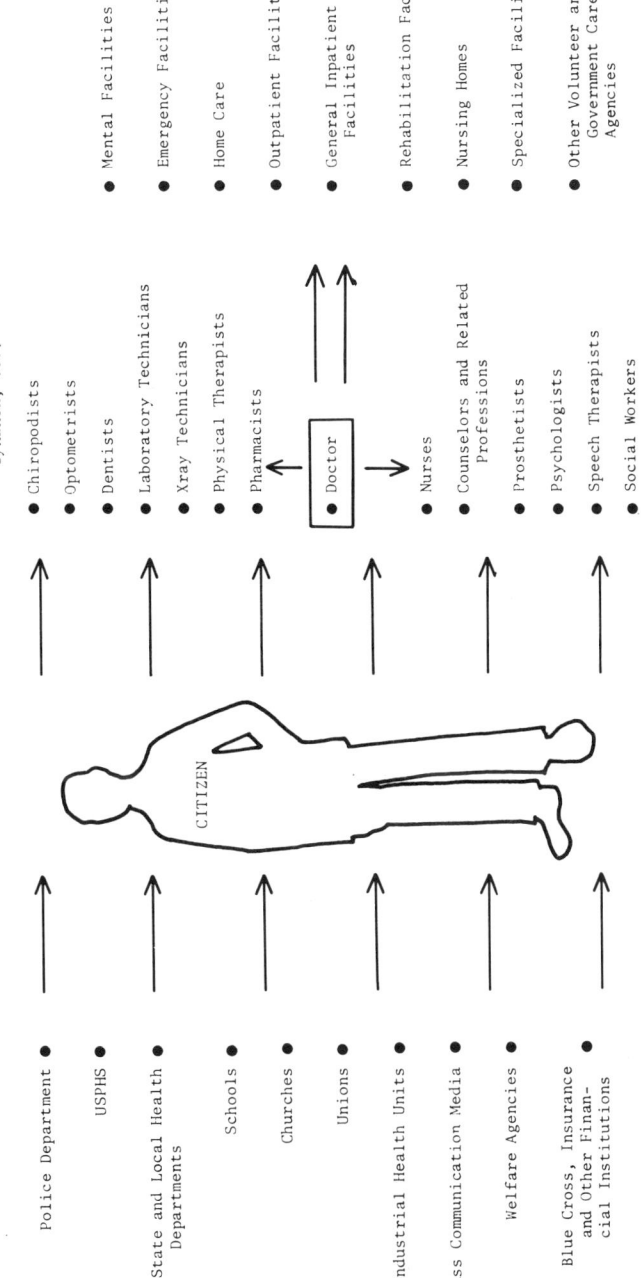

Figure 1-4. The Citizen and Health Care. After "The Complexity of Medical Care," Report of the Commission on the Cost of Medical Care.

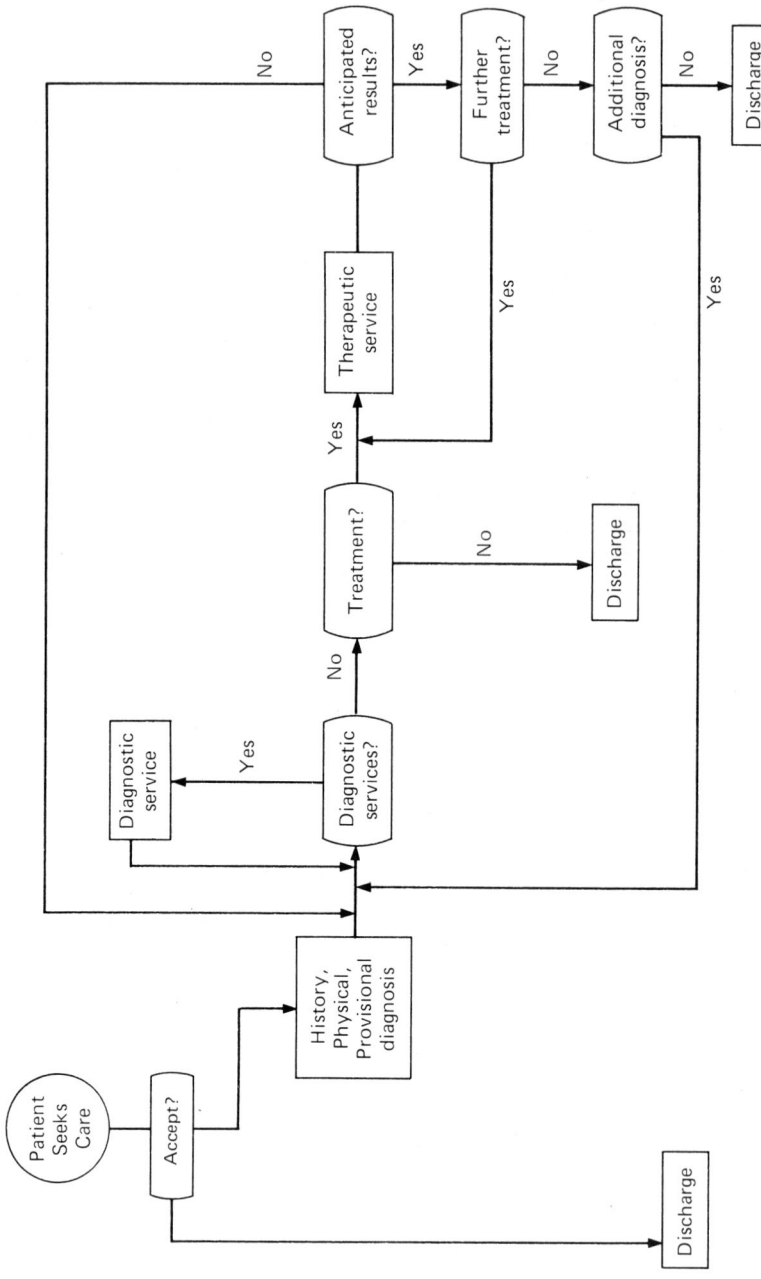

Figure 1-5. Simplified Model of the Medical Care Process.

much beyond the resources he has immediately at hand. As the patient's disease becomes more complex, the process becomes more complicated and the number of additional resources the doctor will need increases. The hospital, as the largest single collection of these resources, soon enters the medical care process.

When the patient presents himself to the physician (the left side of figure 1-5), the doctor's first decision, usually made quite automatically, is whether or not he will accept the patient. (Decision points are shown in figure 1-5 and subsequent figures by the oval-ended boxes.) In a few cases the doctor may decide that there is no medical need or that he is unable to serve the patient and may discharge him from the process at that point. The patient is then free to initiate the process with some other doctor. After the doctor accepts the patient, his first job is to establish a probable diagnosis, which he does initially by careful interview and examination (history and physical). Many specialized diagnostic services are available to aid him in refining and extending this diagnosis. Laboratory and x-ray are commonly thought of, but there are, in addition, electrocardiography, electroencephalography, myography, thermography, and a growing list of others. The second decision box in figure 1-5 raises the question of which diagnostic tests, if any, the doctor wishes to use. He may then either provide these services himself or order them from some outside resource such as the hospital. In either case, the process is diverted to the diagnostic service box. Information from the diagnostic test returns to the physician. He may then use this information to order other tests. Thus the process may involve several passages through the diagnostic test box. (Such a situation in systems analysis is called an *iterative loop*, indicating that the process repeats itself with new information occurring with each circuit of the loop).

At some point the doctor decides that he has obtained as much diagnostic information as he needs. He does not order further diagnostic tests, and the process passes to the next decision box. Here the doctor can select therapy based upon his knowledge of the diagnosis. It is possible that, despite the diagnostic tests, there is no therapy to be rendered. In this case the patient is discharged from the system. Otherwise the doctor may decide a specific course of treatment and may then call on other resources to supply the treatment. He may provide it himself as well. Here again the hospital is frequently the source of the service for the patient.

When the therapeutic service is ordered, certain results are expected, and the next step in the process involves the evaluation of whether or not these results were achieved. If they were not, a second loop is formed as the doctor returns to his diagnosis to review its accuracy and again considers what therapy should be ordered. This process is the feedback loop, or monitor and control process previously encountered. Presumably the selected therapies will eventually be as effective as was anticipated, and the process moves to the last decision boxes. Here the patient's needs are evaluated in terms of possible additional treatment and additional diagnoses. If it is indicated, other iterative loops are formed, with the process moving back to a diagnostic or a therapeutic service. If no further treatment is indicated and no additional diagnosis found, the patient is discharged from the medical care process.

In summary, the model in figure 1-5 shows a process which is basically governed by the patient and his individual physician, which may or may not involve the hospital or any other institution. The hospital is frequently involved, however, and its points of involvement are at the provision of diagnostic services and treatment services. Often the total amount of hospital services which is required is great enough to warrant physically transferring the patient to the hospital and admitting him for a period of several hours to several weeks. It is not always necessary that this be done, however. Many hospitals provide limited quantities of services to patients on an outpatient basis or deliver them to the patient's home through a home care program.

The demand upon a specific service which results from a given patient's problem is obviously conditioned by a large number of more or less independently operating factors, ranging from social and environmental factors through patient-related, doctor-related and disease-related factors. Two key conclusions result from this fact. The first is that "need," i.e., some medically determined condition, is neither a necessary nor sufficient condition for demand. "Demand" and "need" are two quite different measures which can (and should) be compared, but never confused. The second is that many of the factors affecting demand for a given service are chance or random factors, so that it is impossible to predict with certainty that a specific patient will need a service. Such a process is said to be "stochastic," that is subject to random variation of some magnitude. The stochastic nature of demand and the difference between demand and needs have profound consequences for hospital resource planning. These problems can almost never be totally dropped from consideration in hospital management. In particular, they will occupy much of our attention in the next four chapters.

Again, figure 1-5 is simplified several ways. The physician need not follow the order shown. In fact, he can consider both diagnosis and therapy at the same time, and he often does this when the patient has a variety of needs or an emergency of some sort. It is also possible to order several diagnostic tests at once, rather than sequentially, as the iterative loop indicates. The same may be done with therapeutic services. The figure deprecates the importance of the vital and subtle process of hearing the patient's history and of other aspects of the physician's own skills. Particularly within the interaction of the doctor and the patient, diagnosis and therapy may be almost indistinguishable rather than the orderly compartments shown in the figure. Lastly, the figure represents a "textbook" approach to medical practice, which is probably greatly abbreviated in many, many instances. These oversimplifications do not, however, destroy the usefulness of the analysis for the purposes of initial understanding and further discussion.

Role of the Hospital

The hospital has two responsibilities toward the process described in figures 1-4 and 1-5. It must meet the demands for specific services which arise from the medical care process. Secondly, it is responsible for parts of the whole process by which the community seeks care and gets it. There is growing pressure for hospitals to concern themselves with failures in the process of demand generation; that is with patients who did not seek care when they should and patients who received care they did not need. The first responsibility implies that hospitals must be able to understand and predict the demand. The second responsibility implies an ability to look beyond demand as it is expressed to potential demand and to need for health services.

Chapters 2 through 5 will explore techniques related to demand analysis. Once quantitative statements of demand have been prepared, it is possible to make systematic efforts at the optimum arrangement of resources. These possibilities are explored in chapters 6 through 9. Finally, the routine monitoring of expectations, particularly quality expectations, is discussed in chapters 10 through 13.

Additional Readings Chapter 1

Donabedian, A. *Aspects of Medical Care Administration.* Harvard University Press, Cambridge, Mass., in press.

Feldstein, P.J. "Research on the Demand for Health Services." *Milbank Memorial Fund Quarterly*, 44, no. 3, pt 2 (July 1966).

Rosenstock, I.M. "Why People Use Health Services." *Milbank Memorial Fund Quarterly*, 44, no. 3 pt 2 (July 1966).

Sheldon, A. "Toward a General Theory of Disease and Medical Care," ch. 5 in *Systems and Medical Care*, A. Sheldon, F. Baker, and C.P. McLaughlin, ed., MIT Press, Cambridge, Mass., 1970.

Part I
Forecasting Demand

2 The Forecasting Problem and Simple Time Series Analysis

The Logic of Demand Analysis and Forecasting

The hospital supervisor serves as process monitor in the terms of figure 1-3. His job is to continually assess the process for which he is responsible, take action to meet varying conditions, and see that the results conform to expectations. But how are expectations established? And knowing that conditions vary, what are the expected changes? How much change in demand or resources input can be tolerated before changes are made in the operating system? These are the fundamental questions of quantitative management. The supervisor must have some knowledge about the answers to these questions in order to perform his function. *Forecasts* or predictions about demand and about the availability of resources are the main form of this knowledge. From the forecasts, the supervisor can develop other performance expectations.

Hospitals are a world where most processes are *stochastic*, that is subject to chance variation. When this is so, exact prediction is impossible. What must be substituted is probabilistic prediction, giving an expected value and the probabilities or chances of changes of given amounts around the expected value. (The opposite of stochastic is *deterministic*, a process which always yields its expected value and is subject to no chance fluctuation. See the section, "A Procedure for Forecasting".) The *expected value* is the mean or average of the distribution of possible values. Thus the predictions which must be made for hospital processes must be made using the mathematical sciences of probability and statistics. The form of the answer will not be, "we can expect twenty-five operations tomorrow," but rather "we can expect twenty-five operations tomorrow, with a 5 percent chance of getting less than twenty and an equal chance of getting more than thirty-one." Such an answer vastly complicates the management of hospitals. If we provide resources for thirty-one operations, we know that five days out of a hundred, eighteen days a year, we will not have enough. At the same time, over the year we will use on the average only resources for twenty-five, so that efficiency is automatically limited to 25/31 or about 80 percent. Whatever we do to improve one problem will worsen the other.

It is possible and sometimes desirable to treat stochastic processes as though they were deterministic. This is the same as assuming that the process will always generate its expected value. Such an assumption simplifies the analysis and forecasting. It is justifiable whenever the range of probable values does not differ enough to change the management decision to be made from the forecast.

In many hospital situations, stochastic processes should be handled as such. The range of probable values is relatively large, and there are high probabilities of values different enough from the expected value to change the decision which must be made from the information. Random factors affect almost all visits to a hospital to some extent. A number of demand processes, such as emergency visits and obstetrical deliveries, are almost purely random. The expected value of demand for these services is no indication of the quantity of resources needed because demand will sometimes be much less and sometimes much more. Although the expected value alone is a key to the appropriate decision, it is rarely sufficient for an optimum decision.

Despite this difficulty, we must make predictions. If the monitor is to function at all, he must have reasonable expectations on which to base his judgment. Within limitations, the more accurate and the more precise these expectations are, the better job he can do.

The statistical techniques for forecasting are largely independent of what is forecast. Forecasting demand, or absenteeism among manpower resources, or failures to meet quality standards in output are conceptually the same problem. Since demand is the first element which must be understood in the hospital situation, the chapters which follow will deal with the forecast of demand. The student should bear in mind, however, that (with only minor exceptions) what is said in this and the following chapters about demand forecasting is adaptable to any other forecasting problem.

Approaches to Forecasting

There are three basic approaches to demand forecasting for the health care field. The first one is through historical experience: A demand which has occurred in the past can be used as a basis for the future. If the department provided 10,000 units of service last year, one can forecast that the expected value will be 10,000 units next year. To make the accuracy of this projection more likely, data for several past years could be reviewed. These might show that demand had grown by 500 units per year. Thus the estimate for the coming year would be 10,500 units. A series of data for several historical periods in order is called a *time series* and extensive statistical techniques exist for analyzing data in this form. Historical data can be used to infer to one situation from one or several similar situations as well. Thus the demand for given situations in one hospital might be forecast based on the demand experience for similar hospitals.

Estimates of need is the second approach. Although need and demand are not synonymous, it is possible to estimate the need for hospital services by measurement of the incidence of certain diseases combined with assumptions about the kind and quality of the services necessary to treat these diseases. If an estimate of the relationship between demand and need can be made, the expected demand can be derived from a forecast of the expected need. For example, if the expected number of births in a community is 1,000, and it is known that 99% of the births occur in hospitals, the expected demand for obstetrical deliveries can be forecast as 990. Most cases are a great deal more complicated than this. Difficulties are encountered at each step of a procedure: estimating the incidence or prevalence of the disease, reaching agreement on the services which are needed for its treatment, and finding the relationship between need and demand.

The third approach to demand forecasting is through direct subjective estimates of demand. There are sometimes situations in which there is no relevant historical information on demand and no way to isolate need and its relationship to demand. The most common example would be in a new or experimental service which had never been previously offered. In cases of this kind, the only remaining alternative is to obtain subjective estimates from the persons who will be ordering the service in question. Surveys of the opinions of doctors, nurses, or in some cases, patients provide the basis for the forecast.

While what is of most direct concern to the process monitor is the number of events—admissions, x-rays, absenteeisms, etc.—it is often true that the best forecast is based upon two components: a *rate*, the number of events per member of the population at risk, and an independent forecast of the population. Admissions per thousand persons, absences per 1000 employees, or x-rays per thousand admissions are examples. Changes can result either from changes in the rate or from changes in the size of population served. It is not always possible to isolate the population for a given service, but substantial improvements in the understanding, and therefore in prediction, are likely if both the rate and the population can be identified. The "population" in this sense is sometimes a geographically identified group of people, but it could also be persons identified according to some other characteristic such as subscription to a given health insurance plan. By extension, a population may be the census of patients in a hospital or the number of patients admitted over a period of time or some similar grouping. Demand forecasts prepared in this way are common. The use of separate forecasts, one of the rate and the other of the population at risk, allows the forecaster considerably more flexibility and generally improves the accuracy of the forecast. They can be developed through any of the three approaches.

It should be noted that the three approaches to forecasting are not mutually exclusive, but can often be used to advantage simultaneously. It is frequently useful to prepare independent estimates of need from an epidemiologic basis for purposes of comparison with demand estimates prepared in one of the other two ways. When this is practical, the additional information provides a crude check upon the validity of the estimate. It also permits an identification of the relationship between the demand and need which may reveal the areas in which the total system of medical care is failing to meet the needs of the community it serves. For example, if the need for service is estimated at 10,000 units but the demand is estimated at only 8,000 units, the causes of the loss of demand might be explored further in order to see if changes in the system by education of patients and doctors, revision of insurance coverage, or changes in the availability of service might alter the level of demand. Similar analyses might be undertaken if the demand were 12,000 units when a need of only 10,000 units was expected.

Output, Demand and Need Measurement

In practical situations in hospitals, the historical statistics usually measure output rather than the true demand. The time series data which are usually available are in terms of services rendered. Information is rarely recorded on the total number of units of service demanded. In some situations, such as when there is known to be a shortage of supply of a given service, significant fractions of a true demand may remain unexpressed. In order to identify the factors influencing the forecast, it is necessary to view the processes of need and demand in three categories:

Demand is the sum of explicit requests for a given medical care service, either by the patient at the initiation of the medical care process, or by the doctor acting for the patient in the process of diagnosis and treatment. Some demands are implied by others according to convention or hospital policy. For instance, an admission to the hospital carries an implied demand for meals, nursing care, linen, etc., as indicated by the patient's condition and preestablished policies. Unless otherwise stated, these are treated as part of the explicit demand.

Unexpressed demand is the demand for services which is not translated to explicit demand, usually because of resource shortages. Examples are demand for doctors' services which are not expressed because patients are aware of long waiting lists, and requests for hospital admission not made because of crowded facilities, etc. Sometimes such demand is carried elsewhere, and sometimes it simply remains unexpressed and unmet. (Unexpressed demand can create serious forecasting difficulties, for its existence implies that historic statistics on output underrepresent the true demand.)

Need is a concept of health services required by a population to maintain it at a preconceived level of health. It differs from demand in that:

1. It requires a subjective definition of the level of health, the services required, or both. The definitions are usually supplied by some medical authority or panel
2. It excludes those portions of both unexpressed and explicit demand which are unrelated to the concept of health level. For example, demand for hospital care among patients whose need is for domiciliary services

available in homes for the aged or foster homes would be excluded from a forecast of the need for hospital care
3. It includes levels of health care (for instance preventive examinations) which may not be perceived as desirable by either the patient or the practicing doctor, and thus do not appear as either explicit demand or unexpressed demand

Of these three concepts, explicit demand is the easiest to measure and is the closest to output statistics commonly available. Unexpressed demand becomes important in the planning of facilities, because it often converts to explicit demand when the barriers imposed by resource shortages are reduced. It should be noted that the existence of unmet need or unexpressed demand does not imply a change in demand unless the underlying factors preventing the expression of demand are altered. Need and unexpressed demand are merely predisposing factors to changes in demand, and should not be interpreted as automatic in their action. Need is measurable only when agreement is established on its definition. Although the term has been commonly used in the past, (as in "bed need" for a given community) it is becoming less popular with the realization that there is sometimes little professional consensus to support a measurement of need in terms of gross processes like the medical care process or hospital admissions, and little practical chance that demand will conform automatically to the need once it has been estimated.

At present, one major use of "need" evaluations lies in monitoring the *output* of the various aspects of medical care services. It is proposed that the doctor has a role in evaluating need as well as demand once the medical care process has been initiated, and that one dimension of the quality of care is its appropriateness. Specifically the treatment of the individual case can be judged in the light of two questions: (*a*) Did this patient receive all the diagnostic and treatment services which good medical judgment indicates? (i.e., all he *needs*, as defined by some medical consensus.) (*b*) Were all the services received by the patient indicated by good medical judgment? (i.e., were all needed, again as defined by medical consensus.)

To summarize the distinction between demand, unexpressed demand, and need, there are six possible states in which a patient can be: (*a*) with need, without demand; (*b*) with need, with unexpressed demand; (*c*) with need, with explicit demand; (*d*) without need, with explicit demand; (*e*) without need, with unexpressed demand; and (*f*) without need, without demand.

Management data usually are derived from measurement of states (c) and (d) combined (explicit demand, with or without need). The statistics of output, which are commonly substituted for the unknown statistics on demand, most closely approximate the sum of these two states. Particularly in situations where available facilities are operated at capacity, output is likely to be a poor approximation of demand. In these situations it is important to allow for the existence of substantial unexpressed demand, cases (b) and (e). As consensus grows among both doctors and patients as to what constitutes "need," cases (d) and (e)—demand without need—may be expected to decline in importance. At the same time, patients in case (a) who need care but do not request it will presumably perceive their needs and change their state to explicit demand.

A Procedure for Forecasting

It should be clear that forecasting a stochastic demand is a complex procedure involving in most instances measurement, judgment, and statistical analysis. To improve the reliability of the result, we need a procedure which will allow the interplay of these three activities but which will allow us to identify the nature of the specific activities. The end-point of the procedure will be a forecast. Normally it will include all three activities, and no one activity is in itself a forecast. Diagramatically:

$$\text{Forecast} = \text{Measurement} + \text{Analysis} + \text{Judgment}$$

and, by extension

$$\text{Errors in forecast} = \text{Errors in measurement} \\ + \text{Errors in analysis} \\ + \text{Errors in judgment}$$

Since our task is to minimize errors, it may help to keep the activities clear.

A systematic approach to forecasting can be summarized as follows. Primarily:

Measurement { Estimating the population from which demand arises
 Estimating the rate of demand from the population

Analysis { Projecting the population to the time required
 Projecting the demand rate to the same period

Judgment { Investigating the unexpressed demand and the need, and adjusting the demand projection for these factors
 Multiplying the adjusted demand projection by the population projection to project adjusted total demand
 Projecting the variation of demand in the light of the adjusted total demand, by review of the probability of variation in the adjusted demand

It is rare that a given specific problem can be handled according to the steps above with objective and quantified data to support each step. The complete process may be unacceptably costly. Often there are no practical methods for estimating factors such as the need for a service because the consensus on need is unclear or because measuring the need is too difficult. On the other hand, the steps can be followed as a guide. Whenever a step is omitted, the forecaster can recognize that an additional possibility for error has been introduced. Often he can estimate at least subjectively the magnitude and direction of the likely error.

A distinction is being made between technique and judgment. Techniques, such as statistical analysis, are to a large extent objective and free of bias. Their application, however, involves the acceptance of a set of assumptions about the conditions where they are used. This acceptance is a matter of judgment which is inescapable in forecasts. Put another way, simple linear regression, which is discussed in the next section, is a technique which is highly objective. (Any two users will obtain the same results from the same data, barring error.) It results in a *projection*, a statement of what will happen if certain conditions pertain. The acceptance of the likelihood of these conditions is a matter of judgment and only after that acceptance may the projection be properly called a forecast. The judgment of the hospital administrator and others in the hospital is often the most demanding and critical component in the forecast.

The techniques for arriving at demand forecasts can become quite complex. The more accurate the forecast which is needed, the more complex the process is likely to become. Similarly, the more obscure the data, the greater will be the cost of obtaining it. In general the accuracy of the forecast should balance the cost of improving accuracy against the value of additional accuracy in improving management decisions. The sections which follow will show specific applications of some important techniques of demand forecasting for health services.

Forecasting Expected Values of a Stochastic Process from Historic Data on the Same Process

In many situations a time series of data about a process is available for several historical periods. For the analysis itself, it does not matter whether the statistic is demand, output, demand rate, or population. It may be projected using widely recognized statistical techniques. These procedures have many applications in the process of preparing demand forecasts, and are reviewed below.

Projection of Time Series Data

Graphic Methods. Time series data on a stochastic process may be graphed. A visual trend line may be drawn through the points on the graph and extended to future time periods. The values for these time periods may be read directly from the graph. The method is quick and cheap, but has the offsetting disadvantage of being subject to inaccuracies and biases by the forecaster. It also yields no notion of the probable errors associated with the estimate. The data shown in table 2-1 will provide an illustration. These data are graphed in figure 2-1.

The line drawn need not be straight, but may be curved by the forecaster to fit his judgment of what he believes to be the trend in the process. Thus two different forecasts might be made from these data, by accepting either the linear or the nonlinear projection. These will differ by more than 10 percent in a few years time. The principal difficulty with this method is that it yields no measure of the relative accuracy of the forecast. There is no simple way to estimate whether the curved line is more appropriate than the straight, or whether either line is the best possible fit to the data given. *In most situations, objective statistical analysis can be performed at only a small additional cost, and is strongly preferred to visual graphic methods.*

Regression Analysis. Statistical techniques, called *regression analysis* will provide a more objective projection of historic data, and will in addition provide some (not all) further information on the questions of whether a time relationship exists and whether it should be projected as a straight or a curved line. These techniques can be applied manually, and it is desirable for the student to do this to gain a full understanding of what the technique is doing and what the output reported means. As a practical matter, however, computerized regression analysis is cheaper, more accurate, and vastly more convenient for large numbers. The example given in table 2-1 and graphed on figure 2-1 will be treated analytically, but the discussion will emphasize the meaning of the resulting projection and the decisions involving the forecasting assumptions. The calculating formulas, and the numerical calculations are shown in this chapter's appendix.

The statistical method of regression analysis will fit a line to the available data. The line will pass through the mean of all the points at the mean time

Table 2-1
Medical and Surgical Patient Days at ELB Hospital Since Opening of Present Facility—1958

Year	Patient Days
1958	34775
1959	36865
1960	40551
1961	39423
1962	39563
1963	40907
1964	43901
1965	45286

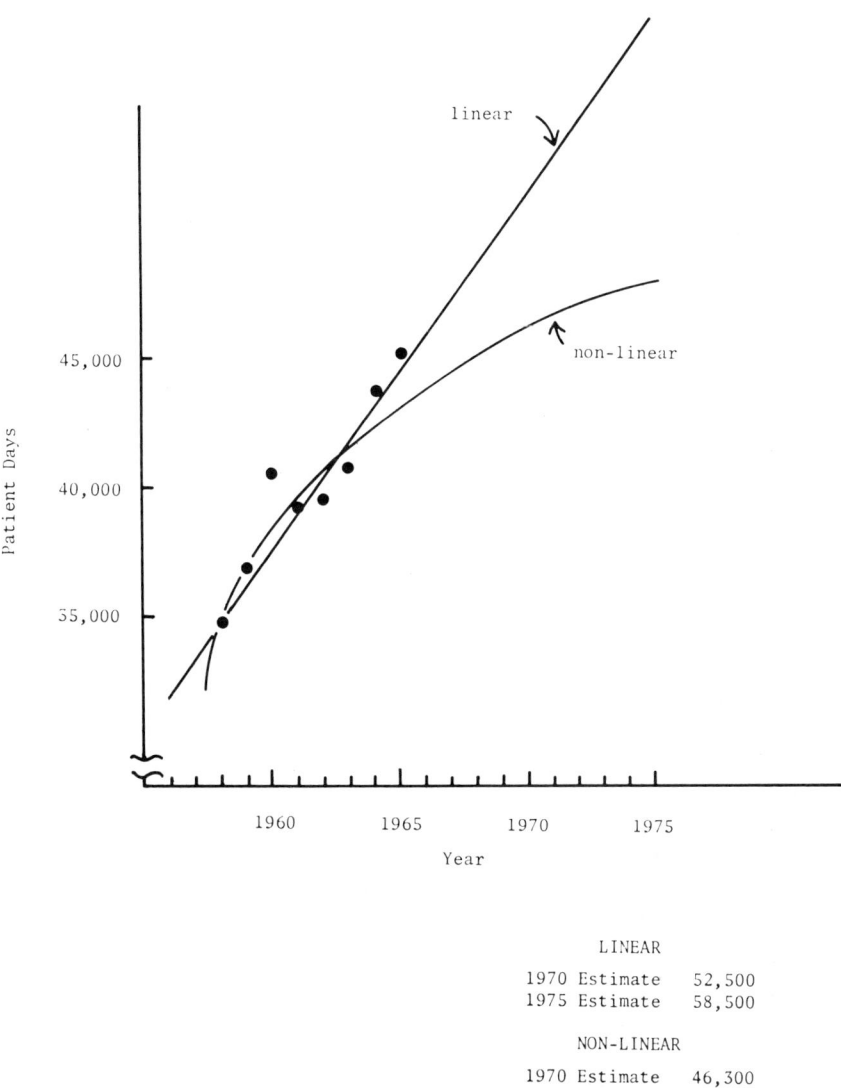

Figure 2-1. Visual Projection of Patient-Day Demand.

period. The slope of the line, or rate of increase per time period, will minimize the distance from the line to the data points. The analyst must select in advance whether the line is to be straight (*linear*) or curved (*nonlinear*). If the line is nonlinear, the method will determine the curvature as well. The method will also produce information on whether the line is significantly different from zero in its slope, and what the probable error is at a future time. The method also gives information on the "goodness of fit" of the line, that is whether the line explains a significant portion of the variation in the original data. Because this variation is measured by the square of the distance of the original data points from the line, the method is called *least squares* regression analysis. If both linear and nonlinear analysis are made, it is possible to compare the "fit," and pick the better one.

The techniques of regression analysis are described in most statistical texts. An example of their application using the data in table 2-1 is given below.

Linear example. The statistic given in table 2-1 can be identified as y, and has the values y_t, from years $t = 0$ at 1957 to $t = 8$ at 1965. The regression line which is to be calculated has the algebraic form

$$\bar{y} = at + B$$

where (in the general case) t is the time from some arbitrary starting point, $t_0 = 0$, to the last available period t_n. There will be n values of y; B will be the value of y at t_0; and a will equal the slope of the regression line, $\Delta y / \Delta t$.[a] Because y is subject to stochastic variation, the measured value of y at any given t will not necessarily fall on the regression line. This situation can be represented by:

$$\bar{y} = at + B \pm E$$

where E is a term representing the residual variation in y after the calculation of the regression line. The line can be calculated by the least-squares method, and the E term can be evaluated for a specific level of confidence.

In addition to the calculation of the line and its error term, two measures of the success of the line in explaining the variation in the dependent variable are important. These are:

- R^2 – the *coefficient of determination*, equal to the sum of squares of deviation remaining around the line, divided by the sum of squares of deviation around the mean of the original data. (The square root of R^2 is called the *correlation coefficient*.)
- F – the *F-statistic*, a tabulated statistic showing the probability that the explanation offered by the line is a chance phenomenon rather than a true association.

---

[a]The symbol $\Delta y / \Delta t$ is the rate of change in y (called Δy) per unit of change in t (called Δt). For a straight line it is the same at all points. For a curved line it differs at different t and is measured by the line tangential to the curve, or, in calculus, the differential, dy/dt.

For the data in table 2-1, the values are:

a the slope = 1309
b the value of $\bar{y}$ at $t = 0$ (1957) = 34,268
$\bar{y} = at + b$, the prediction equation, $\bar{y} = 1309t + 34,268$
$R^2 = .88$
$S.E. = 1275$
$F = 44.3$

The first question is the significance of the explanation. Did this answer result from pure chance, or was there some real association in the data? The high value of R^2, which is never greater than one, indicates that there probably is an association. A more reliable test, however, is provided by the F-statistic. This statistic has been tabulated for the purpose of testing this hypothesis, in terms of the degrees of freedom for the regression, equal to the number of independent variables used in the regression, and the degrees of freedom residual, equal to the sample size, minus one, minus the number of independent variables, or

$$\text{d.f. (residual)} = n - 1 - \text{(number of independent variables)}$$

In this case, d.f. (residual) = 8 − 1 − 1 = 6. Statistical tables of F show that at 5 percent probability that the results are due to pure chance.

$$F_{.05} = 5.98 \qquad \text{for 1,6 d.f.,}$$

and at 1 percent probability,

$$F_{.01} = 13.74 \qquad \text{for 1,6 d.f.}$$

Since our value, $F = 44.3$, is much larger, we can be reassured that the results are not a chance phenomenon.

A prediction can be made from the equation (shown in figure 2-2)

$$y = 1309t + 34,268$$

for any future year. For example, for 1967 ($t = 10$)

$$\begin{aligned} y^{10} &= 1309(10) + 34,268 \\ &= 47,358 \end{aligned}$$

An estimate of the error of this prediction can be made at a desired level of confidence. Using the standard error term, $S.E. = 1275$, and a 95 percent confidence level, (two standard errors):

$$E = 2 \times 1275 = 2550$$
$$y_{10} = 47{,}400 \pm 2500$$

or we are 95 percent confident that *if the association continues as it has been*, the true value for 1967 will be between 44,900 and 49,900. A more conservative way to make this estimate which increases the confidence range as the prediction is extended to the future is given in this chapter's appendix. This calculation yields the curved confidence limits shown in figure 2-2.

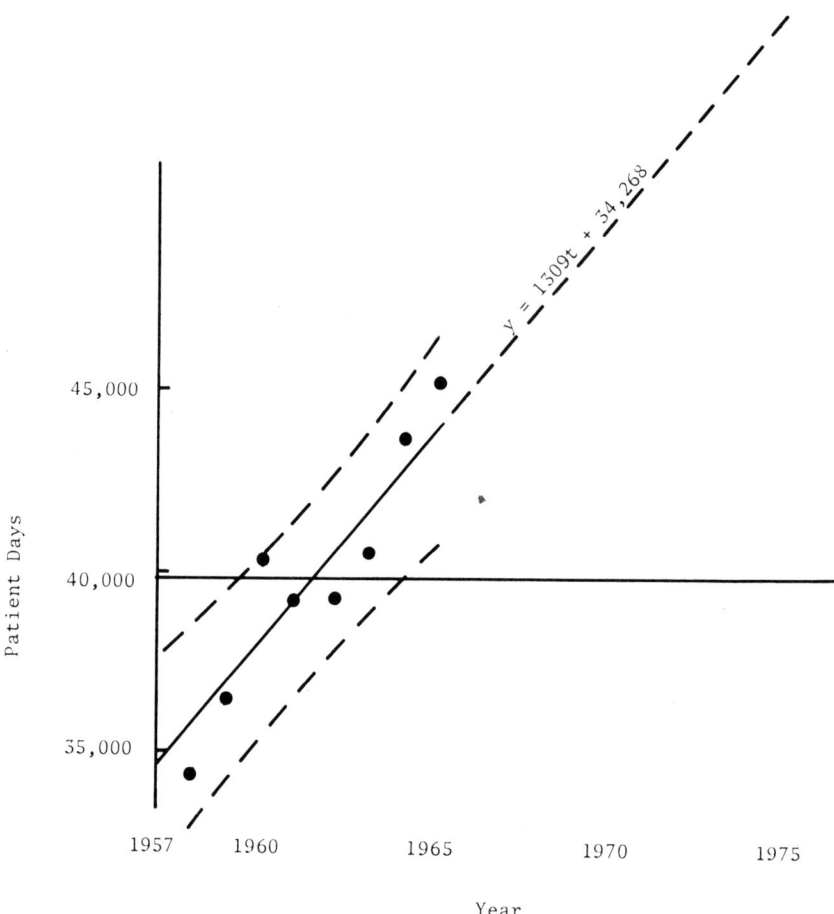

Figure 2-2. Regression Line of Patient Days in ELB Hospital.

Nonlinear case. In some processes, a linear estimate will not be appropriate. Often the best evidence of this is in the process itself. Rapidly changing demand for a service, such as the growth of a recently introduced service, or changes in the usefulness of a service, are a good indication of nonlinear growth situations. Study of the graphic plot of the data may suggest a nonlinear pattern as well. Evidence for similar studies may suggest investigation of nonlinear trends; emergency room demand, for example, has been regarded as nonlinear. Situations where both the use rate and the user population are changing may be better modeled for total demand by a nonlinear regression. This might be the situation for the example. Both the community population and the patient days per thousand population seemed to be increasing at the ELB Hospital. Conceptually, the nonlinear case may be thought of as the assumption, *"if the change in the association continues at the same rate."*

In cases where the logic of the situation suggests a nonlinear analysis, it should be explored. The choice of one analysis or the other is indicated by the measures of goodness of fit. A significant improvement in the value of F justifies switching from a linear to a nonlinear analysis.

A curved line can be represented as a logarithmic equation

$$\log \bar{y} = at + b \pm E$$

This equation can be handled exactly as the linear equation, by transforming the original data to their logarithms. If the new values are designated by y', where $y' = \log y$, the equation becomes

$$\bar{y}' = at + b \pm E$$

the same form as the linear case. (The values of a, b, and E will be different numerically, and an estimate of $\bar{y}'$ will be the logarithm of the original statistic, of course.) Many modern computer programs for regression analysis have a feature permitting automatic log transformation, so that the linear and nonlinear analyses are equally simple to perform. The one yielding the better value of F, or R, is that one the forecaster would prefer, presuming that his notion of the process supported the assumption that it would continue as in the past.

The nonlinear form can be modeled graphically by using semilogarithmic graph paper. The data from table 2-1 are shown in figure 2-3.

The results of the analysis for the example are

log y	= 0.01423t + 4.5384
where t	= 0 at 1957
S.E.	= 0.01403
R^2	= 0.88
F	= 43.2

A slight, insignificant deterioration has occurred in the prediction. The R^2 value at two significant figures shows no change, but the F statistic value dropped from 44.3 to 43.2. The nonlinear model has not proved useful in this situation.

Making the Forecast. The difference between the projection and the forecast lies in the phrase "if the association continues as it has been," in the linear association, and in, "if the association continues at the same rate" in the nonlinear case. If one accepts either of these phrases, then one would accept that projection as a forecast. Suppose, however, you believed that growth of the ELB Hospital would be limited by a shortage of facilities. Then clearly neither association would continue. On the other hand, suppose it were known that growth in population would be much faster in coming years. Then the historic association might be too small. There is clearly an area of judgment here which in many situations is more important than the statistics themselves. These judgments are an area where the hospital administrator can make his biggest contribution, from his knowledge of the process being forecast, the experience reported by others, and the situation in his community. The statistics, however, are likely to sharpen his judgment substantially.

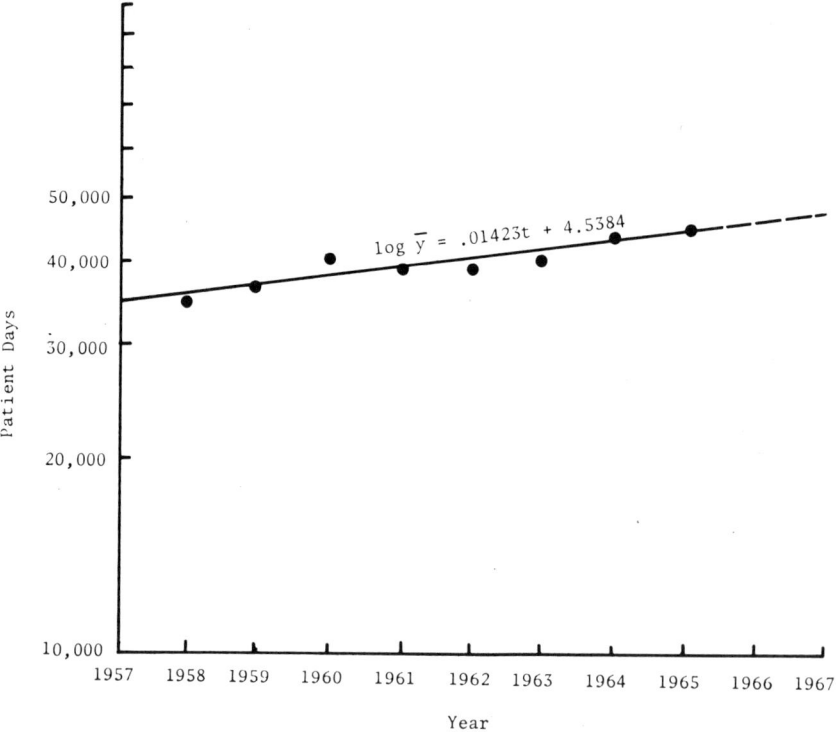

Figure 2-3. Patient Days at the ELB Hospital on Logarithmic Scale, with the Regression Line ($\log \bar{y} = .01423t + 4.5384$).

Chapter 2
Appendix

Equations for the line

$$\bar{y} = at + B \pm E.$$

The data have a grand mean:

$$\bar{\bar{y}} = \frac{\sum_{t=0}^{n} y_t}{n}$$

and an overall variance:

$$\sigma^2 = \frac{\sum_{t=0}^{n}(y_t - \bar{\bar{y}})^2}{(n-1)}$$

The parameters of the regression are:

$$a = \frac{\sum (t-\bar{t})(y-\bar{\bar{y}})}{\sum (t-\bar{t})^2},$$

$$B = \bar{\bar{y}} - a(\bar{t} - t_0),$$

$$E = k \sqrt{S^2 \left[1 + \frac{1}{n} + \frac{(t-\bar{t})^2}{\sum_{t=0}^{n}(t-\bar{t})^2} \right]},$$

where k is the value from Student's table for the desired level of confidence (at $n - 2$ degrees of freedom) and S^2 is the unbiased estimate of the variance of y about the line $\bar{y}$.

$$S^2 = \frac{\sum (y - \bar{y})^2}{n - 2}$$

It is desirable to test the hypothesis that the slope of the regression line, a, is not equal to zero and this is done by the F test, with one and $(n-2)$ degrees of freedom:

$$F = \frac{\sum (\bar{\bar{y}} - \bar{y})^2}{\sum (y - \bar{y})^2 / (n - 2)}.$$

It is common to calculate the correlation coefficient R,

$$R = \frac{\sum (t - \bar{t})(y - \bar{y})}{\sqrt{\sum (t - \bar{t})^2 \sum (y - \bar{y})^2}}$$

Algebraic simplifications can be made for these calculations, and the formulae are as follows:

$$\sum (t - \bar{t})(y - \bar{y}) = \sum ty - \frac{(\sum t)(\sum y)}{n}$$

$$\sum (t - \bar{t})^2 = \sum t^2 - \frac{(\sum t)^2}{n}$$

$$\sum (y - \bar{y})^2 = \sum y^2 - \frac{(\sum y)^2}{n}$$

$$\sum (\bar{\bar{y}} - \bar{y})^2 = \frac{[\sum (t - \bar{t})(y - \bar{y})]^2}{\sum (t - \bar{t})^2}$$

$$\sum (y - \bar{\bar{y}})^2 = \sum (y - \bar{y})^2 - \sum (\bar{\bar{y}} - \bar{y})^2$$

$$R^2 = \frac{\sum (\bar{\bar{y}} - \bar{y})^2}{\sum (y - \bar{y})^2}.$$

These formulae permit the calculation of all required statistics from $\sum y$, $\sum t$, $\sum yt$, $\sum y^2$ and $\sum t^2$

Calculations for the Example, Chapter 2

To apply these equations to the example, the data will be more convenient to handle if $y = y' - 40{,}000$, $t = \text{year} - 1957$. The following presents the statistics necessary for calculation, y, t, $\sum y$, $\sum t$, $\sum yt$, $\sum y^2$, $\sum t^2$, from table 2-1.

t	y	t^2	y^2	ty
1	−5225	1	27,300,625	−5225
2	−3135	4	9,828,225	−6270
3	551	9	303,601	1653
4	− 577	16	332,929	−2308
5	− 437	25	190,969	−2185
6	907	36	822,649	5442
7	3901	49	15,217,801	27,307
8	5286	64	27,941,796	42,288
36	1271	204	81,938,595	60,702

$\bar{y} = 159$
$\bar{t} = 4.5$

Simplified calculations:

$$\sum (t - \bar{t})(y - \bar{y}) = \sum ty - \frac{(\sum t)(\sum y)}{n}$$

$$= 60{,}702 - \frac{(36)(1271)}{8} = 60{,}702 - 5720$$

$$= 54{,}982$$

$$\sum (t - \bar{t})^2 = \sum t^2 - \frac{(\sum t)^2}{n}$$

$$= 204 - \frac{(36)^2}{8} = 204 - 162$$

$$= 42$$

$$\sum (y - \bar{y})^2 = \sum y^2 - \frac{(\sum y)^2}{n}$$

$$= 81{,}938{,}595 - \frac{1{,}615{,}441}{8} = 81{,}938{,}595 - 201{,}930$$

$$= 81{,}736{,}665$$

$$\Sigma(\bar{\bar{y}} - \bar{y})^2 = \frac{[\Sigma(t - \bar{t})(y - \bar{y})]^2}{\Sigma(t - \bar{t})^2}$$

$$= \frac{(54{,}982)^2}{42}$$

$$= 71{,}976{,}936$$

$$\Sigma(y - \bar{y})^2 = \Sigma(y - \bar{y})^2 - \Sigma(\bar{\bar{y}} - \bar{y})^2$$

$$= 81{,}736{,}665 - 71{,}976{,}936$$

$$= 9{,}759{,}729$$

Values of the regression line:

$$a = \frac{\Sigma(t - \bar{t})(y - \bar{y})}{\Sigma(t - \bar{t})^2} = \frac{54{,}982}{42} = 1309$$

$$B = 159 - (1309)(4.5) = -5{,}732$$

$$S^2 = \Sigma(y - \bar{y})^2 / n - 2 = 9{,}759{,}729 / 6 = 1{,}626{,}622$$

$$R^2 = \frac{\Sigma(\bar{\bar{y}} - \bar{y})^2}{\Sigma(y - \bar{y})^2} = \frac{71{,}976{,}936}{81{,}736{,}665} = 0.88$$

$$F = \frac{\Sigma(\bar{\bar{y}} - \bar{y})^2}{\Sigma(y - \bar{y})^2 / n - 2} = \frac{71{,}976{,}936}{1{,}626{,}622} = 44.3$$

at 1, and 6 degrees of freedom,

$$F_{0.05} = 5.98 \ .$$

Therefore the slope, a, is significant at 95 percent confidence limits. At 90 percent confidence limits, $k = 1.94$ for $(n - 2) = 6$ d.f. (from student's t table), the error, E:

For 1965 ($t = 8$)

$$E = 1.94 \sqrt{1{,}626{,}622 \left[1 + 1/8 + \frac{(3.5)^2}{42}\right]}$$

$$E = 2948$$

$$y_{1965} = 1309 \times 8 + 34{,}268 \pm 2900$$

$$= 44{,}700 \pm 2900$$

For 1961.5 ($\bar{t}$)

$$E = 2500$$

$$y = 40{,}000 \pm 2500$$

N.B. The value of E is a function of t, with a minimum at $\bar{t}$

The line which has been derived (after restoring the data to the original form by adding 40,000)

$$y = 1309t + 34{,}268$$

is shown in figure 2-2. The error at 90 percent confidence limits, $E = \pm 2900$ at 1965, is also shown by the broken lines above and below $y = 1309t + 34{,}268$. These limits of confidence are actually curved, approaching the line most closely at t.

Additional Readings

Most basic statistical texts contain discussions of simple linear and nonlinear regressions which will supplement the very limited mathematical discussion given here. The chapter citation for one common text is given below. This work will be referenced in connection with other statistical concepts in later chapters.

Freund, J.E. and F.J. Williams. *Elementary Business Statistics*, Prentice-Hall, Englewood Cliffs, N.J., 1964.

– On curve fitting and least squares regression, pp. 296-308.
– On correlation, pp. 312-18.
– On time series analysis, pp. 320-31, also pp. 347-50.

3 Forecasting by Multivariate Analysis and Techniques for Forecasting Variation

The time series regression analysis developed in chapter 2 develops a model which can be used to predict demand in the form of an equation

$$y = at + b$$

based upon changes in demand (y) associated with changes in time (t). The forecast derived from the model is usually based upon the assumption that whatever the causes of the relationship were, they will remain approximately the same in the future. As discussed in chapter 2, there are a number of situations where this assumption is not justified:

1. Forecasting demand for inpatient beds where it is known that shortages of beds in the past have created large amounts of unexpressed demand, and the only available statistic is an output measure, days of care given
2. Forecasting demand for services not previously available in the community, such as a new coronary care unit or mental health service
3. Forecasting the impact of changes in finance of services, such as the impact of Medicare in 1966
4. Forecasting where demand varies widely, so that the expected value is not in itself sufficient to make the best decision (e.g., situations where demand on a given day is sometimes 2 or 3 times the expected value)

Despite the difficulties which are apparent in forecasting under these conditions, the strategy for management remains the same as before: to reduce uncertainty as much as practical. There are several ways to develop forecasts under these conditions. These techniques will be discussed in this chapter.

In cases where historic data do not exist, or are judged not to be reliable for forecasting, what is needed is a model which will relate the variable of interest (in this case demand) to a set of measurable underlying factors so that knowledge of these factors can be used to develop a forecast. Such models exist and are called *multivariate models*. They are developed by a technique called multivariate analysis or multiple regression analysis. Because they do not depend on time alone, they can be developed from comparison of several different situations at the same point in time as well as data from a single situation which is changing over time. They can be used both for forecasting and for comparing different situations by adjusting for known differences. The development and use of multivariate analysis models for forecasting is reviewed in the first two sections of this chapter.

There are many situations in the hospital where forecasts of monthly or annual expected values are not good enough to make management decisions. Variation from day to day and from shift to shift is so great that short-run forecasts must be prepared before schedules can be prepared or workloads calculated. The techniques for short-term forecasting and for analyzing variation in demand will be presented in this chapter's last two sections.

Multivariate Analysis

The technique of multivariate analysis or multiple regression analysis is a powerful one made possible by modern computers. While it will be discussed here in terms of demand analysis, where most of the health applications have been made, it is also useful in analyzing variations in costs or resource use and variations in quality and efficiency. The logic of the technique is not difficult, and it exactly parallels the simple regression analysis discussed in chapter 2. This discussion will be based upon the assumption that qualified statisticians are available to perform the analysis. The focus here will be upon the logic of the analysis, the requirements for input data, the form of the output and the factors which must be considered in transforming the raw statistical output to a forecast. The statistical operations and computer programs themselves will not be reviewed. The former are well covered in recent statistical texts,[1] and the latter are specific to machine capabilities. There are literally hundreds of multiple regression programs for differing machines and analytic purposes. Consultation with local programmers is usually necessary for specific applications.

Logic

Several of the problems listed above can be approached by the technique. Forecasting demand for beds where time series data are not adequate will serve as an example.

Consideration of the problem might take the following steps:

1. The demand for the community question is likely to be the same as the demand from a similar community
2. A "similar community" might not exist. No two communities are identical, and the exact factors influencing demand are unknown, so that we do not know exactly what we should compare in finding similarity
3. It is known from many prior studies that a variety of factors influence demand. Among those which have been cited are:

Age of population
Income level
Education level
Availability of facilities,
etc.

4. If these factors could be measured for several communities together with their demand for hospital care, the impact of each factor can be estimated. Then by measuring the factors in the community of interest, it is reasonable to use the impact of each to infer the demand. This is exactly analogous to the simple time series regression, where the impact of time was measured and used to infer the demand at a later time

Multiple regression permits the simultaneous study of several factors. The statistic to be predicted is called the *dependent variable*. The factors affecting it are called *independent variables*. The goal of the analysis is a *function* or mathematical statement relating the dependent variable to a given set of values of the independent variables. As in the case of simple regression, the function is arrived at by studying the ability of the independent variables to reduce the variation of the dependent variable. The reduction in the variance of the dependent variable becomes the measure of the success of the analysis.

One simple way to envision multivariate analysis is in terms of partitioning the data according to the factors of interest. In a simple example, considering only two independent variables, age and sex, and doctor visits as a dependent variable, the doctor visits could be calculated from several similar communities on the basis of the use per 1,000 population for each of several groups of age and sex.

Examples of this kind of partitioning, called *age specific rates*, are common. The following data have been used in forecasting neighborhood health center visits. They give visits per person per year.

| | Sex | | |
Age	M	F	Total
0- 4 yrs.	–	–	5.7
5-14 yrs.	–	–	2.9
15-24 yrs.	3.2	3.3	–
25-44 yrs.	3.3	4.1	–
45-64 yrs.	4.5	4.7	–
Over 65 yrs.	6.0	5.9	–

(Obstetric-gynecology visits omitted) Knowing for example, that there were 2000 males and 3000 females aged 25 to 44 in the service population, the number of visits for that age group would be 3.2 x 2000 + 3.3 x 3000 = 16,300 visits/year. The balance of the table could be used to arrive at a total expected workload. Presumably this would be more accurate than simply finding the gross average rate and multiplying it by the total population. Some multivariate analysis programs, called *analysis of variance* programs, work in exactly this fashion. They are particularly useful when it is not possible to express the factors of interest in relative quantitative terms. An example might be insurance coverage, where several different policies were common and the benefits of each were difficult to compare to each other. Use rates would be calculated for the fraction of the population with each kind of coverage.

Another form of multivariate analysis is the multiple regression equation. This form treats the dependent variables as continuous, rather than as separate cells. For example, a continuous variable—percent female—would be used in place of the two cells—male and female—to forecast use for a given population. Average age might be used in place of the six age cells. The regression form would be some relationship between these two variables and the total number of visits, such as

$$y = a \text{ (Average Age)} + b \text{ (\% Female)} + c$$

The possible forms are discussed below. This approach is more common than analysis of variance, which is generally restricted to situations where a continuous variable cannot conveniently be constructed.

The statistical programs for analysis of variance do more than simply calculating the rate for each cell. They also calculate the variance of each cell about its own mean and the variance of the totals. By comparing these, it is possible to estimate how much the variance of the estimate can be reduced and then to verify that the reduction is a significant one (that is, not occurring from chance). If there is no significant reduction in the variance, one would infer that the variables selected do not improve the prediction, and that therefore their use is not worth the added expense to collect the data. In such a case, the forecaster might either use the gross rate or seek other variables.

Input Data Requirements

Large quantities of data are usually required for multivariate analysis. In the example of doctor visit demand, each community is a *data point*. The total number of data points constitutes the *sample size*. Each variable must be measured for each data point. The sample size must be larger than the total number of variables. Selection of the variables becomes an important practical consideration. They must be measurable without excessive cost, or already available through census data or other reliable published studies. The accuracy of the measurement of input affects the accuracy of output. Variables which are only crudely estimated themselves should be avoided, as should heterogeneous collections of estimates from a variety of sources which take different approaches to estimating. If the resulting relationship is to be used for forecasting, predictions of the independent variables must be available for the forecast period as well as for the input data. Independent variables which themselves must be forecast by complex techniques should be avoided if possible. Thus one would not forecast inpatient care by studying outpatient visits, doctor's office visits, and emergency visits unless a simple way to measure and forecast each of these were available. (In most situations, this would not be the case.) Many variables might be considered for developing a multivariate estimate. Some would be abandoned because of measurement difficulties to gain the input data. Others would be rejected because they could not be measured or forecast for the community of interest. The remainder might be tried in the statistical analysis. Finally all but a few which proved to be the best predictors would be dropped.

Form of the Results

Linear form. The most common form of result of multivariate analysis is the *multiple regression equation*, an equation relating the dependent variable to the independent variables. If the dependent variable is designated as y and the independent variables as $x_1, x_2, \ldots, x_n$, the form:

$$y = a_1 x_1 + \ldots + a_n x_n + b$$

called a linear multiple regression equation, is common. The a terms are called the *coefficients of regression* and the b term is a constant indicating the value of y if all the independent variables are zero.

In many computer programs for multiple regression, this form of equation is selected in advance. It assumes that the relationship between y and each of the independent variables is linear, that is that a simple regression equation of the form: $y = a_i x_i + b_i$ can be written for each independent variable. In graphic terms, this equation indicates that each dependent variable is related to the independent variable by a straight line, exactly as was shown in chapter 2. At least this should be the case over the range of values of y that are of interest, even though it may not be true for all values of y. (It should be noted that over narrow ranges a straight line always provides an approximation to a curved one. Whether or not this approximation is satisfactory depends on the nature of the true relationship and the use to be made of the prediction.)

Nonlinear forms. There are other forms of multivariate analysis which do not assume a linear relation, just as there are of the simple regression. These are less frequently encountered because computer requirements and input data requirements increase rapidly and are often impractical. The form:

$$y = a_{11} x_1 + a_{21} x_1^2 + a_{12} x_2 + a_{22} x_2^2 + \ldots + b$$

is one way of presenting nonlinear multivariate regression. Another is the exponential form:

$$y = (e^{a_1 x_1})(e^{a_2 x_2})\ldots(b),$$

where e is a mathematically convenient constant. (e = 2.71828). This form is equivalent to

$$\log y = a_1 x_1 + a_2 x_2 + \ldots + b$$

which is the same form commonly used in simple nonlinear regression.

Measures of the Analysis

Although the prediction equations take the forms given above, a substantial amount of additional information is produced by most multiple regression programs. This information is equally important as the equations themselves. Although the exact output depends upon the specific program, most of the following are usually present, and are useful in interpreting the results.

1. Variances and means: Each of the variables has a sample mean and variance. The sample variance of the dependent variable is of particular importance. If there are N data points

$$\bar{\bar{y}} = \sum_N y_i / N$$

$$\sigma^2 = \sum_N (y_i - \bar{\bar{y}})^2 / (N - 1)$$

The term *SST* is the *total sum of squares* of y.

$$SST = \sum (y_i - \bar{\bar{y}})^2$$

If the analysis results in a predicted value of y, which can be designated as $\bar{y}$, there is a *residual sum of squares (SSR)*.

$$SSR = \sum_N (y_i - \bar{y})^2$$

The difference between the residual sum of squares and total sum of squares is the *regression sum of squares (SSE)*.

$$SSE = SST - SSR$$

The *residual variance*, S^2

$$S^2 = SSR / (N-n-1)$$

if there are N data points, and n variables.

2. Correlation coefficients:

    (a) *Multiple correlation coefficient (R)* or coefficient of multiple determination (R^2)

    $$R^2 = \frac{SSE}{SST}$$

    R^2 is the fraction of the variation of the dependent variable explained by the regression analysis.

    This is the same meaning and definition as the simple coefficient of determination used in chapter 2.

    (b) *Simple correlation coefficients*

      For each pair of variables, there is a simple correlation. These are usually presented in tabular form and are used to check the reliability of the results.

3. F statistic

    $$F = \frac{SSE/n}{SSR/(N-n-1)}$$

    This statistic is the same as has been previously encountered. It measures the significance of the regression analysis. The degrees of freedom are (n) and ($N-n-1$).

4. Standard deviation of coefficients of regression: It is possible to calculate a standard deviation for each of the a terms of the regression equation. This is used to check the significance of the individual terms.

Each of these statistics has its uses. The F statistic can be used to test the statistical significance of the regression. If the regression is not significant, the forecaster does not gain by using it instead of the simpler value, $\bar{y}$. The residual variance, S^2, can be transformed to a standard deviation, S, and used in the usual way to estimate confidence limits of the estimate. As is the case in simple time series analysis, the estimate of the confidence interval may require a complex adjustment to S. The appropriate calculation should be discussed with qualified statisticians in terms of the specific situation.

As noted in chapter 2, the problem of prediction in the future is a slightly different one from that of simply ascribing a confidence limit, for it involves judgment as to whether the relationship of the dependent variable to the independent variables will remain the same in the future as it has been during the time in which the data were collected. As a practical matter, one is frequently forced to assume that it will remain constant because of a lack of any information to justify any other assumption.

The individual simple correlation coefficients are used to select among the independent variables and in some cases to arrange the order in which they appear in the equation. This is discussed in this chapter's next section.

The standard deviation of the individual coefficients of regression is used to check their significance as explanatory variables. The limits of confidence of the coefficient can be established using the standard deviation and the normal or student's t table. As a rule of thumb, a coefficient is considered significant if it is more than twice its standard deviation. Only significant variables should be used in forecasting, because of the cost of data collection. (However, if insignificant coefficients appear in the equation they cannot be omitted without recalculation of the equation from the original data.)

Difficulties of Multiple Regression Analysis

Despite its apparent exactitude, multiple regression analysis is subject to far more human judgment and human interference than are usually found in statistical processes. The basic problem is that there are relationships not only between the dependent variable and each of the independent variables but also between each independent variable and each other independent variable. This network of interrelationships is usually imperfectly understood and it leads to a number of potential problems both in performing the analysis and interpreting the results. The difficulty is most clearly illustrated by considering what would happen in multiple regression analysis if two highly correlated independent variables were used simultaneously. Such a situation should not occur in acceptable research because a researcher would not allow both variables to appear in the equation.

Consider an effort to estimate the demand for hospital care based on two independent variables, one measuring age of the population and the other measuring social security payment of hospital services. Since social security support is almost entirely limited to patients over age 65 it can be seen that these two variables will be highly correlated. That is when the percentage of aged is high, the percentage of social security finance will also be high and vice versa. If a simple correlation analysis is run on hospital admissions per 1000 population versus the percentage of the population over age 65, it is likely to show a significant positive correlation coefficient and a significant regression equation.

If multiple regression analysis is then done using both the percentage over 65 and percentage covered through social security financing as independent variables, any one of three possibilities may occur. The actual result is dependent on the mechanical order in which the independent variables are handled and the techniques of analysis prescribed in the specific computer program. The result may be a high coefficient of regression for age and a low one for social security coverage, the opposite of that, or an approximately equal weight to each of these factors. All three of these equations are likely to be significant according to the F test, since the original significant relationship is still present. The unsophisticated analyst who has made only one calculation of his regression equation and who has not carefully considered the meaning of the dependent variables he had selected may be tricked into some insupportable conclusions about the effect of social security financing on the use of the hospital.

There are specific steps which can be taken to avoid or reduce the possibility of errors of this kind. First is in the selection and ordering of the variables. It is good practice to review the simple correlations between each of the independent variables and between these and the dependent variables. Obviously highly intercorrelated variables, such as the two in the example, would be detected by study of these correlations. Normally one of them would be discarded. In some programs it is also wise to specify the order in which the variables are listed, taking them in decreasing order of simple correlation to the dependent variable (some programs do this automatically). Second, care should be taken in the selection of the data. If one were in fact seeking the impact of social security financing on use of the hospital, one would attempt to restrict the data to exclude populations where this factor was not an issue, such as those under 65. Third, care is necessary in the selection of the analysis program. Some programs have better capability of handling interactions between independent variables than others. The fourth step is the repetition of the analysis and the review of the values for the coefficients of regression under varying conditions. It is possible to do this by repeating the analysis on several different sets of data and also by repeating the analysis with several different selections of independent variables. An important independent variable would be one which tended to appear repeatedly as a significant factor in the estimation of the dependent variable. Other variables, which did not have this characteristic, should ideally be dropped from the equation before it is used for forecasting. Fifth, the conclusion should be written cautiously with full recognition of the extent of the exploration, the limitations of the data, and the limitations of the program. From an administrative viewpoint, it should be clear that an analysis which shows careful attention to these five elements is more likely to be reliable than one which does not. Further, it should be noted that the transferability of results of multivariate analysis is limited. An analysis which is performed for one purpose may not be carefully designed and interpreted for the second purpose. The user who adopts the conclusions for purposes other than those originally intended does so at his own risk.

Multiple Regression Computer Programs

A rapidly growing number and variety of multiple regression programs are available in the libraries of large computers. As computer capacity has grown, the sophistication of these programs has increased and it is reasonable that this trend will continue. Two general programming approaches have been taken in the more elementary programs. The first of these, stepwise multiple regression, proceeds automatically through a list of independent variables adding them to the regression equation in order of their correlation with the dependent variable. That is, a simple equation is calculated using the single independent variable with the highest simple R^2 value, a new set of simple correlations is calculated against this first estimate of the dependent variable, the variable from this set with the highest R^2 is added and a second equation calculated, and the process is repeated a number of times.

Other programs take a more general approach and permit the operator to specify the order in which variables are to be handled. Usually these permit the operator to make a large number of selections of independent variables and to compare and analyze the resulting equations. In general these programs are capable of more revealing analyses than stepwise programs, but they can also be time-consuming. If reasonable care has been taken in specifying the independent variables for stepwise regression, it can yield meaningful results. More advanced regression programs exist which take into account nonlinear relationships, permit the handling of several dependent variables simultaneously, and perform other complex chores. These are beyond the scope of this discussion.

Examples of Multivariate Analysis of Demand for Inpatient Care

The intricacies of analyzing the effect of population and supply factors on demand led many researchers to the use of multivariate techniques when the computer advancements made these available. Despite widespread work with these techniques, analysis of the causes of demand is still unclear, with substantial disagreement among authors. The development of a general model for prediction in terms of the population characteristics of local service areas has not yet come about. In order to be useful for administrative purposes—that is, to predict demand for management decisions—the model will have to fulfill the conditions of careful analysis given above and in addition will have to permit estimation based upon a few easily measurable independent variables. The coefficients of regression will have to have been tested in several locales and shown to yield stable results over a range of values of independent variables. Also, the estimate must be valid when it is compared to actual use in several communities. The principal difficulties which must be resolved are as follows:

1. Many analytic models have been based upon household surveys and restricted by practicality to living civilians not residing in institutions at the time of the survey. Data from surveys of this sort understate actual use by 10 to 30 percent because of underreporting, use by patients who died before the survey, and use by patients in institutions.[2,3,4]
2. Dimensions of the analysis are unsuitable. Dollar expenditures are the dependent variable instead of admissions or patient days. Independent variables are not easily measurable in themselves.
3. Correlations are low, errors of estimate high, significance of the equation is not given, or the models fail to give stable results when tried on different sets of data.[5]
4. Data are derived from limited populations, without evidence that generalization is justifiable.[6,7]

There appears to be good reason to hope for improvement in the future. The problems of weakness of survey data are being studied by the National Center for Health Statistics,[8] which now compiles a continuing series of data on use from family surveys. This series, when corrected for reporting errors, might provide a reliable model for prediction.[9] Although most of the problems listed above apparently can be overcome, the predictive value of the model will have to be tested after it has been developed.

Feldstein and German have suggested that a combination of population characteristics plus past experience will be most useful for the hospital with historical data of its own.[10] Their effort was an attempt to predict statewide hospital use, rather than individual hospital use. Using the fifty states as the sample and patient days of acute hospital care in 1961 as the dependent variable, the resulting equation was:[11]

$$PD/1961 = 248.43$$

$$- 0.039 \text{ (Median Income)}$$
$$(0.019)$$

$$+ 0.391 \text{ (Insurance)}$$
$$(0.082)$$

$$- 5.370 \text{ (Room Rate)}$$
$$(3.020)$$

$$- 0.085 \text{ (\% Urbanization)}$$
$$(0.821)$$

$$- 3.013 \text{ (\% 55 and Over)}$$
$$(3.719)$$

$$- 1.115\,(\%\,\text{Nonwhite})$$
$$(0.997)$$

$$+ 0.893\,(PD/1956)$$
$$(0.052)$$

yielding $R = 0.97$

$R^2 = 0.94$

$S = 43.37$,

where:

$PD/1961$ = patient days in 1961 (or five years after the prediction date)

$PD/1956$ = patient days in 1956 (last available actual data)

S = Standard error of estimate

Parenthetical values are standard deviations of coefficients of regression.

This equation was substantially more satisfactory than any other tried without the PD/1956 term and slightly more satisfactory than those which ignored population variables. Standard errors for population-variables-only equations were about 100; for patient-day-only models, 55 or larger. The equation was developed after exploration of at least eleven others. Although the F value was not reported, one may infer high significance from the R^2 value, combined with the fact that there were 41 degrees of freedom remaining. (R^2 can be high but not significant if the residual number of degrees of freedom ($N - 1 -$ number of independent variables) is low.)

Despite the promise which this finding holds, substantial work must still be done to bring it to a useful state for management purposes. Four of the independent variables are not statistically significant and were included by the authors because economic theory or previous studies of hospital use indicated that they might be significant. The coefficient for the age variable is negative, an unexpected result. The data are pre-Medicare. This change in availability of funds for care might result in a major shift among the coefficients. Lastly, the application has not been made to an individual service area. All of these problems bear investigation.

The model does suggest a promising opportunity, however. A hospital having data for a ten-year period or more could perform analyses upon its own data and derive its own prediction equation, testing its validity upon known past experience and modifying the equation as new independent variable measures become available. In order to do this, it would be necessary to know the service area, annual patient days, and values for the other independent variables. These might be estimated from periodic surveys of the community, however. Variables such as bed supply, number of physicians, and percentage of patient days covered by insurance might be tested as well as those suggested by Feldstein and German.

It should be noted that all the techniques for predicting demands that have been discussed—projections of historical data, estimates based upon population characteristics, and combined population and historical approaches—assume that the future community will resemble the one or ones from which the data were drawn. Even in the case where population projections of both numbers and characteristics of the population are used, the assumptions imply that there will be no abrupt large changes in the nature of the community or its health care system. No matter how sophisticated the estimating equations become, using them to predict the future will imply that the conditions of the future are not startlingly different from those which were used to derive the equations. Only sound professional judgment can be used to evaluate this implication. At least three kinds of situations where the conditions for use of the estimating equations are not met can be imagined. The first of these is where a sudden disruption in the demand for service is occasioned. Such a situation might have existed in the United States in the late 1960s as the impact of Medicare and Medicaid provisions was implemented in communities across the nation. In some communities having large percentages of the population eligible for either one or both of these financing mechanisms, a sudden upward shift in demand may have occurred. Equations based on past experience, whether that of the nation or of the local community, are not likely to predict this shift well. A second condition of this kind will be in an area where rapid growth has occurred in the number of persons or corresponding sudden shifts have occurred in the population characteristics. Such a situation might create substantial unmet demand as both the supply of physicians and that of hospitals are likely to lag behind the population growth. A third case would come about by policy decision, in a situation where the indicated level of utilization of acute facilities was felt to be too expensive, or unnecessary. A deliberate limitation of facilities might be contemplated with the intent of curtailing explicit demand.

In each of these cases and others like them, the use of estimating equations is still of substantial value. However, it is equally important that the dynamics of the situation be carefully studied by people experienced in the prediction of demand, and that they employ their subjective judgment to revise the prediction. Their revision, aided by the statistical techniques, seems likely to be a better estimate than their unaided judgment. Even in cases where statistical estimates apparently have little validity, their preparation and study appears to be worthwhile, for it provides a point of reference for comparison.

Short-Term Forecasting Techniques

There are many situations in the hospital when it would be desirable to know the demand for a given service over a period ranging from 24 hours to several months in advance. For most of these situations it is necessary to know more than simply the expected value based upon past experience generally. A specific forecast tailored to seasonal or weekly variation, or a probabilistic forecast may be in order. For example, for the purpose of nurse staffing, it would be desirable to know what the census of the various units is likely to be twenty-four hours in the future. Many other demand variables, such as meals, laundry, and pharmacy service are related to the daily census. Emergency services sometimes fluctuate by hour of the day, and staffing may be adjusted to the forecast load. Simple methods exist for predicting these values.

Many hospital demand processes are *complex*, that is, the demand is the sum of several different generating processes or *components*. These will have different variation over time and often different rates of growth. In addition, there may be differing priorities associated with each component. For example, operating room demand is the sum of both inpatient and outpatient scheduled demands, and emergency demand. Emergency demand usually represents a life-threatening situation, and is accorded a much higher priority. The first step in refining forecasts of demand is to divide it into components representing reasonably identifiable elements in the total. Each component can then be examined for its special characteristics and forecast independently. The principal characteristics of interest are the stationarity, secular trend, cyclical variation, and random variation. These will be discussed in the following pages.

When demand is stable with respect to time, it is said to be *stationary*. When a detectable pattern of change over time can be detected, the demand is *nonstationary*. Nonstationarity is of two types: secular trends and cyclical variation. Either or both can occur in a given situation. A *secular trend* exists in nonstationary demand when it changes consistently over time. Trends may be either upward or downward, and they are detected by time series regression analysis as described in chapter 2. A secular trend is proven to exist when a regression equation, either linear or nonlinear, is judged significant by the F test.

Cyclical Variation

Cyclical variation exists when a statistic changes periodically in a recurring manner. It is detected by a study of values for comparable time segments of the cycle (days for a weekly cycle, hours for a daily cycle, etc.). The cycle is proven to exist when statistically significant difference is detected for each of the time segments. Although analysis of variance techniques can be used to prove cyclical variation, the more common method is the use of the χ^2 test, as illustrated in the following example.

The data shown in table 3-1 represent two month's experience on the demand for operating room service. The total demand has already been divided into components representing scheduled and emergency portions. The question is whether the forecast of daily expected value of the scheduled work can be refined by a weekly cyclical index. To construct the index, the sum of values for each day of the week must be calculated. This calculation is shown in table 3-2.

The index, I_j, shows some variation, but it is clearly small and may be statistically insignificant. The χ^2 test can be used to test the hypothesis that the variation is not significant. This test measures the cumulative variation from a hypothetical value. In this case the calculations are as follows; where

$$y = \text{sample value}$$
$$y_n = \text{hypothetical value} = 17.4 n_j$$
$$\chi^2 = \frac{(y - y_n)^2}{y_n}$$

Day	y	y_n	$(y - y_n)^2$	$(y - y_n)^2/y_n$
Monday	156	156	0	0.000
Tuesday	148	156	64	0.410
Wednesday	148	156	64	0.410
Thursday	171	156	225	1.442
Friday	142	139	9	0.065
TOTAL	765	765	362	2.327

The values of χ^2 for varying probabilities and degrees of freedom are tabulated. Degrees of freedom are calculated by the following formula:

$$(r - 1)(c - 1) = \text{d.f.},$$

where
$r = $ number of rows
$c = $ number of columns

In this case: $(5 - 1)(2 - 1) = 4$ d.f.

From the tabulated values of the χ^2 statistic, $\chi^2 = 2.327$ for four degrees of freedom will occur more than half the time by chance ($\chi^2_{0.50} = 3.4$), and the value of χ^2 for rejecting the hypothesis at 95 percent confidence, $\chi^2_{.05}$, is 9.5. Therefore, the index I_j is not significant, and will not be of value in refining the daily forecast. If it had proven significant the expected value for the average day could be refined for each day of the week by using the index value. For example, if a forecast was prepared for each week in the future, $\hat{y} = $ ex-

Table 3-1
Operating Room Demand

| | Scheduled | | Emergency | |
Day	Month I	Month II	Month I	Month II
Saturday	0		1	
Sunday	0		1	
Monday	18		3	
Tuesday	14	16	2	1
Wednesday	14	17	1	2
Thursday	18	20	3	1
Friday	19	20	0	1
Saturday	0	0	2	3
Sunday	0	0	4	1
Monday	16	17	3	2
Tuesday	17	17	0	4
Wednesday	20	16	4	2
Thursday	20	20	2	1
Friday	14	15	2	1
Saturday	0	0	6	3
Sunday	0	0	0	2
Monday	17	15	2	3
Tuesday	16	18	3	2
Wednesday	13	13	2	0
Thursday	20	18	3	6
Friday	19	18	1	2
Saturday	0	0	1	2
Sunday	0	0	2	4
Monday	21	19	4	0
Tuesday	19	14	2	3
Wednesday	19	18	1	4
Thursday	18	16	3	2
Friday	19	20	1	0
Saturday	0	0	1	3
Sunday	0	0	2	1
Monday	15	18	1	2
Tuesday		17		3
Wednesday		18		1
Thursday		21		1
Total		765		126

Table 3-2
Scheduled Surgery Demand by Day of Week

Day	n_j	Sum$_j$	Mean$_j$	I_j
Monday	9	156	17.4	1.00
Tuesday	9	148	16.5	0.95
Wednesday	9	148	16.5	0.95
Thursday	9	171	19.0	1.10
Friday	8	142	17.8	1.02
Saturday	–	–	–	–
Sunday	–	–	–	–
All Days	44	765	17.4	1.00

Expected daily sum (hypothetical value) = $17.4 \times n_j$

Index $I_j = \dfrac{\text{Sum}_j}{17.4 n_j}$

pected surgery for a five day week, the value for the j day of that week would be

$$\hat{y}_j = 1/5\,(\hat{y}) \cdot I_j \;.$$

Daily and monthly cyclical variations can be handled together, in sequential operations, if desired. For example, if an annual cycle has been detected, an index I_m can be constructed for each month. For a monthly expected demand, given an annual forecast $\hat{y}$,

$$\hat{y}_m = 1/12\,(\hat{y}) \cdot I_m \;.$$

and for 22 scheduled day month, the daily variation

$$\hat{y}_j = 1/22\,(\hat{y}_m) \cdot I_j \;.$$

Exponential Smoothing

Another approach to short range forecasting under non-stationarity is the exponential smoothing method. This technique has the advantage of very simple calculations, relatively easy adaptability to the computer, and adjustable sensitivity to the immediate past. Experimental applications in hospitals are numerous, and routine use is likely within the next few years.

This approach uses a previous forecast and the actual value from the most recent completed time period to make an adjusted forecast. Where

$\hat{Y}_{t+1}$ = forecast for the desired time period, 1 period in the future
Y_t = actual, last time period
$\hat{Y}_t$ = forecast, last time period
a = weighting factor or *smoothing coefficient,* $0<a<1$

then:

$$\hat{Y}_{t+1} = \hat{Y}_t + a(Y_t - \hat{Y}_t)$$

The forecast is last period's forecast, adjusted by some fraction of the error between last period forecast and actual. The equation permits calculation by only three terms. In computerized projections, only two terms, a and $\hat{Y}_t$, need to be stored for future reference. The initial forecast to start the series can be based on an average of recent values of Y, or on a regression analysis. The forecast is self-correcting. Any initial errors disappear as subsequent forecasts are prepared.

Selecting the value of the weighting factor a is largely a matter of judgment. The larger the value of a, the more weight is given to the current value rather than the old estimate. At $a = 1$, the current value is used exclusively. Conversely near $a = 0$, the old estimate is weighted much more heavily than current experience. The value of a can be checked by trial and error by keeping record of the forecast and the actual and adjusting a to minimize the error over time. One authority suggests a value of $a = 0.1$ for most uses, with higher values, up to $a = 0.5$, for the first few periods of use, or when there has been a sudden permanent change to eliminate errors rapidly. Higher values are also justified when the statistic is *autocorrelated*, that is when near future values are heavily determined by present values. This situation is likely to occur in census prediction, for example. Exponential smoothing can be used to forecast from one to several periods into the future. For longer range forecasts ($k \geqslant 3$), low values of a, near $a = 0.1$ are generally appropriate.[1,2]

A number of modifications can be made upon this simple calculation, including adjustment for cyclic indexes, extra smoothing coefficients, and variable smoothing coefficients. The larger the smoothing coefficient, the more quickly the forecast moves in response to a sudden change. This can be either good or bad, depending on the situation. If the change represents a shift in the underlying process which is likely to recur for the next several periods, it is good, but if it represents a random effect which is not likely to recur, then the forecast should ignore it.

The measure of effectiveness of exponential smoothing forecasts is the difference between forecast and actual. Various arrangements of smoothing coefficients and their values are generally tried on past data to find the one which fits local needs the best. This is not always the one which gives the minimum absolute error. Sometimes the forecaster would rather be high than low, or he can accept many small errors but is seriously troubled by a few large ones, etc. All this tends to make exponential smoothing models a "cut and fit" proposition.

Work at the University of Michigan has been directed to the evaluation of several model variations and smoothing coefficient values in preparing monthly forecasts for all the departments of a single hospital. Preliminary results indicate that the best models usually include a seasonal index correction, and that different departments require different models and smoothing coefficients. The final selection of the model is also a function of the kind of error which can be tolerated.[13]

Analysis of Randomness

In many hospital situations, forecast of the expected value is not sufficient. This is true generally when demand must be met without appreciable delays and demand varies by an important amount from day to day due to random factors. Obstetrics and emergency services of all kinds are the most obvious examples, although they are not the only ones. If resources are made available only to meet the expected value of demand, these resources will be overtaxed about half the time. It is obvious that additional resources must be provided to meet peak loads in demand. What is desired is a known level of confidence about the size of these peaks, and this knowledge comes from an analysis of the variation in demand. A similar problem can exist when the amount of resources available varies. The most common example is manpower, where absenteeism creates apparently random variation in the number of persons reporting for work. The techniques described below are applicable to either situation.

Empirical Inference

The simplest approach to problems of this kind is to analyze past experience and to forecast with the assumption that future behavior of the process will be the same as the past. To do this, historic data must be arranged in a frequency distribution showing the relative number of occurrences of values of the event in question. For example, analysis of the absenteeism records of a small hospital show that of 150 employees absenteeism was as follows.

Number Absent	Days Occurring	Percentage of Days
less than 2	3	0.4
2-3	20	2.7
4-5	75	10.3
6-7	150	20.6

Number Absent	Days Occurring	Percentage of Days
8-9	200	27.4
10-11	137	18.8
12-13	98	13.4
14-15	32	4.4
over 15	15	2.0
Total	730	100.0

The frequency distribution can also be graphed, as shown in figure 3-1. Such graphs are called *histograms*.

The probabilities can be read directly from this table and can be used as a forecast. Absenteeism will be less than 5 percent (7.5 persons) 34 percent of the time, or one day in three. It will be 10 percent or greater 2 percent of the time, or seven to eight days a year. The assumption accepted in the forecast is that the process generating absenteeism will remain the same.

In making the forecasts about the probability of relative frequency of absenteeism, the *empirical* distribution was used. That is, inference was made directly from the data themselves, and no attempt was made to describe the frequency distribution mathematically or to ascribe any theoretical shape to it. The groups of the frequency distribution were accepted as is. No effort was made to estimate individual values within the group, as for example, the frequency of exactly fourteen persons absent. A variety of arbitrary techniques exist for estimating individual values within grouped empirical data. These are

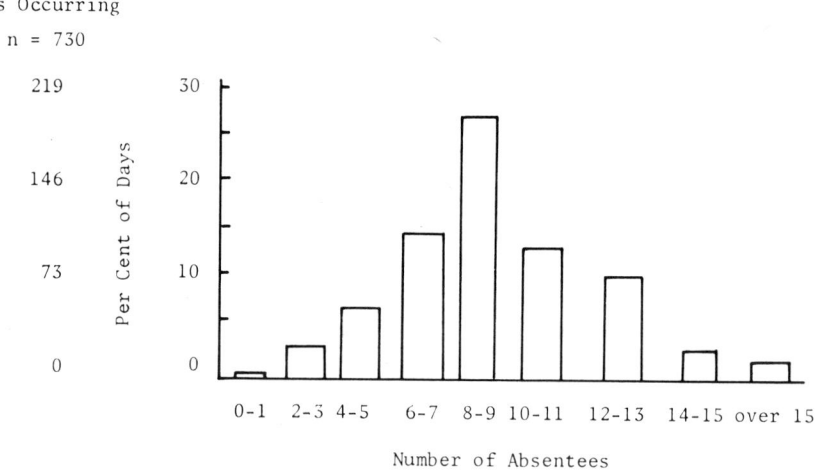

Figure 3-1. Histogram of Absenteeism.

called *smoothing* techniques and involve interpolations between adjacent groups. The smoothed empirical data are frequently used to prepare a forecast. For example, one might assume the average value for eight and nine absences is 100, and for ten and eleven, 68. Then the value for 10 might be set at $(100 + 68)/2 = 84$. The value for 11 would be $137 - 84 = 53$. This technique gives the same result as drawing a smooth curve through the midpoints of each group on the histogram and dividing the scale on the vertical axis by the group size.

Inference from Known Distributions

Another approach to forecasting variation is to demonstrate that an empirical frequency distribution is congruent with a known, tabulated theoretical distribution. Once a particular generating process has been shown to take the form of a known theoretical distribution, it is convenient to assume that it can be approximated by the theoretical value. In this way, much of the tedious and expensive work of data collection can be avoided. The distributions themselves can be manipulated mathematically to estimate what would occur if various changes were introduced. The theoretical distributions are usually described in three ways: by name, by mathematical function, and by tabulated values. A growing number have been identified by operations researchers. The three most common in hospitals will be described here, in terms of their applications rather than their mathematical derivations.

Binomial distribution. The binomial is an ancient distribution which theoretically describes most chance or random situations having the characteristic of two and only two states. Thus it describes coin tosses (heads or tails), lottery draws (winning tickets versus nonwinning tickets) dice throws, and playing card deals. (The latter of course must be broken down to binomial situations as spades versus no spades, "boxcars" versus other possibilities.) Other than in games of chance, the binomial describes any situation where a number of independent trials or draws are made with equal likelihood that each trial will have one of the two possible states. The distribution describes the probability that any given number of the trials actually are in the desired state. If, for example, the probability of death is considered equally likely for any patient with a given disease, and twenty-five patients have been admitted with the disease, the binomial theorem will predict the probability of specific numbers of deaths, from zero to twenty-five. If falling out of bed is equally likely among a certain group of patients, and fifteen of these patients are on a ward, the theorem predicts the number of falls.

The conditions which must be met, stated without mathematical rigor, are:

1. Two states and only two states. Many problems can be structured to this condition even if they do not seem so immediately

2. Equal likelihood of a given state for all members of the population
3. Independence of trials. There can be no "linkage" between the individual cases of the desired state. Thus each death must be independent of every other, each fall, and so forth

The processes which generate trials meeting these conditions are sometimes called *Bernoulli processes* or Bernoulli trials.

The practical uses of the binomial distribution are to test the conditions of independence and to forecast demands of a certain type. In testing independence, the expected frequency forecast by the binomial theorem is compared to the actual. A significant difference indicates a high probability that the process is not a Bernoulli process. Either the equal likelihood condition or the independence condition, or both, are not being met by the process.

Investigation is likely to reveal some linkage between individual trials or differing probabilities of being in the desired state. If the possibility of a given patient demanding a certain service is equally likely among all patients, then the total demand for that service is estimated by the binomial. An example is the nurse call light. If there are ten patients, and each has an independent 30 percent chance of putting the call light on in one hour, the binomial theorem gives the probability that a given number of call lights will go on in the next hour.

The algebraic statement of the binomial theorem is

$$P_k = \frac{n!}{(k!)(n-k)!} p^k q^{n-k},$$

where P_k = probability of k trials out of n occurring in the desired state
p = probability of the desired state in a single trial,
$q = 1 - p$.
The term $n!/(n-k)!$ is sometimes written $\binom{n}{k}$:

The expected value of the binomial is

$$\bar{x} = pn$$

and the standard deviation

$$\sigma = \sqrt{pq/(n-1)}.$$

The major difficulty with the binomial theorem is that the probability equation cannot be solved when n gets large. Tabulated values are available for small n (less than 50). Approximations are used in other cases. The theorem allows the estimation of the standard deviation, in cases where the process applies, without empirical data. Thus a situation is fully described in a probability sense by saying it is a Bernoulli process, with a given probability p.

Poisson Distribution. Another common theoretical distribution dealing with the probability of random events is called the *Poisson* distribution. It describes special cases of the binomial or Bernoulli process covering events where the probability, p, for any individual member of the population is very low. The conditions of independence and equal likelihood among all members of population which are required of Bernoulli processes are also required for Poisson processes. In addition the condition must be met that the probability of any individual member of the population having the desired characteristic is low. This condition plus the three conditions of the Bernoulli process define a *Poisson process*. The process is measured by the Poisson distribution, which is expressed mathematically as

$$P_k = \frac{e^{-\alpha} \alpha^k}{k!}$$

where $e = 2.71828$
k = the number of occurrences of the desired event
α = the expected value of occurrences

By definition the expected value of a Poisson distribution is α. The variance of a Poisson distribution is also α.

$$\bar{x} = \alpha$$

$$\sigma = \sqrt{\alpha} \ .$$

This characteristic of the Poisson distribution, that $\bar{x} = \sigma^2$, is very convenient for the solution of practical problems. In terms of a given population or number of trials of size n, with a probability of ocurrence in each member of p, it is also the case that

$$\alpha = pn \ .$$

Many practical examples of Poisson processes in hospitals have been uncovered. Accidents and illnesses meet the conditions under some circumstances. So do pregnancies. Thus demands for emergency room, coronary care unit, intensive-care unit, labor and delivery rooms, and emergency admissions can usually be described by the Poisson distribution. Each case must be considered individually because the conditions of independence and equal likelihood are not always met. Some illnesses are caused by factors such as epidemics which link members of the population. Accidents are often subject to cyclical variation by hour of day or season of year. The process is nonstationary, and the assumption of equal likelihood can only be made for corresponding parts of the cycle.

Although variations from independence are insignificant in the occurrence of pregnancy, the demand for delivery room service can be scheduled in some cases. When this occurs, independence has been lost.

Certain processes do not meet the conditions for Poisson but have been shown empirically to be close enough that the distribution provides an adequate approximation. These are usually compound processes combining several simpler processes. If there is independence between the simpler processes, the total can be sometimes treated as independent even when some of the simple processes are strongly linked in themselves. An important example of this is the hospital census, when it is not curtailed by a restriction on its upper limit. (That is, when there is never a shortage of available beds.) Even though it combines both scheduled and random elements in both admission and discharge, the combination of multiple processes follows the Poisson distribution.[14] Considering all its known applications, the Poisson distribution is more common by far than the binomial. Values for probabilities of Poisson distributions are tabulated through $\alpha = 30$. For larger expected values, the normal distribution is used as an approximation. If the assumption of a Poisson process is proven, the standard deviation need not be calculated empirically, but can be assumed to be.

$$\sigma = \sqrt{\alpha}$$

(The reverse is not true. That is, just because $\sigma = \sqrt{\alpha}$ one cannot assume a Poisson process.)

Proving Congruence to a Poisson or Binomial Distribution. If a process is suspected to follow a known process such as the binomial or the Poisson, and an empirical frequency distribution is available, it is a simple matter to test the fit of the empirical distribution to the theoretical one. The test used is the χ^2 test, and the proof is of the null hypothesis, that the empirical distribution is not significantly different from the theoretical one with the same expected value. The statistical proof, which is illustrated in the example below, should be corroborated by comparing the conditions for the Poisson or the binomial against the actual process wherever possible.

The emergency surgery data given in table 3-1 can be used as an example. The processes generating this demand are multiple, but most of them appear independent. While accidents can lead to linked multiple occurrences and might be nonstationary on a seasonal basis, there are apparently no other epidemic type links, and the Poisson process looks promising.

The statistical test is as follows.
If:

h = hypothetical frequency (from a Poisson table)

f = observed frequency (from table 3-1)

k = number of values of y

$$\chi^2 = \sum_k \frac{(f-h)^2}{h}$$

for $k-1$ degrees of freedom,
the values are as follows where the hypothetical distribution is Poisson, with mean = 2.0.

y	f	h	$(f-h)$	$(f-h)^2$	$\frac{(f-h)^2}{h}$
0	6	8.4	−2.4	5.76	0.686
1	18	16.8	1.2	1.44	0.086
2	18	16.8	1.2	1.44	0.086
3	12	11.2	0.8	0.64	0.058
>3	8	8.8	0.8	0.64	0.072
Total	62				0.988 = χ^2

$\bar{y} = 126/62 = 2.03$ $\chi_{.05}^2 = 7.8$ for d.f. = 3,

and the conclusion is that sample values do not differ significantly from the hypothetical distribution. In applying the χ^2 test, the usual formula for calculating degrees of freedom (d.f. = $(r-1)(c-1)$) has been modified. Because one row of the distribution contains more values than the others (the row ">3" contains values for 4, 5, and larger values in both the actual and the hypothetical distribution), an extra degree of freedom has been sacrificed. The remaining degrees of freedom are

$$(r-2)(c-1) = 3.$$

Collapsing the upper end of the distribution is necessary because the χ^2 test is appropriate only when there are five or more cases in each cell.

With the additional information derived by the assumption that emergencies follow the Poisson distribution, the maximum demand at a given confidence level can be specified. Thus 95 percent of the time from the Poisson distribution, $\bar{x} = 2.0$, there will be four or fewer emergencies in a day. Six emergencies can be expected only slightly more than 1 percent of the time.

The χ^2 test can be used to test congruence with other theoretical distributions, such as the binomial or the normal, when desired.

The Normal Distribution. By far the most frequently encountered tabulated distribution is the *normal*, which is familiar to every student of elementary statistics. There are three major reasons why this distribution is so useful:

1. Many statistics from natural processes are themselves normally distributed. Frequency distributions of height, weight, intelligence scores, and count-

less other measures of human performance can be approximated by the normal distribution.
2. Both the binomial and the Poisson distribution approach the normal distribution under certain commonly encountered conditions. For the Poisson, this occurs when α becomes large ($\alpha > 30$). For the binomial, the normal distribution is commonly substituted when n (the number of trials) becomes large ($n > 30$).
3. The distributions of values of repeated samples from a single population follow the normal distribution even if the original population is not normally distributed, according to a mathematical statement called the *central limit theorem*. This theorem is used most extensively in statistical quality control and is also useful in other estimating problems.

Values of the cumulative probability under the normal distribution are generally tabulated according to the z statistic, where

$$z = \frac{x - \bar{x}}{\sigma}$$

where
x is the value of interest
$\bar{x}$ is the mean of the distribution
σ is the standard deviation

It is useful to recall that values of x greater than $\bar{x} + \sigma$ occur with an approximate cumulative probability of 1/6 (0.17) and values of x greater than $\bar{x} + 2\sigma$ occur with a probability of 1/40 (0.025). The normal distribution is symmetrical, so that values of x less than $\bar{x} - 2\sigma$ and greater than $\bar{x} + 2\sigma$ occur with a combined probability of 1/20 (0.05). Thus the range $\bar{x} \pm 2\sigma$ includes 95 percent of the probable values of x, and is said to be the 0.95 confidence interval.

Additional Readings

Fox, Ezekiel and K.A., *Methods of Correlation and Regression Analysis*, John Wiley and Sons, 1965

Freund & Williams, *Elementary Business Statistics*
- On one-way analysis of variance, pp. 384-89.
- On χ^2 tests of variation in proportion, pp. 278-80, 284-86.
- On χ^2 tests of goodness of fit, pp. 287-92.
- On seasonal (cyclical) variation, pp. 335-44.
- On frequency distributions and histograms, pp. 10-20.

- On the normal distribution, pp. 195-211, also see index entries.
- On the binomial distribution, pp. 136-39.
- On the Poisson, pp. 141-42, exercises 11 and 12. This description is very limited. A better discussion is usually found in elementary operations research texts, or C.H. Springer, et al. *Statistical Inference*, vol. 3, Mathematics for Management Series, R.D. Irwin, Homewood, Illinois, 1966, pp. 143-48.

4 Determining Population Service Areas and Calculating Use Rates

The Concept of a Service Population

The philosophy of a community hospital includes by definition a notion of a specific community or population group to be served. This population generally can be related to a geographic area, which is referred to as the *service area* of the hospital (the corresponding term in the United Kingdom is "catchment area"). In a conceptual sense the service area population is the group of people who turn to the hospital to meet their needs. Conversely, it is the "public" to whom the hospital is immediately responsible. Its size and special needs will influence the quantity and variety of services the hospital will provide. Its monetary resources are the underlying source of both capital and operating funds. Its human resources and leadership are the most important source of manpower for the hospital, from trustee to unskilled employee. It follows then that identifying and analyzing this service area population is a primary requirement for sound planning.

The concept of a service area population is easier to visualize in a nonmetropolitan setting, where small cities or towns are dispersed from each other geographically. Each contains a community hospital which serves the city and some fraction of the surrounding rural area. It is clear that as long as people have a free choice of hospital or doctor, other factors than geography will influence their choice, and the geographic definition will be less than perfect. In all likelihood, there will be no geographic area which turns entirely to one hospital for care, but the farther the patient is removed from one hospital, the more likely he is to select some other hospital. Thus between any two hospitals in reasonably distant towns there is a high probability that patients in one town will use the hospital in that town, and that the patients between the towns will have some tendency to use the nearer hospital. There is no perfect dividing line for a service area; rather there is some relationship between distance, or geography, and the proportion of patients going to each hospital. One usual solution is to select as the service area limit that point at which there is an *equal likelihood* that patients seeking admission will turn to the study hospital, versus all other hospitals combined. The area so defined is called the *equal likelihood service area*. Another is to plot the proportion, or *density* of use of each hospital by each small population and to sum the product of density and population. Such an approach is called a *relevance index service area*.

The exact measurement of service area involves the cooperation of neighboring hospitals and detailed analysis of the residency of several thousand admissions. In one of the largest-scale applications of the equal likelihood technique, in Kansas and Missouri, the cost was estimated to be $5,000 per service area in 1960, if each were defined individually.[1] However, in individual projects done by the author for several Michigan hospitals, it appeared that the cost of the definition could be kept to less than $1,000 per hospital. Large savings are possible if several areas are done at one time. In the Kansas-Missouri project, the actual cost of definition of 153 service areas simultaneously was $200,000.[2] The cost was probably increased in that project by the extreme care which was taken. Several planning agencies are now defining service areas for all their member hospitals. These generally cost less than $1,000 per hospital.

In addition to the cost, there are certain other difficulties:

1. In urban areas, geographically close areas, and in areas where the offices of doctors are intermingled, the service area tends to be relatively diffuse because patients select from several nearby hospitals with nearly equal frequency despite the difference in distance. Thus large numbers of patients in metropolitan areas do not go to their nearest hospital. In this context, the equal likelihood service areas of individual hospitals do not exist. No hospital captures as much as 50 percent of a given geographical area.
2. In certain cases where a few hospitals are close together, patterns of use depend on other factors than geography and there are no individual service areas. There is a service area for the combined set of hospitals, however.
3. The service area is subject to change in itself, particularly in response to changes in doctors' admitting practices. A doctor serving a village between two hospitals may direct his patients to either hospital or to both. If one hospital adds new beds and attracts the doctor to closer affiliation, it may enlarge its service area at the expense of the other.
4. The hospital may draw relatively large numbers of patients from beyond its service area. This is particularly true of university hospitals and other large institutions with many specialist physicians.
5. The hospital may serve a group of people without geographic definition. Hospitals constructed by group practice plans, such as the Kaiser-Permanente hospitals in California are an example. Veterans Hospitals are another.

The first and second of these difficulties can be met in part by taking hospitals in groups and finding the group service area. The roles of individual hospitals can then be assigned according to the total plan. The third difficulty cannot be met except by recalculation of service areas after changes have occurred. The fourth and fifth require the definition of population groups, either in addition to a geographic service area or instead of it.

The combination of the difficulties and the cost leads some planners and hospital administrators to substitute more arbitrarily defined service areas than those indicated by actual patterns of use. The Joint Committee of the American Hospital Association and the U.S. Public Health Service, on area-wide planning for hospitals, offered the following definitions for planning regions (essentially a logical grouping of service areas) and service areas:

Planning Region – The particular geographic unit for which comprehensive coordinate hospital and related health facilities (hospital, nursing home, other long-term care, rehabilitation, outpatient, home care and public health centers) are planned. . . .
An urban region should include central city, suburbs, and that portion of the surrounding territory which may be expected to become urban in the foreseeable future. A region in less urbanized areas should include trade centers and rural territory normally associated with each Center.
Service Area: A geographic subdivision within a planning region which, by virtue of its population and economic and sociological character, is or can be expected to support a facility offering at least the basic hospital services.[3]

It is not unusual for a hospital to take a set of nearby townships, or other small political subdivisions and assume that this approximates its service area. Similarly a planning agency may take a state or region and divide it into service areas, either arbitrarily or based upon other patterns than hospital use. (Retail trading areas, postal delivery areas, telephone exchanges, and other commercial service areas have been used.) Such procedures are subject to two weaknesses.

1. No comparison of the use rates or demand derived in this manner can ever be made with any other service area because the population base is subject to unknown error. (Studies by the Bureau of Hospital Administration of The University of Michigan of several Michigan communities indicate the error can be far from trivial. Particularly in the cases of Traverse City (1966) and Albion (1961), the actual service area proved to be notably different than expected, by factors of more than 20 percent.)
2. The selection is justifiable for internal use within the institution only if there is evidence that the actual service area and service area population are similar to the assumed ones and in particular are subject to the same trends in characteristics affecting the demand for medical care services. Such evidence might be obtained by analysis of the geographic location of admissions. For example, a hospital might draw 90 percent of its admissions from a few nearby towns, villages and townships, and the use rate calculated on the basis of this population might approximate regional averages very closely. From the first evidence, it can be inferred that *no other* communities lie in the service area, since only 10 percent of demand comes from outside in total, and the amount from any single outside

community will be very small. From the second evidence, that the use rate approximates the regional average, one might infer that the hospital does in fact serve all those places on the arbitrary list. The dangers of the second inference are obvious. The assumption on which it is based is the same as that for which the data are collected; namely that the use rates are in fact equal.

Equal Likelihood Service Areas—The Poland-Lembcke Procedure

Data Collection

The essence of a service area defining procedure is an effort to obtain a complete survey of all general admissions by geographic location. Poland and Lembcke used these data to estimate equal likelihood service areas.[4] The technique is easier to understand than the relevance index approach, but is useful only in rural or near rural areas. Newborn admissions and those to specialized facilities as like nursing homes are excluded. Postal addresses or discharged patients are obtained from hospital records. A survey is taken of all discharges except newborn over a substantial period of time, usually one year. Admission ledgers and annual admission files are the usual source of the data, under the assumption that admissions and discharges are nearly equal. The data are collected from the study hospital and from all surrounding hospitals within reasonable traveling distance. Previous experience in Michigan shows that service areas of small hospitals rarely exceed ten to fifteen miles; thus hospitals with service areas impinging upon the study hospital's are unlikely to be more than twenty to thirty miles distant. This dimension is likely to vary with population density; in thinly populated areas the distance may be much greater. Special care must be taken with larger referral hospitals, which may draw over larger distances. Figure 4-1 shows a hypothetical situation typical of much of the U.S. Midwest. All the hospitals in cities H_1, H_2, H_3, and H_4 would be included in the data collection, and use by post offices "a" through "g" would be determined. Town "h" would normally be excluded because it is much farther from S than either H_2 or H_5. H_5 would not be used in the data collection unless there were reason to think that patients from "h" area used the hospital. Evidence for including "h" and H_5 might be:

— doctors from "a" or "h" admitting to the study hospital S
— significant numbers of patients known to come from "h" to S
— highway routes favoring the trip from "h" to S rather than some other hospital

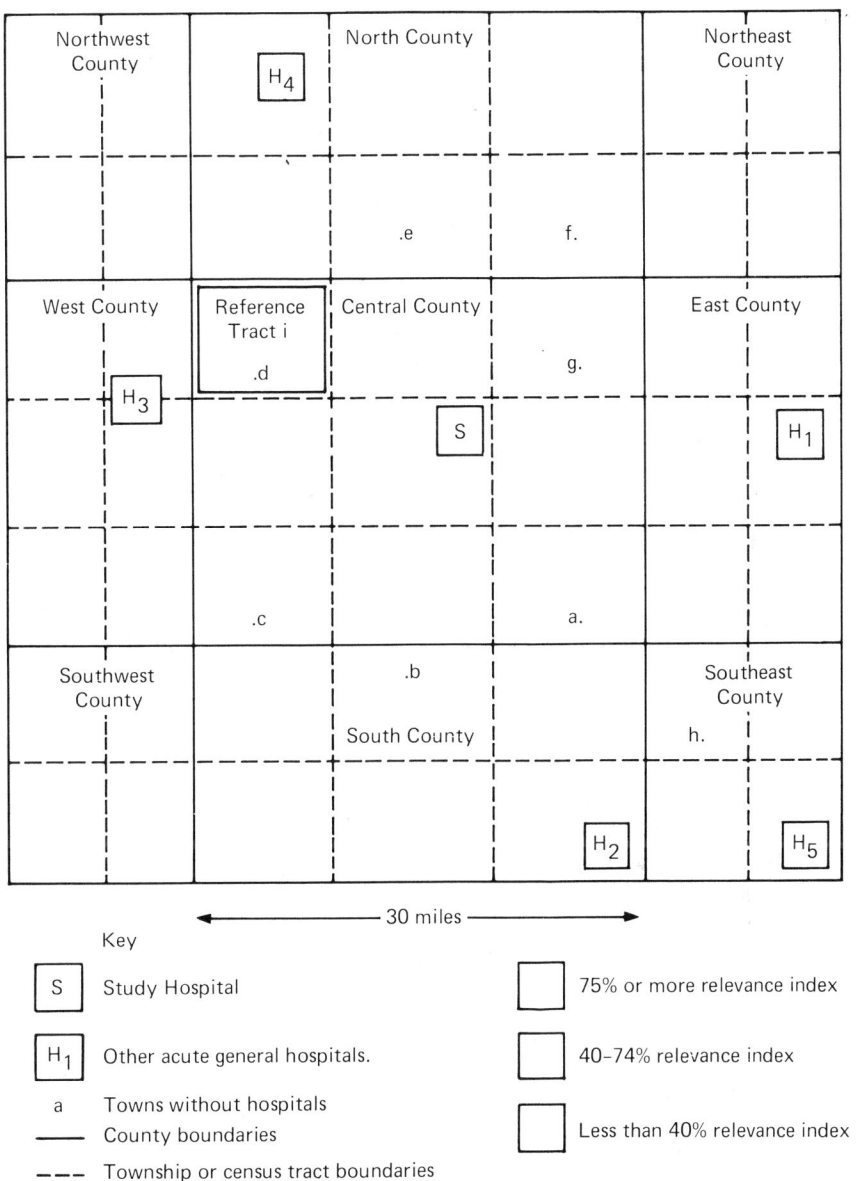

Figure 4-1. Hypothetical Geographic Region.

Identifying Service Area

The Poland-Lembcke procedure translates postal address to township or minor civil division because census information is maintained on this basis. This transformation involves careful study of addresses and census tract boundaries, often with the aid of maps and actual plotting of locations. In metropolitan areas the U.S. Bureau of Census has developed computer programs to translate street address to census tract.[5] In rural areas manual methods may still be required. At this point all admissions from each township are known, and the fraction of admissions to the study hospital can be calculated. The following cases can occur:

1. The township under study has a clear majority (greater than 50 percent) of its patients admitted to the study hospital, and all townships between it and the hospital also have a majority. In this case the township lies within the equal likelyhood service area
2. The opposite of 1. is true. That is, the township does not have a clear majority of admissions to the study hospital, and is adjacent to similar townships. In this case the township lies outside the service area
3. The township divides equally or nearly equally between the study hospital and one or more other hospitals, and adjacent townships show both a majority and less than a majority. In this case the equal likelihood line passes through the township
4. The township has no admissions to the study hospital
5. The township has a clear majority of admissions to the study hospital but is not adjacent to a township having a similar majority, or the converse, the township has a clear majority to another hospital, but is surrounded by townships with majorities to the study hospital

The fifth case is a theoretical possibility which has never been reported in a rural situation. The fourth is treated by grouping the township with a nearby one, depending on post office and travel patterns, and treating the two as one.

Drawing Geographic Boundaries

The equal likelihood line must lie either on the boundary between two townships, or more likely, within the townships of the third case, those not having a clear majority to any one hospital. The rules for drawing the boundary, as set forth by Poland and Lembcke, are as follows:

1. A service area must have one continuous line for its boundary. That is, service area boundaries cannot cross each other or include more than one enclosed area

2. Enclaves (service areas which lie entirely within another service area) are possible for very small hospitals. These are judged to be rare and did not occur in the Kansas-Missouri study
3. The township in which the study hospital is located is assigned to the hospital with very rare exceptions
4. Dividing lines are drawn through townships by judgment, evaluating road networks and population centers. Poland suggests, "It is helpful to draw a line through a populated [village or town] because [it] shows that patients from that place spread to both districts."[6]

Modifications to the Poland-Lembcke Procedure

The University of Michigan Bureau of Hospital Administration studies simplify the Poland-Lembcke procedure by working directly with post office addresses rather than the more detailed study of exact addresses which are translated to townships. Rural population is prorated to the adjacent post offices as follows:

1. The general areas of postal rural routes are determined by discussion with the local postmaster
2. Populations served by rural routes are estimated by taking the number of rural delivery stations (RFD and Star Route boxes) and multiplying by the average family size in the area (from U.S. Census reports). The number of delivery stations is published annually by the Post Office Department.[7] (This technique is useful only where there is no "city" delivery.)
3. Data are collected by post office only, rather than by exact address
4. The service area boundary is drawn to include all post office delivery areas having more than 50 percent admissions to the study hospital, to divide all post office delivery areas where admissions divide equally or nearly equally, and to exclude all post office delivery areas having less than 50 percent admissions to the study hospital. The rules for drawing the boundary (above) are followed

Figure 4-2 shows a hypothetical equal-likelihood service area. The data supporting the line which has been drawn would be like that shown in table 4-1.

It can be seen that considerable judgment is used in drawing the line. It represents at best an approximation of the true situation. (For example, consider that to the south the line clearly falls short of the county boundary, but there is little evidence to show exactly how it should be drawn within the south central township of Central County.)

Calculating Service Area Population

In addition to the geographic map of the service area, it is necessary to have an estimate of the service area population. This can be obtained by summing the

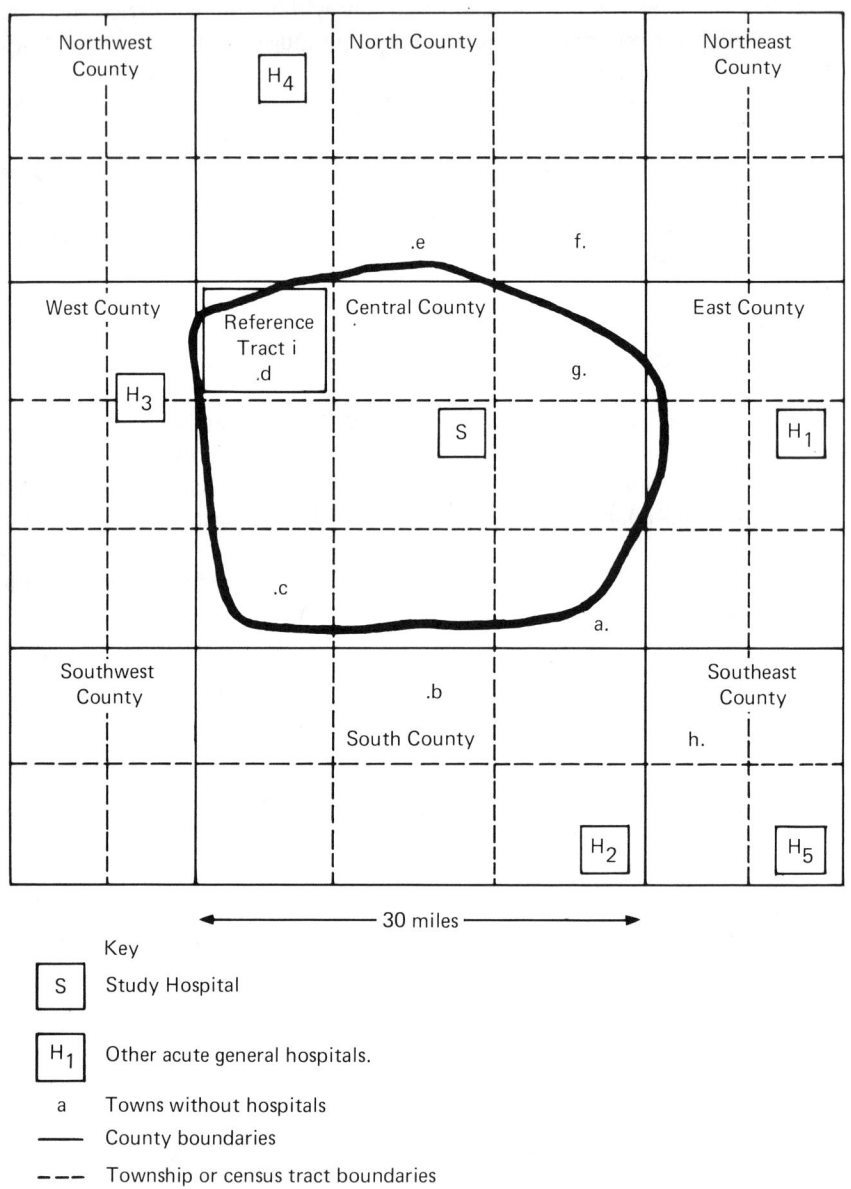

Figure 4-2. Hypothetical Geographic Region Showing Equal Likelihood Service Area.

Table 4-1
Usage of Area Hospitals: Central County and Environs (Hypothetical)

Post Office	Percentage of Admissions					
			Hospital			
	S	H_1	H_2	H_3	H_4	Total
Central County						
S	87	3	–	8	2	100%
a	45	50	5	–	–	100%
c	65	–	–	35	–	100%
d	70	–	–	20	10	100%
g	65	35	–	–	–	100%
North County						
e	35	–	–	–	65	100%
f	10	60	–	–	30	100%
West County						
H_3	10	–	–	90	–	100%
South County						
b	20	–	80	–	–	100%

populations of townships or post office delivery areas and parts of these, as divided by the service area line. Populations of areas on the service area lines are divided in proportion to their admissions. In the Michigan procedure, the total population served by the post office is used for the division. In the Poland-Lembcke procedure, the population of the geographic area is divided according to the land area and villages included or excluded.

Correction Factor for the Equal Likelihood Service Area Population Estimate

The population estimate is subject to two sorts of errors. First, the boundary is drawn subjectively to a certain extent. Second, the nature of traffic across the boundary is not uniform. Some hospitals draw heavily from civil divisions adjacent to their primary service area. Others in contrast "lose" patients even from the town in which they are located. In order to adjust for these errors and permit a more accurate estimate of the service population, the following procedure can be used.

First, calculate the following sums from the original data:

A = sum of all admissions from within the service area to any hospital
B = sum of all admission from within the service area to hospitals in adjacent service areas

C = sum of all admissions from adjacent service areas to study hospital. (In practice this is usually the admissions from towns having hospitals adjacent to the study hospital and all towns in between the study hospital and the next hospital but not in the service area)

In this procedure, admissions from townships or post offices along the line are counted as from the service area to which admission occurs. (That is, there are neither B nor C admissions from boundary line communities.)

Second, calculate an adjusted population P' by multiplying the crude population (P) by the ratio:

$$P' = P \frac{(A - B + C)}{A}$$

This population P' is the estimated *primary service area population*.

Secondary Service Area

It is important to note that certain admissions, namely those to adjacent service areas, have been used in the adjustment, while others, to other hospitals beyond the adjacent service area, have been treated in the same manner as admissions to the study hospital. In other words, no adjustment has been made to deduct admissions from the study service area to distant hospitals, nor to add admissions from distant areas to the study hospital. These admissions, involving travel to distant hospitals, generally fall into three classes: (*a*) emergencies occurring away from home, (*b*) travel for social or nonmedical purposes, (*c*) care requiring specialists or services not available in the study hospital. It is difficult to differentiate among these causes. The estimate is based on the assumption that for small hospitals travel because of emergencies, social or other reasons will remain approximately the same over time, in each direction.[8] Long-distance admissions to the study hospital are counted in the data collection but excluded from the population estimate and the use rate. Long-distance admissions from the service area to distant hospitals are not included in the data-gathering mechanism and thus are never counted.

In certain circumstances, this assumption may prove incorrect because the hospital has a substantial portion of its demand occurring outside its own and adjacent service areas. In this case, a *secondary service area use* is calculated. This use is simply the total number of admissions to the study hospital from outside its own and adjacent service areas. It is possible in some cases to ascribe a geographic area and a population base for this use and from this to calculate a secondary use rate. Such an estimate is difficult and highly subjective, however. More commonly the secondary use is taken in itself and projected as a total demand. This need for a secondary service area occurs most frequently in connection with large hospitals which serve as referral centers. It may also occur in rare cases where large volumes of accidents are treated.

Relevance and Commitment Indices for Service Area Definition

Definition and Calculation

Both philosophical and practical problems exist with the equal-likelihood service area approach. As the practical problems of data collection and the assignment of addresses to geographic areas are solved, the basic weakness of the concept will become more apparent. This is that the procedure approximates by a dichotomous decision (in the service area or out) what is actually a much more fluid reality, a continually decreasing tendency to use a given hospital as the distance from it grows. This tendency can be at least crudely measured with data from the example in table 4-1 (see column 1). This statistic, the percentage of all admissions from a geographic area which go to a given hospital, can be defined algebraically. The numbers of admissions used to generate table 4-1 are placed in a simple matrix form; identifying the various hospitals as $j = 1, 2, \ldots, m$, where 1 is the study hospital, and tracts or geographic areas as $i = 1, 2, \ldots, n$. Then a_{11} will be the number of admissions per year to hospital 1 from tract 1, etc.:

Tract \ Hospital	1	2	3, ..., j, ..., m			Total
1	a_{11}	a_{12}	a_{13}	$a_{1j}, \ldots, a_{1m}$		$\sum_j a_{1j}$
2	a_{21}	a_{22}	a_{23}	a_{2j}	$\vdots$	$\vdots$
$\vdots$	$\vdots$	$\vdots$	$\vdots$	$\vdots$	$\vdots$	
i	a_{i1}	$\cdots$		a_{ij}	$\cdots$	
$\vdots$	$\vdots$					
n	a_{n1}	$\cdots$			a_{nm}	
Total	$\sum_i a_{i1}$	$\cdots$				$\sum_{ij} \sum a_{ij}$

Using this matrix, it is possible to construct two indices of planning importance. The first, the *relevance index*, is the percentage of total admissions from the tract (the row total) which go to the study hospital. Algebraically, if the study hospital is identified as $j = 1$,

$$R_{11} = \frac{a_{11}}{\sum_j a_{1j}} \qquad R_{i1} = \frac{a_{i1}}{\sum_j a_{ij}}$$

There will be a set of these values R_i for all the tracts under study. The data shown on table 4-1 are measures of the relevance indices for the study hospital, and the areas on the equal-likelihood boundary are those areas where the relevance index was 50 percent.

The second index from the matrix is the *commitment index*, the percentage of total admissions to the study hospital (the column total for $j = 1$) which come from the ith tract. Algebraically:

$$C_i = \frac{a_{i1}}{\sum_i a_{i1}}$$

The set of commitment indices is available from data at the study hospital only and thus has tended to find more use in hospital planning than the relevance index. It is actually the less useful of the two, however.[9]

The set of relevance indices shows the tendency of each tract to use the study hospital. In situations which resemble the hypothetical one geographically, and where the surrounding hospitals are of approximately the same size as the study hospital, R_i values will be high for the tracts near the study hospital and will decrease with distance. By shading the tracts on a map it is possible to show the communities of high relevance and moderate relevance, thus defining the geographic service community. This has been done for the hypothetical study hospital in figure 4-3.

The contribution of each tract to the total service population can now be calculated easily, by multiplying the tract population by the relevance index. Algebraically, if P_i is the ith tract population,

$P_i \times R_i$ = contribution to study hospital service population

and the sum of these values is the *service area population*;

$$\sum_i P_i R_i = \text{service area population.}$$

Both of the measurement questions have now been solved at least in a theoretical sense. The map of R_i values identifies the service area geographically,

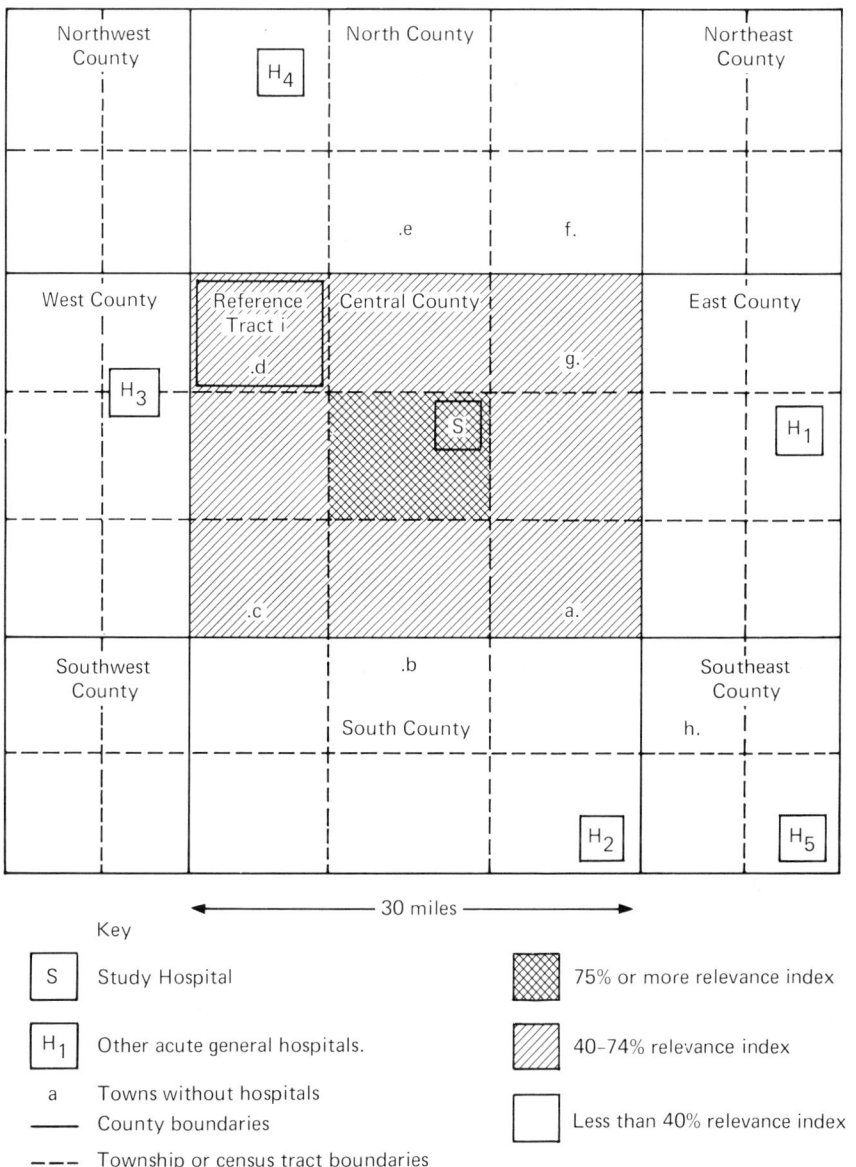

Figure 4-3. Hypothetical Geographic Region Showing Relevance Index Values.

and the sum of the tract populations weighted by the R_i values is the service population. The method has a clear advantage over the equal-likelihood approach in that it is more flexible. This will be of particular use in cities and urban areas, where many tracts will divide among three or more hospitals, leaving no equal-likelihood solution. Even in the rural example, the relevance index gives more information and eliminates the need for adjustments such as the P' calculation. With minor adjustment (creating a dummy "all other" tract), it also includes the concept of a secondary service area.

Problems of Data Collection and Implementation

As might be expected, the data required for the relevance index and population calculation must be more complete than the equal likelihood approach, and the opportunities for serious error are greater. For example, see the west central township of Central County. This township probably divides in some way among S, H_1, and H_3, but particularly because it has no post office, it will require precise analysis to determine its relevance index. Another problem is presented by the northwest township of South East County (near "h"). Residents of this area may go principally to H_5. In the equal-likelihood analysis, this hospital was not included in the data collection. A few, however, may go to the study hospital or to H_1 or to H_2. Only these few will appear in the data as collected for the equal-likelihood service area. The relevance index will be completely inaccurate because it omits many hospital admissions in the denominator. While such a case may be dropped by careful judgment, the possibility of error is high. The relevance index approach is useful only (a) where accurate geographic assignment of patients' addresses can be made and (b) where data collection extends well beyond the study hospital's anticipated service area. These conditions are most likely to be met in studies of large metropolitan regions, with computer assignment of addresses to tracts. Where they are met, the relevance index and the weighted population summation are the preferred way of defining the geographic area and the service area population.

Data Collection for Service Area Population Estimates

Both the equal-likelihood or the relevance-index approaches to service area definition require data on geographic addresses of hospital admissions and population data on relatively small geographic areas. The population data are generally accumulated by tracts, which are groups of approximately 4000 persons living in a reasonably defined area. The Census Bureau establishes tracts and provides both descriptions of tract boundaries and changes with the decennial census. In recent years attention has been devoted to the postal zip code region as a population element because it is so convenient for data collection. The Bureau of the Census has computerized conversion of much population data from tracts to zip code region, making calculation of basic service areas straight forward. There are, however, several drawbacks:

1. Zip codes do not exist for all rural areas
2. Zip code territories are larger than tracts and arbitrarily bordered. (They follow delivery routes rather than political boundaries or traffic patterns)
3. Zip codes are subject to change by the post office, for reasons quite extraneous to population measurement. Correction of the population characteristics may lag several years behind the actual change
4. Some socioeconomic data (income, etc.) of interest in planning studies may never by translated to zip code areas because of concern over confidentiality and nuisance-mail problems

The preferred basis of calculation of service area is clearly the tract, and in some unusual situations still finer subdivisions such as the census block face. It is however clearly more costly, and is often avoided for that reason.

Estimates of admissions from each geographic area can be obtained by sampling procedures to reduce cost. The technique of calculating sample size and suggestions for accurate manual data collection are in the appendix to this chapter. With computerized patient record summaries, however, it is often possible to collect data on all admissions. The Commission on Professional and Hospital Activities in Ann Arbor and other centralized data-processing services will tabulate data on geographic origin of patients by zip code or other manually supplied classification. These data permit only commitment index calculations, however, until several hospitals' data are pooled.

The costs and difficulties of data collection have caused most applications of service area population estimation to be to general acute hospital care. It is likely, however, that some hospitals have several different reference populations. Their obstetrics, their outpatient services, and their uniquely specialized services may each have reference populations. This is most likely to be true for large metropolitan hospitals. Precision of this sort is unlikely until routine computerized data analysis is available.

Birth and Death Rates as Service Area Indicators

Work by the Commission on Hospital Care in the 1940s indicated the possibility that demand estimates might be based upon population estimates derived by comparing deaths or births in the study hospital to the total rates of these occurrences in a relatively large surrounding population.[10] Their work was expressed in terms of demand for beds rather than the statistics of patient days or admissions which have been used more recently. Commission studies indicated that the demand for beds was stably related to the number of inhospital deaths. By extension, then, the population served, P, can be derived from the area crude death rate, D_R, by the formula

$$P = \frac{D}{D_R},$$

where D is the total number of deaths in the time period (usually annually). D can be calculated if the percentage of deaths occurring in the hospital, p, is constant over time. Under this assumption,

$$D = \frac{D_H}{p},$$

where D_H is the number of inhospital deaths. Unfortunately, the percentage of inhospital deaths, p, is not constant. When p is unknown, it becomes impossible to complete the calculation of the population. There is no way to measure p without first determining P, the population value desired.

A similar line of reasoning may be adopted in regard to births. Since the percentage of births in the hospital is very high, it is likely to remain constant, permitting use of the reasoning above. This early work was further developed by Drosness and Lubin in connection with the Hospital Utilization Research Project in California. The project studied in detail the patterns of admissions from census tracts to each of ten hospitals in Santa Clara County. Computer analysis compared use of hospitals relative to auto travel time. Tendency to use the hospital for obstetrical delivery closely paralleled tendency to use for all purposes. This finding was consistent among all hospitals. Differences between the geographic pattern of obstetrical use and of all use were insignificant except in the case of one 445-bed hospital, where the tendency to use the hospital from distant locations was understated by the obstetrical use by 10 percent. This hospital was the largest in the area, and the distant use might easily be attributed to demand from the secondary service area. Obstetrical demand is almost entirely met within the primary service area.[11]

Birth data can usually be obtained with substantially less effort than the addresses of all admissions. In some areas, addresses of mothers may be centrally available in local health departments, together with information on the place of confinement. If the Drosness-Lubin findings hold true in other areas, the data-handling procedures for calculating equal-likelihood service areas can be substantially reduced.

If it is believed that births are uniformly distributed among the population of a geographic area, and data are available on the number of births per year at the hospital and the number of births for the region (usually a county), the service population from the region is:

$$\text{Service area population} = \frac{\text{Births in hospital}}{\text{Births in county}} \times \text{County population}.$$

The assumption that births are uniformly distributed is a dangerous one, however. The birth rate of small populations is known to be affected by age, ethnic, and racial factors which are not often uniform.

Use Rates

Given an estimate of the primary service area population and data on the number of admissions generated by that population, it is a simple matter to divide the two and calculate the *admission use rate* in admissions per thousand population. Where time series data for both these statistics exist, the rate can be calculated for each year and forecast by regression analysis. The population forecast can be obtained independently, and the expected number of admissions can be forecast by multiplying the two independent forecasts. This method is preferred to direct forecast of admissions.

The measure of demand for inpatient care is the *patient day use rate*, expressed in patient days of care per thousand population. It should be possible to calculate the number of patient days used by the primary service area population. However, such a calculation is usually difficult with current record keeping. Hospital records which show the addresses of all patients admitted within a given time period are often business office or admitting office records which do not contain accurate patient stay information. Medical record data which show the patient's stay are not organized by time period. Thus the necessary information in conventional hospital systems is inaccessible. (Electronic data systems will probably overcome this difficulty.)

The usual way in which this problem is overcome is to assume that the length of stay of patients is independent of their distance from the hospital. Under this assumption, the equal likelihood boundary will be the same for patient days as for admissions, and the use rate in patient days will be:

$$R_D = R_A \times (\text{average length of stay}).$$

There is some evidence that this assumption is incorrect.[1,2] It is particularly likely to be invalid in large hospitals with substantial secondary service areas. In this case the most accurate approximation is to calculate two separate averages for length of stay for the primary and secondary service areas. A sample of admissions can be drawn for this purpose, and sampling errors can be calculated from the normal distribution, for each of the two populations. (The errors may be different in each population because the variance of each may be different as well as the mean.)

Application to the Urban Setting

The Poland-Lembcke technique, the relevance index, and the Drosness-Lubin technique are all means of establishing the geography and population of the hospital service area. They have been discussed so far in terms of the single hospital, small city situation. While this is the actual situation of most U.S. hospitals, the majority of beds is in the multiple hospital cities, ranging from two hospital cities with populations under 100,000 to megalopoles like Chicago, Los Angeles, and New York which have more than 100 hospitals each.

There are three important uses of the service area information: to identify a specific population for forecasting; to allow calculation of a use rate and its projection or deliberate modification in planning; and finally, to identify the group or groups of people to whom management is responsible in a social or political sense. These uses can all be met in the rural, small city, single hospital case by any of the three methods. As the cities get larger and more and more hospitals are located in them, the problems of defining the service area become more difficult. Useful estimates of equal likelihood service areas can be reached for moderate sized cities containing a few essentially similar institutions. In the major metropolitan areas, however, only the relevance and commitment indices are useful. Relevance indices are likely to be substantially less than 50 percent for any tract.

For the smaller multiple hospital community there may be little point to treating the hospitals individually. In this case the set of hospitals can be treated as a unit in defining the primary service area and the use rate. After forecasts have been made for the total demand, it is allocated to individual hospitals based upon the best results for the total community. This approach implies the existence of a community planning agency to make these decisions. It is probably the most practical solution to long-range planning problems for cities up to a million population, which do not have a medical school hospital or some similar anomaly.

The metropolis cannot make so easy a decision. There are on the order of 100 institutions, ranging in size from a few dozen beds to over 1,000 and having a variety of commitments to political and social groups as well as special purposes such as medical education. The most thorough analysis to date of a metropolitan situation has been done by deVise, Morrill, Earickson, and others for Chicago. Using an area of forty-mile radius from the center of the city, they studied 123 hospitals ranging from the inner city to distant "satellite" cities like Gary, Joliet, and Waukegan. Ninety-nine separate factors were measured and studied by multivariate analysis in terms of their effect upon use rates by individual communities and upon the relevance indices of specific hospitals. By combining correlated measures into components, they grouped the hospitals according to their positions on these dimensions into the following: (a) city and near suburban medium size, moderately high scope of services; (b) two groups of satellite city and medium-to-large suburban; (c) two groups of small city hospitals; (d) small far suburban hospitals; (e) very large teaching and research hospitals with medical school affiliation. (There were a small number of hospitals which remained anomalous. These included among others Veterans Hospitals, a children's hospital, and the 2700 bed charity hospital, Cook County Hospital.)[13]

Using these characteristics, Morrill and Earickson have developed models explaining the frequency of admission from communities to hospitals by distance, similarity of the community to the hospital, and the number of intervening hospital beds, together with other variables further refining size and scope of services.[14] The models generally give good results, predicting volumes of traffic with correlation coefficients of 0.8 or better. The analysis supports the conclusion summarized below:

	Group	Rate of demand decline	Inner proportion[a]	Extent of demand
A	Medium competitive	Low to moderate	Moderate	Moderate
B	Satellite, medium isolated	Moderate to high	High	Moderate
C	Small city	Moderate	Low	Low
D	Small suburban	Moderate	Moderate	Moderate
E	Research or special-purpose	Very low	Low	Very large
	Cook County Hospital	Moderate	Very high	Very large

[a]"Inner Proportion" is the density of traffic from the area immediately surrounding the hospital. "Rate of demand decline" is the rate at which demand falls off with distance, and "Extent of demand" is the area over which patients are spread.

Source: Morrill and Earickson, "Hospital Variation and Patient Travel Distances" *Inquiry*, 5, no. 4, December 1968.

From this it can be seen that only the hospitals in the satellite cities and the medium to large, remote suburban hospitals have the characteristics which might yield an equal likelihood service area. Other hospitals will not capture large fractions of any identifiable geographic area, with the exception of Cook County Hospital. The research and special purpose hospitals have no primary service area, but serve the entire region as a second service area. The medium sized to small hospitals have a pronounced geographic relation to their service community, but compete in each community without dominating any one. The communities are not homogeneous. They include a wide variety of urban and suburban neighborhoods and vary in their racial, religious, and income characteristics with resulting differences in their demand and need for health care services.

The problem of forecasting community demands with sets of competing hospitals is at the moment unsolved. Morrill and Earickson are working on the development of a large simulation type model which can be used to study the impact of changes on the system, whether they result from changes in the population or are imposed by changing the facilities which are available. For this purpose they are developing predictive models for demand.[a]

In the meantime, there appears to be definite value in collecting geographically related information which will permit understanding the extent of a metropolitan hospital's service to surrounding communities. Certain communities may be in a primary service relation to the hospital. (That is, more than 50 percent of the admissions are to the study hospital.) Forecasts of individual neighborhood growth and use rate may give improved estimates of total future demand. And finally, the knowledge of the composition of the service population may be important in major policy decisions concerning trustee selection, hospital size, services, and location. The collection and preliminary analysis of geographic information on patients is feasible only through metropolitan planning agencies. The results should be important, however, at both local and citywide levels.

---

[a]The most successful to date appear to be general nonlinear relationships of the type:

Model 1 ($r = 0.807, r^2 = 0.651$) — Medical-surgical cases:

$$\text{MC cases} = \frac{(15.8 \text{ Pop.}^{0.423})(\text{Beds}^{0.507})(\text{Similarity}^{0.367})(\text{Pop.65+}^{1.238})(\text{MDs}^{0.203})}{(\text{Inter. Pop.}^{0.425})(\text{Inter. Beds}^{0.298})(\text{Facilities}^{0.42})}$$

Model 2 ($r = 0.810, r^2 = 0.656$) — Percentage of hospital's medical surgical patients from community:

$$\text{\% Hosp.} = \frac{(131.2 \text{ Pop.}^{0.291})(\text{Interns}^{0.104})(\text{Pop. 65+}^{0.142})(\text{Similarity}^{0.197})}{(\text{Interv Pop.}^{0.307})(\text{Interv. Beds}^{0.277})(\text{Facilities}^{0.436})}$$

Model 3 ($r = 0.785, r^2 = 0.616$) — Percentage of community's medical-surgical patients to hospital:

$$\text{\% Comm.} = \frac{(108.7 \text{ Beds}^{0.343})(\text{Physicians}^{0.209})(\text{Similarity}^{0.249})}{(\text{Interv. Beds}^{0.276})(\text{Interv. Pop.}^{0.320})(\text{Facilities}^{0.242})(\text{Pop.}^{0.215})}$$

Source: Morrill and Earickson, "Variations in the Character and Use of Chicago Area Hospitals," *Health Services Research*, 3, no. 3, fall 1968, p. 224 ff. These models can be transformed to the more conventional appearance by taking the logarithm of every variable.

Forecasting from Use Rate and Service Area Population

The principal planning advantage of identifying a service area and calculating population-based use rates is that it permits each of these two statistics to be forecast independently. If time series data can be developed on the use rate, it can be forecast by regression analysis. If sound multivariate models are developed which relate use to population characteristics, these can be used in forecasting the rate. If neither of these conditions can be met, subjective forecasts can be prepared. In any event, the problem of forecasting population growth is isolated for separate study.

Population prediction is a difficult problem which fortunately is of interest to many other people in the community than the hospital. Although it is possible to make population forecasts by simple trend extrapolation or other methods of estimating based on historical trends in the total population, such procedures are subject to two profound weaknesses: (a) they fail to provide information on changes in the composition of the population, such as age and sex percentages (these changes affect the demand for care); and (b) they neglect cyclical and economic factors in population growth and movement and thus are frequently inaccurate.

The general interest in population forecasting has resulted in substantial effort by government and voluntary groups serving all segments of the community. State populations are now projected by the U.S. Bureau of the Census, which also prepares estimates annually between the decennial census. State governments, regional planning offices, local groups and commercial services such as *Sales Management*[15] provide estimates and forecasts for smaller units. The best of these projections have the following characteristics:

1. Total forecasts are based upon independent projections of the three factors affecting them: births, deaths, and net migrations
2. Local area forecasts are logically related to state and national totals
3. Estimates within the ten-year (or in some cases five-year) census counts are verified by comparison with available data known to relate closely to census

The Population Studies Center for the University of Michigan forecast the population of Michigan and its counties by age group through 1980 and provided estimates of the years after the 1960 census. Their analysis, which involved extensive multivariate analysis, viewed the change of population in terms of three factors: births, deaths, and net migration. The first two are available for estimates of past years. They were projected by age cohort application of birth (fertility) and mortality rates. Birth-rate cohorts include estimation of birth spacing and completed family size. Net migration presents a more complex problem. It is influenced by economic factors and is estimated by a "ratio correlated method." This method is a regression analysis of the relationship of selected indicators which measure the impact of known statistics upon the population and are used to estimate population between census years. Births, auto registrations, school census, voters and sales tax returns were used in Michigan. Forecasts are derived by considering the trends in each of the three factors, plus an adjustment for statewide growth, derived from the trend in percent of the state total and the projected state total (available from U.S. Bureau of Census).[16]

Work by the Hospital Utilization Research Project of the California Department of Public Health cites migration information as the major weakness of population projection and indicates that school census which is available annually, is one of the more reliable indicators of migration.[17]

Despite the intricate methods of population forecast used by experts, the validity of projections may be low. In Lenawee County, Michigan in 1960, sophisticated projections indicated a decline in population, but actual school census, new housing, and various local estimates through 1965 indicated an increase. Projections to 1970 apparently could be inaccurate by as much as 10 percent in a population of 80,000 or more. The source of the inaccuracy appears to be the impact of economic factors; population in the county has tended to grow in spurts.[18]

The best solution for hospitals appears to be to use the most sophisticated forecasts and interim estimates available, checking them frequently against known local data, such as school census reports. The projection should include estimates of the age distribution. Often the projection will be in terms of counties and cities rather than for the exact service area. The service area population can be derived by taking the percentage of the county or city populations falling in the service area and projecting this percentage. Care must be taken to see that the expected growth will be proportionately within the service area. In many instances migration is centered in one to two small geographic areas. The effect of this situation must be judged and appropriate adjustments made, largely on a subjective basis.

Chapter 4
Appendix—Data Collection Aids for Service Area Definition

Sampling for Service Area Definition

The work described so far has relied upon full counts of all discharges (excluding newborns) over a period of one year. Obviously many thousands of individual discharges must be reviewed, and tallied at least by post office delivery area or township. One possibility for reducing the work involved is by systematic sampling. It is also possible to reduce workloads by nonsystematic sampling, as for example, reducing the number of months' records surveyed from twelve to six. But this has the disadvantages of possibly introducing bias, and not permitting unbiased estimates of precision. In order to apply sampling techniques, however, some assumptions must be made about the precision of the estimate that is desired. The following example will illustrate the procedure.

Example

Consider Hospital A serving an unknown service area. Hospital A has 120 beds and 5,000 admissions yearly. Some distance away lies Hospital B, with 250 beds and 11,000 admissions annually. There are no hospitals between A and B, and roads are good between the two towns in which the hospitals are located. Between the two hospitals assume a hypothetical village or census tract, t, whose service area assignment is unknown. Figure 4-4 illustrates the geographic relationship.

If the tract t has 2,000 inhabitants, it can be expected to generate approximately 280 admissions and 2,000 patient days of care annually based on

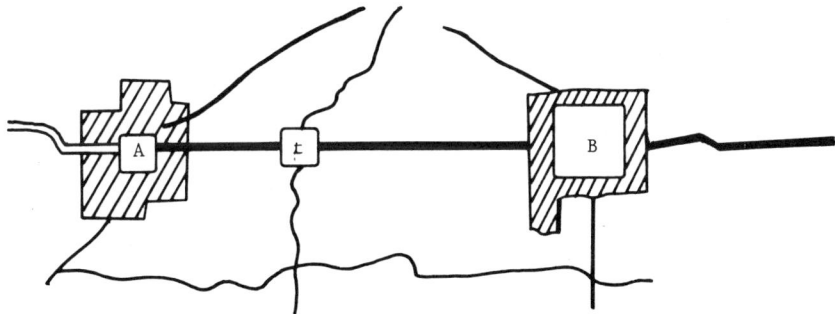

Figure 4-4. Hypothetical Road Map, Showing Location of Town A, Town B and Village t.

national averages. Thus if t is wholly excluded from the A service area when in fact it should be wholly included, an error of slightly over 5 percent (280/5,000) in the A service area will be incurred. Let us assume that the relevance index for Hospital A, R_{tA} should show a sample value of 0.5 whenever the true value is between 0.4 and 0.6. We can be 95 percent confident that this will occur if twice the standard error is equal to 0.1. At 95 percent confidence, where σ_R is the standard error:

$$R_{tA} \pm 2\sigma_R = 0.5 \pm 0.1$$
$$\sigma_R = 0.1 \div 2 = 0.05 = 0.1 R_{tA} .$$

At this condition, the number of admission from t to A, a_{tA} will be:

$$a_{tA} = 0.5 \times 280 = 140 ,$$

and the commitment index C_{tA} will be

$$C_{tA} = 140/5,000 = .03 .$$

The standard error of C_{tA} will be

$$\sigma_C = 0.1 C_{tA} = .003 .$$

Using a common formula to estimate sample size, n:[19]

$$n = \frac{NC_{tA}(1 - C_{tA})}{N\sigma_C^2 + C_{tA}(1 - C_{tA})}$$

where C_{tA} is the proportion to be detected, and N is the size of the sampling universe. Solving this gives:

$$\sigma_C^2 = (.003)^2 = 9 \times 10^{-6}$$
$$n = \frac{5,000 \times 0.03 \times 0.97}{(5,000 \times 9 \times 10^{-6}) + (0.03 \times 0.97)}$$
$$n \sim \underline{3100}$$

Thus 3,000 of the 5,000 annual non-newborn admission at Hospital A must be sampled.

For Hospital B:

$$C_{tB} = 140/11{,}000 \sim 0.01$$
$$\sigma = 0.001; \sigma^2 = 10^{-6}$$
$$N = 11{,}000$$
$$1 - C_{tB} = 0.99$$
$$n = \frac{11{,}000 \times 0.01 \times 0.99}{(11{,}000 \times 10^{-6}) + (0.01 \times 0.99)}$$
$$n \sim \underline{\underline{5{,}200}}$$

In establishing the equal likelihood boundary, the village t (and any other geographic area of the same size on the Hospital A boundary) will be split if the sample proportion to Hospital A is more than 40 percent and less than 60 percent. It is important to recognize that *the village t is hypothetical, and is used only to establish the sample precision.*

After the data have been collected, it is possible to estimate the accuracy of the boundary for any real town by studying the numbers of admissions to each hospital in terms of the sample size of that hospital.

The confidence limits of a given real value of R_{ij} can be calculated from the sample size involved in its calculation. Where

$$R_{ij} = a_{ij} / \sum_j a_{ij}, \quad \text{and} \quad \sum_j a_{ij}$$

is the sample size, n. The universe from which the sample is drawn, N, is the expected number of admissions from the ith tract population, equal to the average admission rate per person times the tract population. The formula for standard error of a proportion for finite samples may be used:

$$\sigma_{Rij}^2 = \frac{R_{ij} \times (1 - R_{ij})}{\sum_j a_{ij}} \left(\frac{N-n}{N}\right)$$

Summary

The following generalized notation will summarize the important sampling formulae.

Problem: to determine the relevance index R_{ij}, the proportion of patients in each tract $i = 1, 2, \ldots, n$, to a selected hospital from the set $j = 1, \ldots, m$.

Let a_{ij} = number of admission to j from i

A_i = total admission from i = $\sum_j a_{ij}$

$R_{ij} = a_{ij}/A_i$

σ_R = standard error of R_{ij}

N_j = number of admission to jth hospital = $\sum_i a_{ij}$

$C_{ij} = a_{ij}/N_j$

σ_C = standard error of C_j

n_j = sample size for jth hospital

To determine sample sizes n_j:

First, estimate A'_i, a value of A_i for a hypothetical population K, such that ½K is equal to an acceptable level of precision for the final population of the service area in question.

Then, assume $R_{ij} = 0.5$, $\sigma_R = 0.1 R_{ij}$

(95% conf: $0.4 \leqslant R_{ij} \leqslant 0.6$)

$C_{ij} = a_{ij}/N_j = 0.5 A'_i/N_j$

$\sigma_C = 0.1 C_{ij}$

And then calculate n_j for each i

$$n_j = \frac{N_i C_{ij}(1 - C_{ij})}{N_i(\sigma_C)^2 + C_{ij}(1 - C_{ij})}.$$

Manual Data Collection Procedures

Drawing the sample in each of the hospitals is not a difficult procedure, although some guidelines are helpful.

1. The sample size is converted to a fraction, n_j/N_j. In Hospital A of the example, this would be $3100/5000 = 0.6$
2. A randomly arranged list or file of admissions for the year is used. It is usually assumed that a file in either chronological or alphabetical order is random for this purpose

3. A sample interval is selected to draw a sample at least as large as n_i. In the case of the example, a convenient interval would be 3, and the procedure would be sample 2, skip 1
4. The admissions file is entered at a convenient point. A random number less than the sample interval is selected and this record is sampled first. In the example either the first or second record is sampled
5. In proceeding through the file, care must be taken to: (a) ignore duplicate copies, if any (but not readmissions of the same patient); and (b) ignore newborn entries, if any
6. If the sample is drawn correctly the sample size will closely approximate

$$\frac{S}{I} \times N$$

where I is the interval, S the number of records sampled in the interval.

In following the procedure for equal-likelihood boundary determination, it is important to make sure that there is no unusual tendency for the individual admissions to be linked. Such a tendency would be present if there had been an epidemic or a disaster in the town in question. Should such an event occur, it is wise to sample all records and consider deletion of the unusual event if it appears to distort the boundary determination. As an alternative, one might exclude the unusual period from the sample population.

5

Demand Forecasts in Specialized Situations

There are a number of specialized demands generated in a hospital which must be forecast with varying amounts of historic knowledge. This chapter will review methods for preparing these forecasts, covering the use of specialized demand rates, analysis of variance techniques to identify sources of demand, and the estimation of potential demand for a service not yet in existence.

Demand Rates

The technique described in chapter 4, where demand, both patient day and admission, was expressed as a rate per 1000 population is one which finds very broad application.

Rates Based Upon General Population

These rates can be calculated for any demand, by dividing the number of units demanded by the population by its size. Two important hospital demand processes can be related to the population at large: admissions and emergency visits. The demand for physicians' services is closely related to population size. Various outpatient demands—x-ray, lab., and so on—might also be analyzed in this way.

It should be clear that careful definition and measurement of the service area population is necessary. The range of confidence in the population estimate determines the confidence in the rate, since in most applications the numerator is taken from major output statistics which are well recorded in hospitals. Differences in primary service-area use rates are often quite large. In Michigan communities studied by the Bureau, differences of over 50 percent in patient day-use rates have been determined. (From 800 to over 1200 patient days per 1000 population in relatively similar communities in the late 1960s.) Differences of this magnitude will easily exceed errors in service area definition or population estimation if the techniques in the preceding chapter are followed.

In dealing with inpatient demand rate forecasts, it is appropriate to apply normative judgments before accepting the forecast. For example, one would forecast an increase of patient day utilization up to 1600 patient days per 1000 population only in unusual situations and with great reluctance. Prepaid group practice plans use at less than half this rate, and many healthy communities show rates under 1000. Hospital utilization is costly, and 1600 days will cost 60 percent more than 1000 days per 1000 population. Deliberate efforts might be undertaken to control the increase, such as reduction of the inpatient bed supply and substitution of ambulatory and home care services. Forecasts would then be based on judgment of the likely success of those efforts.

Demands for hospital admissions, doctor visits, emergency treatments, and similar services can be viewed as analagous to the epidemiologic concept of *incidence rates*, which are rates based on the occurrence of new cases of disease over a specified time period, usually one year. The demand rates discussed above are new cases of demand—admissions per 1000 people per year, doctor visits, etc. It is also common in epidemiology to calculate *prevalence rates*, rates expressing the number of people per 1000 population with a given disease or condition. The prevalence rate has only limited usefulness in demand analysis. It is frequently considered in relation to chronic disease. If a known fraction of the population has a disability which confines them to their home (a prevalence rate) this may be used in planning home care service, home meal delivery, and so forth.

The notion of attempting to forecast hospital use by calculating incidence rates of every common disease has been suggested repeatedly. Extensive work was done on this concept by Lee and Jones.[1] Essentially, there is an incidence rate for every hospital condition (appendicitis, gall bladder disease, pregnancy, heart attack, etc.). The sum of all of these should be the admitting rate, and the sum of each rate times the average length of stay for that disease should be the patient day rate. Life is not so simple, however. Not all gall bladder attacks are hospitalized. Even among those going to surgery, there are two different procedures, with different lengths of stay. Some heart attacks are immediately fatal and the patient is never admitted. Some diseases are quite different among the old than among the young. When all of these kinds of problems have been taken care of, there are several thousand distinct conditions, making calculation unwieldy and perhaps impossible. But the final problem is more serious: the incidence rates, the treatment patterns, and the diseases themselves are interrelated with each other, and with the supply of doctors, hospitals, and other resources. The incidence, the treatment, and even the definition of a disease tend to vary in a way not easy to predict. The cure of acute infectious diseases, for example, has permitted higher incidence and better care to chronic degenerative diseases. The result is that no one has ever made a forecast by this method which improved upon other, more direct, estimates.

Rates Based on Special Populations

Often a demand rate is related to a specific population rather than the general population, and a specific rate is calculated based upon this group. The most common example is the fertility rate, used in forecasting the demand for obstetrical facilities. The *fertility rate* is an incidence rate, the number of births divided by the number of women in the population age 15-44. National and international data on the fertility rate have been tabulated for many years. It has ranged in the United States from a low mean of 70 per 1000 women to a high mean of 120 over the past four decades. Since it adjusts for the number of women who are likely to get pregnant, it is believed to be a better forecaster of births than the *birth rate*, which has the same numerator (births) and the general population as a base.[2]

Another example is the use of the population over age 65 as a base for a chronic disease facility demand rate. This is common because a large preponderance of the demand for these facilities is from this group. As in the case of the fertility rate, the rate is usually calculated as the total demand (regardless of age) divided by the population within the special group. While there are more refined ways to make the rate calculation, they are expensive and not rewarding in improving accuracy of the forecast.

Another common example is the calculation of pediatric inpatient demand based upon the young population. This is sometimes done for three or more age groups, reflecting the age restrictions of pediatric wards for infants, preschool, and other children.

Age Adjusted Rates

If the calculation of rates based on specific populations is carried to its logical conclusion, there will be a demand rate for each age group using the hospital. Preparing demand forecasts by using these demand rates was suggested in 1961.[3] Admission and patient day rates would be calculated for each 15-year age group:

0-15	(Pediatric)	
16-30 non-OB	+ OB	
31-45 non-OB	+ OB	(Fertility rate)
46-60		
60-75		
75+		

Each rate and each population would be independently forecast. The sum of the products of the individual forecasts would provide the total forecast. A comparable rate, using national or other average rates for each age group, could also be calculated. This would be an *age adjusted* hospital use rate which could be compared with the local rate. Similar procedures are used to adjust for population differences in other incidence and prevalence rates, notably the death rate.

Unfortunately, this method is largely untested as a demand predictor. No one has offered evidence that it yields an improved forecast. To apply it, statistics on both the demand and the population must be available by age category. While many centralized computer services for medical record abstracts, such as PAS (Professional Activity Study),[4] can produce at least output data on an age specific basis, few hospitals have coupled this resource with the necessary study of their service population. There are some obvious questions centering on the interval of fifteen years. It would seem, for example, that finer division of pediatric demand is important, while little will be gained by splitting the two groups over and under thirty.

Demand Rates on Bases Other than Population

Demand rates can be constructed on a variety of bases other than a geographically identified population. The base can be any statistic which is logically related to the demand being studied, even another demand. For example, the following rates are commonly used: exams/admission, meals/patient day, operations/doctor, admissions/doctor, live births/delivery, EKGs/medical service admission.

Combinations of rates can be used to prepare a forecast. An electrocardiographic unit with several kinds of demand might be analyzed as follows:

$$\begin{aligned}\text{Total EKGs} &= (\text{EKGs/med. admission})(\text{No. med. admiss.}) \\ &+ (\text{EKGs/executive physical})(\text{No. exec. phys.}) \\ &+ (\text{outpatient EKGs}/1000 \text{ pop.})(1000 \text{ pop.}) \\ &\div (1 - \% \text{ all other EKGs})\end{aligned}$$

Each term can be forecast independently. The final term assumes that increase in all other demand, which is presumably only a small part of the total, will change proportionately to the more closely identified items. The rate used is the rate of "all other" EKGs per itemized EKG.

Analysis of Variance to Evaluate Demand Rates

It is sometimes desirable to calculate rates for components of demand by reviewing a sample of some kind. For example, EKG statistics may not be available by service, and to measure the rate of EKGs per admission, a sample of discharges will be drawn. In the simplest case, a general random sample of n discharges would be drawn and for each discharge in the sample, a demand for the service y_i would be measured.[a] (For example, y might be the

---

[a]The sampling problem for patient days, rather than admissions, is more difficult. Note that a sample of n admissions which stayed a total of N patient days is *not* a random sample of N patient days because many of these days are linked by the patients themselves. Samples of patient days must be drawn directly and over large time periods to minimize this linking problem.

number of EKG examinations in each discharge record.) The sample will then have a mean demand per admission, $\bar{y}$, and an unbiased estimate of the sampling variance σ^2.

$$\sigma^2 = \frac{\sum_i (y_i - \bar{y})^2}{n-1}$$

The rate is equal to y plus or minus an error of estimate. The error of estimate would be calculated from σ using the normal table.

Collection of data of this kind presents the opportunity for analysis of variance to measure which of the various components of demand are significant contributors to the variation in the total. Thus a sample might be drawn of sufficient size to permit calculation of several different demand rates and their internal variances. At the same time, the overall rate and its variance can be calculated. Each individual rate contributes some reduction in the total variance. The significance of the contribution can be tested by the F statistic, and those making significant reductions can be considered for forecasting. The technique is similar to multivariate analysis, described in chapter 3.

With large samples and computer analysis, large numbers of possibilities are presented, including multiple arrays such as age × sex × service. Reasonably careful application of the technique is necessary to avoid spurious results and unnecessary data collection in the forecast. The question is not merely one of significance, but rather of utility. Although a specific rate may yield a significant improvement in a forecast, it may be a small one which is purchased at high cost. Some statisticians feel that only the few best variables which make pronounced contributions to the forecast should ever be considered.

Without attempting to cover the subject of analysis of variance or make any comment about the more complicated situations, the following example will illustrate the role of significance testing and the principles upon which the analysis proceeds.

Consider a demand for a service which is related to the number of admissions and is expressed as R = rate/admission. A sample of N admissions reveals that

$$\bar{R} = \sum_i R_i / N$$

$$\sigma_R^2 = \sum_i (R_i - \bar{R})^2 / N-1$$

The sum of squares of the deviation about the mean is of interest. This can be designated *SST* (Sum of Squares Total):

$$SST = \sum_i (R_i - \bar{R})^2 = \sigma_R^2 (N - 1).$$

Now suppose that review of the data suggests that admissions to the medical service are important. We take these from our sample and find

$$\bar{R}_M, \sigma_M^2, \text{ and } SS \text{ (Medicine)};$$

for the remaining admissions we have

$$\bar{R}_0, \sigma_0^2, \text{ and } SS \text{ (Other)}.$$

Our analysis is significant if the two categories reduce the deviation sufficiently. The new deviation SSR, will be the remaining deviation

$$SSR = SS \text{ (Medical)} + SS \text{ (Other)}.$$

The deviation explained by the analysis will be

$$SSA = SST - SSR.$$

The test of significance is the F test

$$F = \frac{SSA/n}{SSR(N - n - 1)},$$

where n is the number of explanatory analyses made. In this case, $n = 2$ (medicine and other). The coefficient of determination, r^2 can also be calculated:

$$r^2 = \frac{SSA}{SST}.$$

Let us assume for a moment that the F test has proven significant, that r^2 is high, and that the possibility of a third individual rate, for surgery admission, is being considered. Since the original medical admissions rate is still included, a new F test with medicine, surgery, and other is likely to be significant. A separate test can be made of surgery and the new "other" against the previous "other" category, and this also may be significant. Should the surgery rate then be included in the forecast? Only if the improvement in r^2, the coefficient of determination, is worth the cost of data collection and analysis. If r^2 was already quite high, the improvement may be very small. Conceivably, the cost of gathering data to make the forecast could be quite high. Under the conditions, it is best not to pursue the refinement.

Forecasting Demand for Nonexistent Services

Hospitals frequently add new services for which they have no historic demand data. Some of the services added to many hospitals for the first time in the 1960s included intensive care units, isotopic diagnostic services, coronary care units, and physical medicine and rehabilitation services. There are three ways to prepare forecasts in such situations: from measures of need, from demand experience of others, and from surveys of intention.

From Measures of Need

Incidence rates of specific diseases can be related to the demand for a service. The work of Lee and Jones, discussed above, was one effort to relate hospital inpatient demand to disease incidence. But it and other similar general attempts have failed. However, the methods may be useful for smaller groups of diseases and more limited services. For example, there should be a clear relation between the incidence of heart attacks and the demand for coronary care services. In all applications of disease incidence rates there are two major concerns:

1. All those patients who have the disease may not be referred to the service. (Some heart attacks may be judged too mild to require the unit, doctors may be reluctant to use it, patients not like it, etc.)
2. Some patients who do not have the disease will be referred to the unit. (Some suspected heart attacks will be admitted to the unit, but later not classed as heart attacks.)

As a practical matter, both of these situations will occur, particularly in the early years of the service. Since they act in opposite directions and are not consistent either among services or hospitals, forecasts based solely on incidence rates and other measures of need should be treated with great care. Raw incidence rates should be adjusted by independent estimates of both these tendencies.

From Experience of Others

Sometimes forecasts can be derived from the experience of other hospitals. Usually demand must be expressed as a rate, based either on population or institutional size (beds, admissions, days, etc.). While this is preferable to forecasts based solely on incidence rates, it is also subject to certain dangers. Most of the services which must be forecast in this manner are ordered by the doctor, not by the patients. Doctors' attitudes toward new services are not consistent. What some staff members refer patients to enthusiastically others will ignore. When most doctors are enthusiastic, demand is high, otherwise it is not. Data on home care demand from four relatively small hospitals, shown in table 5-1, reflect the magnitude of the problem.

The problem of how heavy the referrals will be must be handled subjectively. Often it is necessary to guess whether the service will be instantly popular or not. There are dangers, of course, in both high and low estimates. Generally, however, low estimates are less costly for new services. Once some actual experience has been accumulated it is usually possible to adjust to that experience. Physical facilities might be planned on higher estimates assuming the development of new and favorable attitudes, but initial staffing decisions should be based on much lower forecasts.

From Surveys of Intention

When more accurate forecasts are required, surveys of the expected demand can be taken. These can range from simple questionnaires to the medical staff, covering such items as the demand for space in the doctors' office building to elaborate surveys of patient condition and possible demand for long-term care, home care, and other alternatives to acute hospital services. The more elaborate surveys involve criteria for classifying patient demand in the proposed situation and the application of these criteria by either doctors or nurses. Delphic forecasting, a new technique not yet common in hospitals, may come into greater use.

Table 5-1
Comparative Demand for Home Care

	Sheldon Memorial Hospital (Albion)	Newton Memorial Hospital	Pekin Memorial Hospital	McPherson Community Health Center (Howell)
Home Care Census	13	10	10	26
Census per 100,000 Population	55	32	17	74
Number of Home Care Discharges	63	78	46	109
Percentage of Hospital Discharges	2.1%	1.9%	0.6%	2.5%

Source: J.R. Griffith, *Taking the Hospital to the Patient*, W.K. Kellogg Foundation, Battle Creek, 1966, p. 21.

Surveys of Doctor's Intentions. Strictly speaking, these surveys are sometimes not of intent because they ask questions of the type "Could this patient be treated? ... " rather than "If such and such were available to this patient, would you order it?" At any rate results have been less than fully satisfying. Browning reported a survey where two panels of physicians independently examined over 1,500 hospital records to see if good long-term care could have been substituted for hospital care.[5] Both panels gave positive responses for about 10 percent of the patients. However, when the individual cases were reviewed, it was found that only one-third of the cases selected had been chosen by both panels. As Dr. Browning stated, such a study "raises more questions than it answers."

The findings cited by Browning led to a series of methodological investigations aimed at finding the reliability of survey evaluations of demand. The original findings have generally been reiterated. The availability of additional information (direct patient observation, interview with physician, etc.) did not significantly improve agreement. There is better agreement on long-stay patients, than on patients in early portions of hospital stay.[6] Nurses may have slightly better reliability than doctors, but they tend to judge more patients as needing lower levels of care. Local doctors have about the same performance as outside doctors imported for the survey.[7] The authors point out that consistency on all cases, including those who were judged not to be candidates for long-term care by the reviewing team is quite high. It would seem that the method of physician review of cases is reliable enough to aid in planning, although its imprecision should not be forgotten.

The survey is taken of a sample of patients, with previous understanding by the surveyors as to the purpose of the survey and the use of the form. The details of these procedures are similar to those described in detail below. The survey form itself is similar to the one shown in figure 5-1. Questions 1 through 7 are for description of the demand. Questions 8 to 12 serve two purposes. They can be used (a) to construct profiles of the expected population of proposed facilities; and (b) for estimating staffing requirements and other considerations. They also serve as a logical device to direct the reviewer's attention to relevant aspects of patient needs. This presumably improves the care with which the central decision is made and recorded in question 13.

A study conducted by White and Preston included both a 100 percent sample of patients over several weeks who were surveyed by nurses for their patient care needs, and a 10 percent sample surveyed by resident physicians and classified by them into ten levels of inpatient and ambulatory care.[8] According to the unpublished paper by White, the two led to different classifications of inpatients.

Level	100 Percent Sample by Nurses	10 Percent Sample by Doctors
Intensive	13%	12%
Intermediate	70%	55%
Self	17%	33%
	100%	100%

(NAME)	(NUMBER)	(FACILITY)

Patient's home address:	1. Current date: ___/___/___	3. Sex and marital status
(Street)	Pt. admission date: ___/___/___	Male | Female
	2. Patient's age:	0 ( ) Single ( ) 1
(City) (State) (Zip)		2 ( ) Married ( ) 3
		4 ( ) Widowed ( ) 5
		6 ( ) Divorced ( ) 7
		8 ( ) Separated ( ) 9

4. Source of payment:
   Self   ( ) 1   Pension   ( ) 5
   Medicare   ( ) 2   V.A.   ( ) 6
   Medicaid   ( ) 3   Other_____7
   BC–BS   ( ) 4   (Specify)

5. Prior living arrangements:
   Alone   ( ) 1   Institution   ( ) 5
   With nonrelatives   ( ) 2   With spouse   ( ) 6
   With relative   ( ) 3   Other_____( ) 7
   Foster home   ( ) 4   (Specify)

6. Primary admitting diagnosis:

7. Other diagnoses or complications:

8. Physical status since admission:
   Deteriorating   ( ) 0
   Stationary   ( ) 1
   Improving   ( ) 2

9. Current ambulatory status:
   Bedfast and/or chairfast   ( ) 0
   Independent in wheelchair   ( ) 1
   Ambulates with human help, crutch,
      cane, walker or other aid   ( ) 2
   Ambulates independently   ( ) 3

10. Current mental status:
   Does not make needs known or
      understand instructions   ( ) 0
   Only able to make needs known   ( ) 1
   Only able to understand instructions   ( ) 2
   Able to make needs known and
      understand instructions   ( ) 3

11. Current self-care status: (Toilet, dressing, eating, bathing)
   Completely dependent in self-care   ( ) 0
   Needs much assistance in self-care   ( ) 1
   Needs little assistance in self-care   ( ) 2
   Independent in self-care   ( ) 3

12. The patient is now receiving the following care:
Occasionally   *Regularly*
1 ( )   Personal care   ( ) 1
2 ( )   Nursing care   ( ) 2
3 ( )   Physical therapy   ( ) 3
4 ( )   Occupational therapy   ( ) 4
5 ( )   Speech therapy   ( ) 5
6 ( )   Diagnostic tests   ( ) 6
7 ( )   Therapeutic procedures   ( ) 7

Reviewer:

13. Doctor to review items 1–12 and complete the following:
Should this patient continue receiving the present level of institutional service?
      YES ( )   NO ( )
If "no" check the appropriate service needed
   Foster or boarding home   ( ) 2
   Own home with isolated services   ( ) 3
   Own home with organized home care   ( ) 4
   Nursing home or infirmary   ( ) 5
   Extended-care service   ( ) 6
   Rehabilitation service   ( ) 7
   Acute general hospital   ( ) 8
                                    , M.D.

(NAME)	(TITLE)	(DOCTOR'S SIGNATURE)

Figure 5-1. Form for Survey of Expected Demand. Source: Zimmer and Groomes, *Medical Care*, 7, n 1, p. 15.

The nurses' sample did not include any ambulatory patients; while the data shown above for the doctors' survey could be supplemented by similar surveys of outpatients and emergency room patients. Apparently for this reason the nurses' survey was abandoned, and conclusions were based upon the doctors' classification. The Preston paper gives the sample means and standard deviations for six levels of care.[9]

Level	10% inpatient sample	Out-patient sample	Emer-gency Room	Total	Percentage
	$(X \pm \sigma)$	$(X \pm \sigma)$	$(X \pm \sigma)$	X	
Intensive	23.8 ± 15.1	0 ± 0	1.3 ± 3.8	25.1	10.4
Intermediate	106.5 ± 27.8	9.8 ± 9.3	2.4 ± 4.7	118.7	49.3
Self	65.1 ± 20.6	4.1 ± 6.9	0 ± 0	69.2	28.7
Long-term	17.0 ± 13.3	1.1 ± 0	0 ± 0	18.1	7.5
Observation	0 ± 0	1.4 ± 0	0.5 ± 0	1.9	0.8
Overnight	2.9 ± 4.9	5.0 ± 7.9	0 ± 0	7.9	3.3

Standard errors are quite large. Ninety-five percent confidence limits of inpatient survey will exceed the mean for intensive overnight and long-term care. "Overnight care" is for ambulatory patients who cannot return home. Usually because of travel difficulties. Care could be provided in selfcare facilities.

It would appear that surveys of doctors' opinions are more expensive and only marginally more reliable than nurses' surveys. The difficulties of reliability of opinions, cited by Browning and Zimmer, are one factor. Large sampling errors weaken the results. The σ values are in part due to observer variation, but they also relate to the small sample size which is in turn related to the difficulty of getting cooperation from physicians.

Nursing Estimates. A method of estimating demand that is derived from detailed nursing evaluation of patient condition is set forth in detail in "The Progressive Patient Care Hospital, Estimating Bed Needs," by the U.S. Public Health Service.[10] Characteristics of patients which appear to determine their nursing care needs are used to classify patients to four inpatient (intensive, intermediate, self and continuing) services. These are derived from work done by Connor[11] and tend to have been supported by application elsewhere.[12] Techniques of this type have proven useful both for forecasting demand for physical facilities[13] and for establishing nursing staffing requirements. Connor's original work was an analysis of staffing rather than facilities. Surveys of the type described below appear to be justified for either purpose. There are variations in the demand for various levels of care for different hospitals. Among the causes are differences in definition of services like "continuing care." The survey technique tends to bring consensus on the more important definitional problems as well as to provide a forecast. It also can be used to create a participative approach to planning by using study teams. While the detail applies to PPC, the criteria and instruments could be changed to a number of other demand situations, and the systematic approach can serve as a guide as well as an indication of the amount of effort required. Following is the methodology outlined by the Public Health Service:

Phase I—Evaluation of Patient Census Based on Care Requirements

Four major steps are to be considered under Phase I:
1. Designate a patient evaluation team.
2. Develop a patient-condition checklist.
3. Determine criteria for patient classification (i.e., intensive care, intermediate care, or self care).
4. Evaluate and classify patients.

STEP 1—*Designate a Patient Evaluation Team*

A preliminary step is to appoint a patient evaluation team consisting of members of the nursing and medical staffs. The hospital administrator may also be included on this team which will be responsible for steps 2 through 4. The final step includes orienting the nurses in the application of the checklist.

STEP 2—*Develop a Patient-Condition Checklist*

The intensity of a patient's illness is usually reflected in specific conditions calling for specific kinds of treatment. Thus it is necessary that a patient-condition checklist be developed which would readily indicate the kind of care required by the patient. (It is presumed that the hospital has already clearly defined the principles, objectives, scope, and responsibility of each patient care unit as noted.)

The patient-condition checklist should be sufficiently detailed to enable the team to reach an objective decision as to the unit in which the patient would be provided the most appropriate care. The checklist should incorporate the broadest aspects of the patient's needs which should then be related to specific conditions. As a first step, for example, the following general needs might be considered:
1. Need for nursing observation of physical signs and changes in clinical conditions.
2. Need for physical assistance.
3. Need for special medical or nursing skills and/or special equipment.

Within each of these basic patient need factors are different degrees of need which are then related to specific patient conditions. In this fashion a patient-condition checklist can be produced which will enable the patient to be classified, on the basis of his condition, for assignment into the most appropriate care unit. Items which would be included under the three need factors noted above follow:

1. Need for nursing observation of physical signs and changes
   a. Temperature, pulse, respiration (and/or blood pressure)
   b. Hemorrhage
   c. Consciousness
   d. Orientation
   e. Isolation
2. Need for physical assistance.
   a. Bathing   b. Mobility   c. Dietary
3. Need for special medical or nursing skills and/or special equipment.
   a. Oxygen therapy
   b. Transfusion and/or infusion
   c. Suction
   d. Pacemaker, defibrillator, or respirator
   e. Stimulants

While this list is somewhat comprehensive, it is by no means exhaustive, and the individual hospital may wish to add to or delete conditions from it.

Some of the patient conditions exist in varying degrees of intensity. For example, hemorrhage may or may not be present; stimulants (Levophed or Aramine) may or may not be needed; or a patient may or may not need to be fed. The different levels of intensity for each of the patient conditions should be incorporated into the checklist. One method for setting up such a checklist is shown in chart 1 [figure 5-2].

STEP 3—*Determine Criteria for Patient Classification*

The patient evaluation team should agree on those patient conditions, or combination of conditions, which will constitute the criteria for admission to, or discharge from, a patient care unit. The team should regard each patient condition as a factor to be considered in determining the most appropriate care unit to assign a patient. For example, the requirement that temperature, pulse, and respiration be measured every 15 minutes may be considered sufficient reason (i.e. compelling indicator), for assignment to the intensive care unit. On the other hand, if a patient should be found to need oxygen, this requirement would contraindicate assignment to the self-care unit.

Three weights may be used in classifying patients: compelling indicator, moderate indicator, and contraindicator. One of these three weights should be assigned to each patient condition and level of intensity. The team should ask the question: Is the intensity of the condition a compelling, moderate, or contraindicator for assignment to the intensive care, intermediate care, or self-care unit? When the entire list of patient conditions is thus weighted, it is then possible to establish rules for the admission to, and discharge from, a specific unit.

The following criteria are suggested as a basis for determining patient assignment:

a. One compelling indicator for intensive care is sufficient reason for assignment to the intensive care unit.
b. Four or more moderate indicators for intensive care constitute sufficient reason for assignment to that unit.
c. If there is no justification for assignment to intensive care, and in the presence of a contraindicator for self-care, the patient is automatically assigned to intermediate care.
d. In the absence of moderate indicators for either intensive or intermediate care, and in the absence of a contraindicator for self-care, assignment is to self-care.

The above criteria may be modified to meet the needs and practices within a hospital as determined by the patient evaluation.

STEP 4—*Evaluate and Classify Patients*

Upon development of a satisfactory patient classification checklist, the nursing personnel should be trained in its use and application.

To effectively use the checklist, each patient should be observed and his condition noted on the checklist at some designated hour convenient to the nursing staff. The form shown in chart 1 can be used as a checklist if a record of the patient's condition during his entire hospitalization is desired. The factors listed are not intended to give a definitive description of patient condition, but only to be the lowest number of factors which are determinants of classification.

Evaluation Criteria	Patient Number or Name									
	Date									
TPR and/or BP	Q5min. to Q2h									
	Q4h to QD									
HEMORRHAGE	Present									
	Not present									
LEVOPHED/ ARAMINE	Needed									
	Not needed									
CONSCIOUSNESS	Unconscious									
	Conscious									
ORIENTATION	Disoriented									
	Oriented									
BATH	By nurse									
	Bathes self									
MOBILITY	Confined to bed									
	Ambulatory in room only									
	Ambulatory unlimited									
DIETARY	Fed by nurse									
	Feeds self									
OXYGEN	Needed									
	Not needed									
SUCTION	Needed									
	Not needed									
INFUSION or TRANSFUSION	Needed									
	Not needed									
PACEMAKER or RESPIRATOR	Needed									
	Not needed									
ISOLATION	Yes									
	No									
Unit Assignment										

Figure 5-2. Patient Condition Checklist.

If patient observations are to be made only once in 3 or 4 days, such a form can be used by listing the patients on the date line at the top so that all patients are classified on one form. The checklists should be forwarded upon the patient's discharge, or daily to the data processing center within the hospital. Processing may be normal or mechanical.

The method outlined by the PHS suggests a team approach to the evaluation criteria, which is undoubtedly desirable. In addition to improving reliability by using a team (which should remain constant during the survey), the method uses the team to teach the nursing staff the preestablished criteria for classification. This also is designed to make the result more reliable, by preventing the observers from changing their opinions as the sample progresses. Without criteria which are as clear and detailed as possible at the start of the survey, individual judgments will differ more on a given case, and they will also differ as the survey progresses.

Sample Size for Patient Care Determination. Determinations of the type described above are used in two ways, either for long-term forecasts of facility needs or in daily or short-term estimates of nursing staff requirements. In the latter case, reports are usually solicited upon each patient (a 100 percent sample), but in the former smaller samples are often possible. The results are in the form of proportions (a percentage of the patients will fall into each class). Under the assumption of independence of patients, a Bernoulli process may be said to exist, and sample sizes may be estimated utilizing properties of the binomial distribution.

For each class of patients, i, the proportion of the total census expected is p_i, the expected average census will be Cp_i, where C is the total hospital census. The standard deviation of the estimate p_i will be[b]

$$\sigma_{p_i} = \sqrt{\frac{p(1-p)}{n}}.$$

This will be largest for $p = 0.5$, but largest relative to p for small p.

The smallest expected value of p will be for intensive care services. This class also requires the most care, so that for two reasons it is the one which is critical. According to the work at the McPherson Community Health Center in Howell, Michigan,[15] the average ICU census will be only 5 percent of the total. The sample size need not be any larger than necessary to detect a difference of one in the mean census. (One cannot build half a bed.) If Δp is the difference in the census as a proportion, and C is the census, then

$$\Delta p \times C = 1$$

At the same time Δp is related to σ_{p_i} by the normal distribution:

---

[b]To be precise, the denominator should be $n - 1$, not n. However, n will be in the thousands, and this correction will be insignificant. The -1 has been dropped to simplify calculations.

$$\Delta p = Z\sigma_{p_i} = Z\sqrt{\frac{p(1-p)}{n}}$$

Substituting and solving for n gives

$$n = Z^2\, p(1-p)\, C^2$$

It should be noted that in selecting Z, only the upper limit of the normal distribution is of interest. Thus, where α is the probability that the true p exceeds $p + \Delta p$,

Z	α
1.96	0.025
1.645	0.05
1.282	0.10

As an example, where $C = 100$, the expected value for $p = 0.05$, the acceptable $\Delta p = 0.01$ (or one bed), and 95 percent confidence is desired,

$$n = (1.645)^2\,(0.05)(0.95)(100)^2 = 1{,}285$$

Thus a sample of approximately 1300 patient days will yield an estimate of p which will not exceed 0.05 + 0.01 more than five percent of the time. The same hospital can expect to find about 70 percent of its beds required for intermediate care. For $p_i = 0.7$,

$$\sigma_{p_i} = \sqrt{\frac{p(1-p)}{n}} = \sqrt{\frac{(0.7)(0.3)}{1285}} = 0.013$$

The average daily census will be $p \times C$, and the precision at 95 percent confidence will be

$$p_i = 0.7 \pm 1.96 \times 0.013 = 0.7 \pm 0.025.$$

This accuracy is well within that of other planning estimates used to derive C.

Sampling should be done in such a way as to avoid bias due to seasonal variations in disease patterns and also to avoid linkage by multiple samples of the same patient. The Public Health Service recommends sampling calendar days over a three-month period including the heaviest use months during the year. On the selected sample days, all patients on the adult medical and surgical service will be sampled. (Assuming obstetrics and pediatrics will not be affected by the PPC organization.) Thus assuming a sample of 1285 patient days is required, and that the average medical-surgical census of the hospital is 100, then 1285/100 =

13 calendar days must be sampled, or every seventh day in the three-month period. One sample day should occur each week. A simple sample interval of seven days should not be used because all samples will fall on a given day of the week. The days can be randomly assigned within each week, however. The linkage problem is not entirely avoided. Certain long-stay patients will be over-represented in the sample because it has been limited to 90 days. However, the loss is probably not significant.

Delphi Forecasting

Delphi forecasting, a technique for situations where historic or comparative data are lacking, was developed in the early 1960s by members of the RAND Corporation.[16] The technique is adaptable to forecasting *when* an event will occur (e.g., when a pollution free automobile will be marketed), *how many* of something will be demanded or produced, or *whether* a given strategy is desirable. The last is not strictly a forecast but really a policy decision and is outside the scope of this discussion. The source of the forecast is the opinions of several experts. (Thus the reference to Delphi, an ancient Greek oracle and pagan worshipping place).

The forecasts must be collected according to certain rules. The panel of experts should be diverse enough to provide different views on the problem (e.g., several different medical specialists, a nurse, and a social worker on questions of how many patients will demand service from a long-term care unit). They do not meet but are individually provided with a detailed and thorough description of the problem to be estimated. Working alone, they give their best guess as to the questions at hand. Answers are then anonymously circulated. Quantitative responses are frequently rank ordered, and the highest and lowest 25 percent are asked to justify why their response differs from the median. Their justifications may be circulated to the others, who then may change their estimates. Nonquantitative answers may be pooled and reevaluated by the panel in terms of likelihood. By these successive evaluations, it is claimed that the knowledge of the panel is effectively comingled, without the status and personality problems, band-wagon effects, and other difficulties which afflict committee activity. There has been some independent validation of the method by using it on known but "obscure" bits of technical information (the number of oil wells in Texas, or board feet of lumber in the United States, etc.). Results were satisfactory to the authors.[17]

Health and hospital applications of the method have been limited. The Harvard Medical School has used the technique to explore the future of medical care and medical education.[18] A commercial drug house has used it to forecast innovations in medical care. The panel predicted, among many other things, worldwide immunization against bacterial and viral disease by 1993.[19] Williamson has used the technique for forecasting medical statistics and for the cost-benefit analysis of alternative treatment patterns of chronic diseases. An extensive study of pediatric atopy (an allergy related syndrome in children) was conducted using modified delphi techniques. Results estimated both decades of "preventable impairment units" and dollar measures of the quantities of resources required. Included in the work were evaluations of the details of the method. The estimates would be of considerable use in long-range, community-wide planning, but less useful in specific applications to hospital or clinic planning.[20]

Summary

Chapters 2 through 5 have presented the various techniques for forecasting demand—time series analysis, multivariate analysis, the description of short-term variation, the calculations of service area populations, the construction of demand rates, the use of surveys, questionnaires, and Delphi techniques. Most of these techniques have other analytic uses. They are used to forecast other statistics (such as the supply of resources) and to make analyses for control purposes.

The major questions in most students' minds at this point may be, "How do you fit the technique of forecasting to the problem?" and "When are the more elaborate techniques appropriate?" There is no simple answer to the first question. You use the best technique you have data for, in general, and where you have enough information you use several techniques to gain more certainty of your answer. The second question is easily answered. The technique is appropriate whenever it may change a management decision by a larger dollar amount than it costs. Thus for forecasting the demand for beds, at $50,000 each average cost, substantial sums are justified for the forecast. In fact, it could be said that any institution that planned to add 100 beds and related services and did not spend several thousand dollars in forecasting was irresponsible. On the other hand, forecasting for home care, which may take one small office and cost $25,000 per year is not worth such precision and expense. There comes a point when it is cheaper to try than to forecast. That point/comes when the errors are relatively cheap and the cost of eliminating them relatively expensive.

Forecasts of the types described in these chapters will be used in the planning and control decisions in the following chapters. Their potential value should then become somewhat clearer.

Part II
Models for Resource Allocation

6 Total Value Analysis

Nature of Resource Allocation Problems

There are two basic questions in planning hospital facilities and services which can sometimes be answered by the application of techniques developed in systems analysis and operations research. These are, "What quantity of a service should the hospital be prepared to provide?" and "What are the best policies and processes for the service at the expected volume?" The techniques which are useful in answering these questions are described in chapters 6 through 9. These techniques involve various forms of *modeling*, the representation of the real world in an abstract form which permits study over a range of conditions not easily studied directly in a real-life situation.

The models are usually mathematical in form and are analyzed by mathematical calculations which suggest the most rational decision and the cost of deviating from that decision. Models, of course, do not make decisions, and the construction and solution of models is only one aspect of the planning process. They do, however, greatly enhance understanding of the results of decisions, clarifying both assumptions and consequences which might otherwise be overlooked. Therein lies their value; they are complex, abstract, and often difficult to understand, but less so than the processes they represent. Chapters 2 through 5 have already reviewed one form of modeling—forecasting models. Several examples were discussed. These were aimed at answering principally questions of demand ("How many patients will request admission?") and occasionally of arrival at uncertain resources ("What will the absenteeism rate be?"). The models which we are about to discuss deal with the resource allocation questions: ("How many nurses should we hire?" and "How many operating rooms should we build?"). Like the forecasting models, these models only provide assistance in making decisions. They are based on the notion of *rational decision making*, that the decision maker wishes to gain the maximum return for each dollar he spends, according to his evaluation of that return.

Concepts

Selecting Policies and Procedures. The cost of providing a service (production cost) does not change smoothly with the number of units of service provided. A very substantial expenditure may be necessary to provide even a single unit of service, because most hospital services require space, equipment, a skilled professional team, and supplies. A laboratory service, such as blood chemistry analysis, is a representative example. To perform one unit of service, at least a laboratory, an inventory of reagents, a centrifuge, microscopes, and other equipment must be available. Also, one must have a pathologist and a trained technician. These personnel must be hired in advance, and a sizable annual budget must be committed. These are *fixed costs*, incurred independent of how many units of service are performed. There are other costs—often minor in the operations of hospitals—which depend directly on the number of units performed. These usually include supplies. Disposable syringes are one such cost in the blood chemistry example. These are *variable costs*, increasing by the same amount with each unit of service.

At some level of output, the initial fixed costs will be insufficient. Additional personnel must be hired, more equipment purchased, and so forth. When this point is reached, there will be a sharp jump in total costs. Figure 6-1 shows fixed and variable production costs over a range covering such a situation for a hypothetical laboratory service. If the costs are now viewed as a cost per unit of service, it can be seen that this cost will be a function of the number of units of service and will be much lower at some output volumes than others.

Figure 6-2 shows the cost per unit, obtained by dividing the cost in figure 6-1 by the output. The production cost is the function of the method or process used to supply the service as well as the volume of service. If an autoanalyzer is used instead of manual methods for blood chemistry determinations, the initial fixed cost—for most of the original resources plus an autoanalyzer—will be much higher. But the process will accommodate a much larger volume before additional fixed costs are necessary. Figure 6-3 shows the configuration of total cost and figure 6-4, the unit cost for the alternative process using the higher initial fixed cost.

If planning for the hospital is aimed at minimizing cost for a given service, then the planning process must include actual analyses of fixed and variable costs over the range of output which is forecast. Thus part of economical planning for the laboratory is the search for the lowest cost solution which provides the desired service. Figure 6-5 superimposes the unit costs of the two alternatives used as examples. Clearly, the autoanalyzer is the method of choice if the volume is expected to exceed 10,000 units. (The figures are *not* actual.)

This kind of analysis, extended and improved in accuracy, will provide information for a number of decisions. Total value analysis, which follows this approach almost exactly, can be used to compare alternative processes and decision rules. It can be extended in some cases to stochastic as well as deterministic decisions. This method of analysis is the least complicated, and it will be discussed in the balance of this chapter.

Selecting the Quantity of Service. *Total value analysis* is the modeling of total costs of service for alternative processes over a range of possible service volumes.

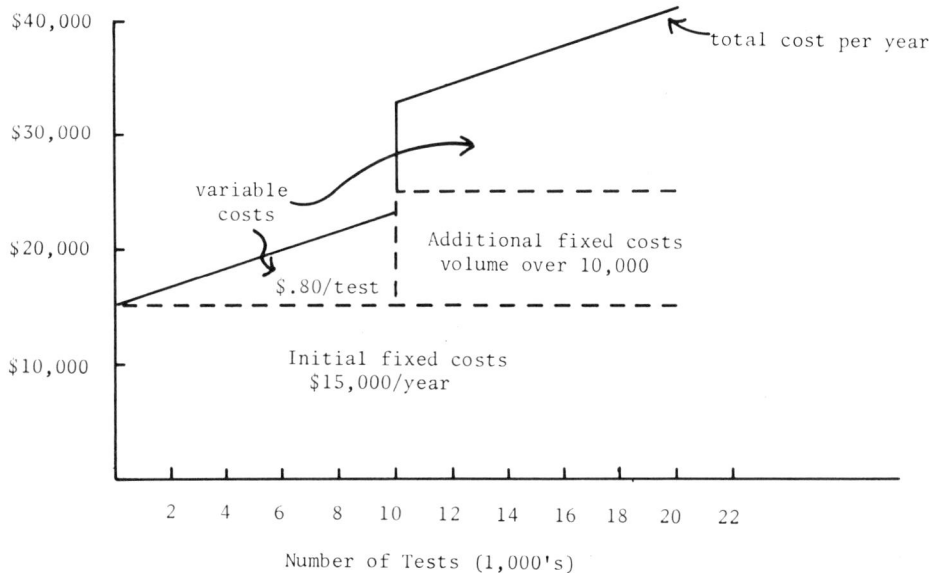

Figure 6-1. Total Costs of a Hypothetical Laboratory Service, Manual Method.

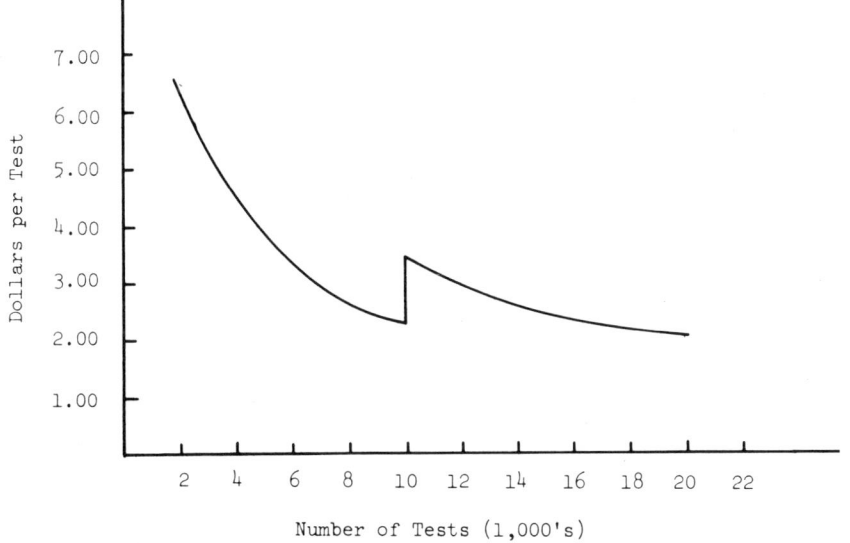

Figure 6-2. Costs per Unit, Manual Method.

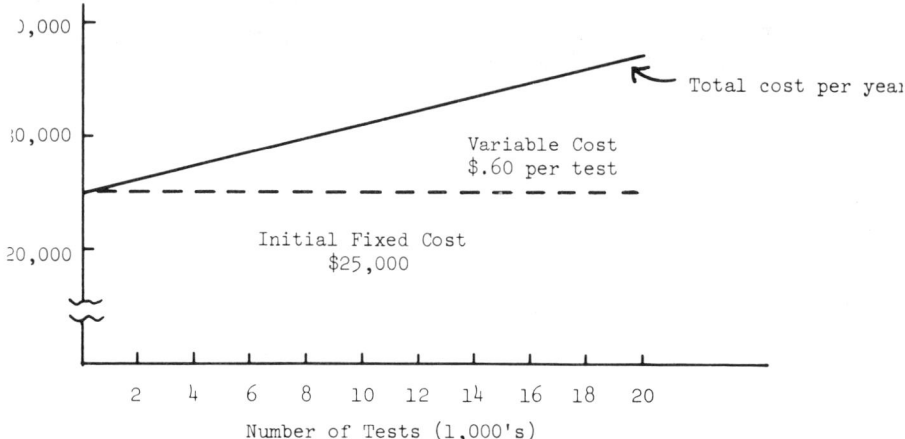

Figure 6-3. Total Cost of a Hypothetical Laboratory Service Auto Analyzer.

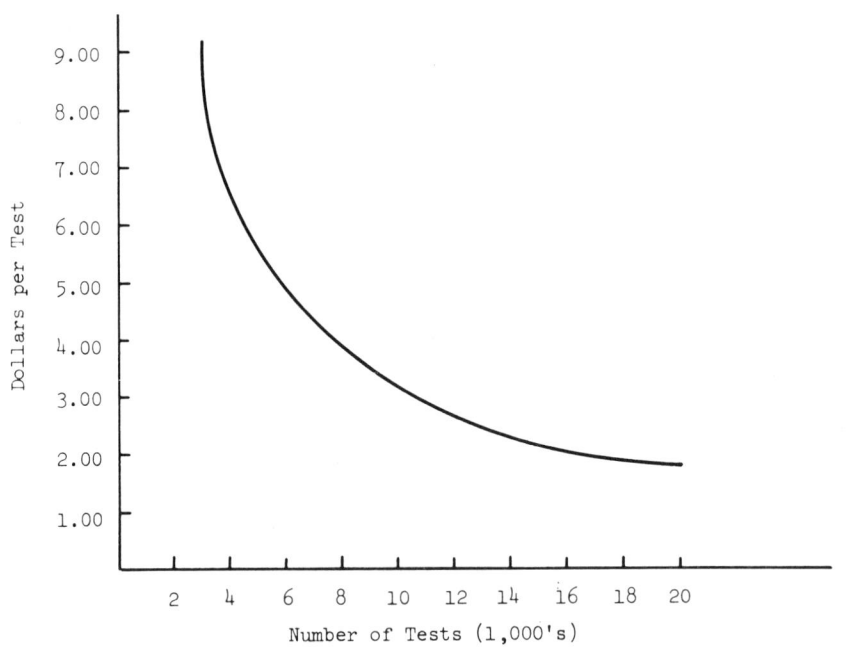

Figure 6-4. Cost per Unit, Auto Analyzer Method.

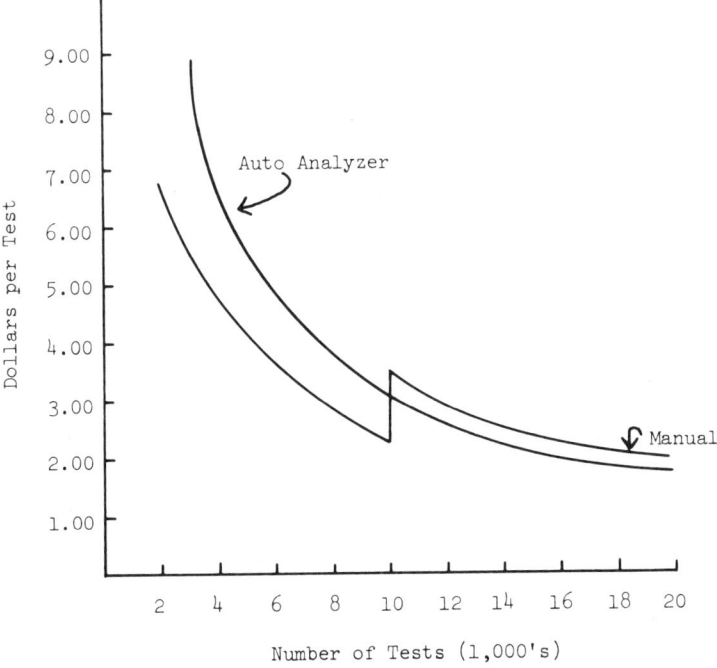

Figure 6-5. Cost per Unit, Auto Analyzer Method; Cost per Unit, Manual Method.

It permits the identification of the least cost alternative and the comparison of other alternatives. It says nothing, however, about a second, and equally important kind of decision: how many units of a given service the hospital should provide. This question is answered in profit-making situations by estimating the demand at varying prices and comparing this schedule to the total cost of production to determine profit. For a variety of reasons, such an analysis is often not appropriate in hospitals. Some substitute procedure must be devised to allow a rational decision. This often involves a concept of *value* or *benefit* of a service provided. The value of a medical service is its contribution to the patient's health and well-being. It is related to the costs which would be incurred if the service were not provided. These are the costs of illness: pain, death, loss of productivity, etc. There is usually no direct market at work for these, and therefore no price readily available. They are called *intangible* or *nonmonetary* costs for this reason. Intuitively each new unit of service would reduce this cost. However, as more units are available, the contribution of additional units of service might tend to be less. A point would come for any service where all possible use had been made, an additional unit would make no contribution at all and would have no value.

Many persons in the health field would choose to provide resources until there were no further benefits from additional units of services. Such a decision is unrealistic, however. For most practical situations, there are not enough resources to permit this, and the cost of the necessary resources mounts to exorbitant levels. The concept of balancing the cost of resources against the value provides the key to a more acceptable solution. Figures 6-6 and 6-7 show the two kinds of costs which must be considered. Figure 6-6 shows the production costs, the costs of the resources which must be expended to provide a given quantity of services, while figure 6-7 shows the value, or the costs of illness which are avoided by providing given quantities of service. At any particular level of service, the total costs will be the sum of these two kinds of costs. This curve is shown in figure 6-8.

The answer to the question of how many units to provide now becomes clear, if the costs can be accurately measured. Additional units of service would be provided as long as the total cost is reduced, or until the production cost of the next unit exceeded the value of the service it would provide. The costs of the next unit are called the *marginal costs* or the *marginal return*. The marginal cost for the nth unit can be defined as the difference between the cost of providing $n-1$ units and providing n units. It is usually represented as ΔC if C is the total cost:[a]

$$\Delta C(n) = C_n - C_{n-1}$$

If the two costs in figures 6-6 and 6-7 are designated as C_1 and C_2, then resources would be supplied until

$$\Delta C_1(n) = -\Delta C_2(n)$$

or

$$\Delta C_1(n) + \Delta C_2(n) = 0.$$

All quantitative solutions to resource allocation problems are approached by variations of this conceptual analysis.

Procedure

Resource allocation procedures are designed to do systematically what the intuitive criterion would suggest, extending to more complex situations where intuitive solution is inaccurate or impossible. Given a problem of resource allocation, the first step to its solution is the clear description of the process involved. This includes demand, outputs, present resources input, and present

---

[a]The marginal costs can be represented graphically as the slope of the curves. For continuous functions of costs, this is the first derivative dC/dU, if U is the number of units.

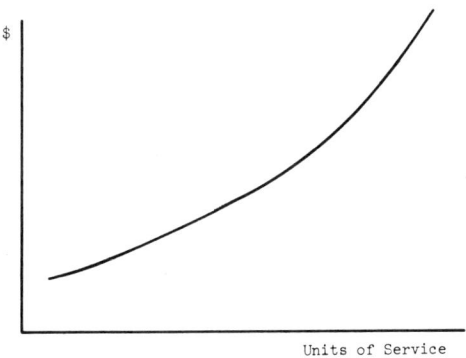

Figure 6-6. Cost of Resources Used in Providing a Health Service.

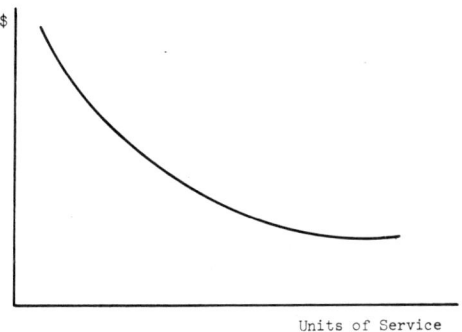

Figure 6-7. Cost of Illness versus Units of Service Provided.

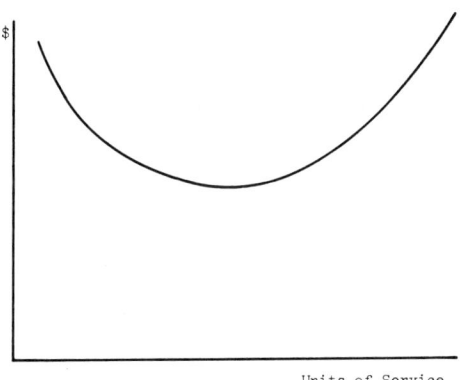

Figure 6-8. Total Costs versus Units of Service.

levels of efficiency and quality. Second, a model is constructed which allows the various parts of the process to be altered, so that the impact on input requirements or output can be studied. Third, the model is studied over the range of relevant present and future conditions. Fourth, the results are evaluated. Lastly, a recommendation is made. For relatively simple problems, such as the inventory size application of total value analysis which is described in this chapter, the work is simple enough that one man may perform the bulk of it. In other cases, where demand is stochastic and many values are nonmonetary, the assistance of many different skills will be necessary.

Difficulties

The problem of resource allocation is not in conceptualizing the best decision but in finding it. As problems become larger and more complex, techniques must be developed to aid in measuring costs and returns and finding the point where minimum cost gains the satisfactory returns. Other than sheer problem size, there are three kinds of difficulties which must be overcome: *uncertainty*, the known chance that the situation will vary; *risk*, the unknown chance of variation; and *value*, the consensus judgment of the relative desirability of goods and services.

Uncertainty is measured by the stochastic nature of the process. A stochastic process contains uncertainty; a deterministic process does not. Resource allocation is more difficult when the process is stochastic. If patients' needs were constant, the problem of nurse staffing would be trivial.

Risk is the unknown chance of change. It cannot be measured, obviously, by known distributions. One example which distinguishes risk and uncertainty is the demand for cobalt radiation therapy. The demand is subject to variation because it is a function of the number of people with certain forms of cancer. That variation is uncertainty. However, there is also some unknown possibility that a new form of therapy will make cobalt treatment obsolete. That is risk.

The techniques described in the following discussion vary in their ability to handle risk, uncertainty, and value. Some are suited primarily to deterministic, monetary problems. Others are capable of handling stochastic situations and nonmonetary situations. One technique, cost-effectiveness, can be applied to almost any combination, including high risk. In general, the more a technique moves away from the deterministic, risk-free, monetary problem, the less precise its answer becomes and the more subjective the resulting decision. These techniques are still useful, however. The process of model building, testing, and evaluating the component costs provides much greater insight to decisions, even if it does not perfectly answer the questions.

Inventory Control Problems—Deterministic Model

One general method of solving management problems is to attempt to describe the total value of each alternative decision. *Total value* consists of all costs which result from a given decision. Estimating total value is not easy, even in industrial situations which are at first glance clear-cut. In hospital situations where one element of "cost" may be a delay or omission of a critical service to a patient, measuring total value may be very difficult.

A simple example of inventory decisions can be used to illustrate the technique and also some of the measurement difficulties encountered. In this situation the model will be deterministic, and non-monetary costs will be excluded.

Total Value Analysis

Consider a problem of selecting the appropriate quantity to order on a supply item used routinely in hospital operations. For simplicity, assume that the item is used in a nonclinical area and that the use rate is constant. The hospital purchasing agent buys a quantity Q which is delivered and placed in inventory at time t_0. When it is almost gone, he reorders Q. The shipment arrives as the last of the first batch is used, at t_1. The inventory of the item over time is as shown in figure 6-9.

The decision which must be made is the quantity Q to be purchased. A model must be devised to test various Q to find the minimum total cost. The elements of the cost which should be included are:

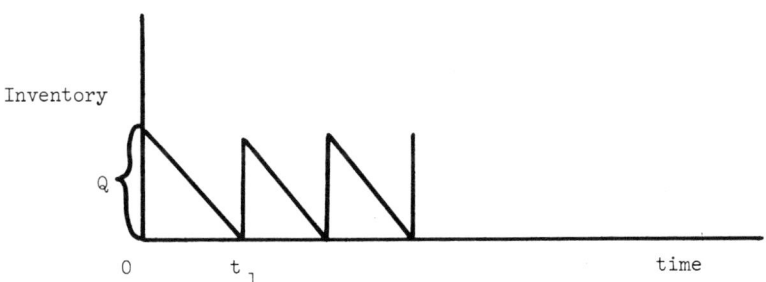

Figure 6-9. Inventory of a Routine Supply Item over Time.

p — price per item (this may vary with the order size)
S — cost per order (cost of preparing an order, paying an invoice, etc.)
W — cost of storage space per item
I — cost of capital invested in inventory (interest)

The average investment, over the year, will be 1/2 Q. The number of orders per year will be the total usage U, divided by Q.

$$\frac{U}{Q} = n$$

The total value will be the sum of each of the four elements of cost, expressed in annual terms. For the purchase cost of the item, assuming that the price remains constant, this will be pU, the price per item times the total number used. For the cost of placing orders, this will be Sn, since S is the cost of processing an order, and there will be n orders per year. For the warehousing cost, space must be set aside for the maximum quantity, Q, that will have to be stored, and the cost will be WQ if it costs W to make space for a single item for a year. The cost of capital invested will be the average amount of the investment, 1/2 Q, times the price per unit, p, times the interest rate I: $IpQ/2$. The total annual cost will be the sum of all these terms:

$$TC = pU + Sn + WQ + \frac{IpQ}{2}.$$

The following simple examples will illustrate the use of this formula to find the minimum cost quantity.

Example 1A.

U = 10,000 units per year
S = $10 per order
W = $.05 per unit per year
I = 5.0 percent
p = variable, as shown. Quantities are minimum for each price.

Model Calculations for Various Q

Q	5,000	3,000	2,000	1,000	500
n	2	3.3	5	10	20
p	$ 0.960	$ 0.967	$ 0.975	$ 0.985	1.00
pU	$9,600	$9,670	$9,750	$9,850	$10,000
Sn	20	33	50	100	200
WQ	250	150	100	50	25
$IpQ \div 2$	120	72	49	25	12
Total cost	$9,990	$9,925	$9,949	$10,075	$10,237
Unit cost	$ 0.999	$ 0.992	$ 0.995	$ 1.008	$ 1.024

Clearly the best decision within the range studied is $Q = 3,000$.

Example 1B. Suppose that the manufactuer's price is constant, that is, the item costs $1.00 no matter what the order quantity. Then the term pU becomes a constant which no longer affects the outcome. The calculations are:

Q	5,000	3,000	2,000	1,000	500
n	2	3.3	5	10	20
Sn	$ 20	$ 33	$ 50	$ 100	$200
WQ	250	150	100	50	25
$IpQ \div 2$	125	75	50	25	12
Total cost TC'	$ 395	$ 258	$ 200	$ 175	$237
Unit cost	$ 1.04	$ 1.026	$ 1.020	$ 1.018	$ 1.024

where
$$TC' = TC - pU$$
TC' min= $175.00 for $Q = 1,000$.

In this case, a check might be made for $Q = 1,500, n = 6.7$

$$TC' = \$67 + \$75 + \$38 = \$180, \text{ for } Q = 1,500$$

In figure 6-10, the resulting values have been plotted to visualize the problem.

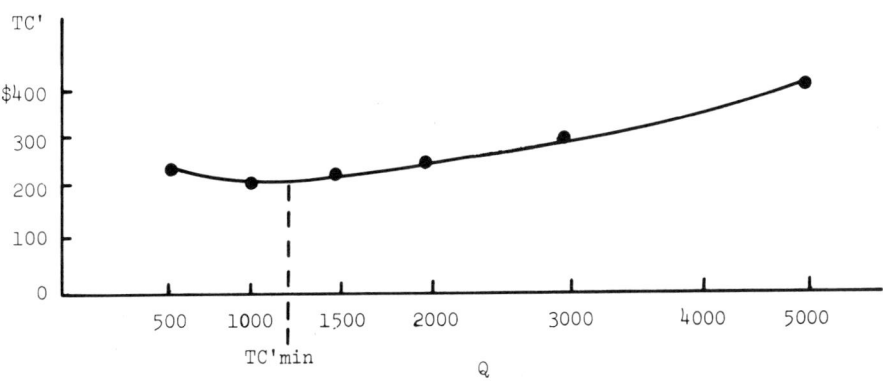

Figure 6-10. Annual Costs of Varying Order Quantities.

Successive approximations could be used to determine TC_{min} exactly. However, the curve seems to be flat around 1,000, and this value would probably be accepted. Many problems can be solved by graphic approaches like this. More exact solutions can be obtained using calculus, but such techniques are beyond the scope of this book.[1]

Marginal Value Analysis

It is possible to consider the problem in terms of the change in cost as the decision variable is altered. This change can be calculated in simple cases by subtracting adjacent values of the total cost. The *marginal cost per unit* change in the decision variable can be calculated by dividing the marginal cost by the change in the decision variable. The notation ΔTC is used to indicate the marginal cost; ΔQ, the change in the decision variable Q; and $\Delta TC/\Delta Q$, the marginal cost per unit. For example 1B:

Q	TC	ΔQ	ΔTC	$\Delta TC/\Delta Q$
500	$237			
1,000	175	+500	$-62	$-0.124
1,500	180	+500	+ 5	+0.010
2,000	200	+500	+20	+0.040

In general two important characteristics about marginal cost permit its use in finding TC_{min} with less effort than would otherwise be required. First, TC_{min} is always at the point where $\Delta TC = 0$. That is, lower values of Q are associated with $\Delta TC < 0$ and higher values with $\Delta TC > 0$. Not all points where $\Delta TC = 0$ are TC_{min}, however. Thus any value of $\Delta TC = 0$ should be checked against the actual behavior of TC near that value of Q. ($\Delta TC = 0$ for TC_{max} as well, and this possibility must be ruled out.)

Second, the terms in the total value equation which are independent of the decision variable do not affect $\Delta TC/\Delta Q$, and may be ignored in determining the minimum. (For example, the unit price in example 1B, although not in example 1A.) This permits considerable simplification in the data collection for some problems.[b]

---

[b] The student who had calculus should note that these two conditions stem directly from the notion of the derivation

$$\Delta TC/\Delta Q \rightarrow dTC/dQ \text{ as } \Delta Q \rightarrow 0$$

and

$$dC/dQ = 0 \text{ if } C \text{ is a constant with respect to } Q.$$

What is said above, is that the total value equation can be differentiated with respect to the variable of interest. The derivative can be set equal to zero and solved for the variable of interest.

$$TC = pU + \frac{SU}{Q} + WQ + \frac{IpQ}{2}$$

$$\frac{d(TC)}{dQ} = W + \frac{Ip}{2} - \frac{SU}{Q^2} = 0$$

$$Q_{min} = \pm\sqrt{\frac{SU}{W+\frac{Ip}{2}}}$$

Measurement Problems

Measurement of the terms in the total value equation presents a number of problems.[2] The cost of placing an order, S, is often a minor factor in the equation, and may be one which is very difficult to determine. Rarely would one wish to construct the exact processing of orders for a given item and price each step by time study or other method. However, the functions of order processing and receiving and of paying accounts for all items in inventory can be estimated with reasonable accuracy. This value, the average cost for processing an order and invoice, could be substituted as an approximation. In the example 1A, where price of the item was a dominant factor, this term might have been assumed to be constant and eliminated. In the second case, however, the cost per order is the largest term near the minimum, and a more careful investigation of it would be in order. This investigation should go at least as far as determining that there are no unusual factors about this item that would make it significantly different from the average order in terms of processing costs.

The storage space cost term presents another type of measurement difficulty. So long as storage space generally is well utilized and neither overcrowded nor frequently vacant, one may assume that the space required for this item is the cost per cubic foot or shelf-foot of maintaining the storeroom. However, if a large idle storage area is available at all times, then the cost of using it may be nearly zero. In this situation Q may be increased, based on investment cost limits versus price and reorder costs alone. The result, as intuition predicts, is a much larger Q_{min}. The opposite of this case is the crowded storeroom. It may be impossible to store more than a given number of units of Q. If this is so, then the minimum must be found from those possibilities of Q less than this limit. In a realistic case of storing several hundred items, there would always be space for the item in question at the expense of some other item or items. In this situation, the theoretical solution would be to formulate the total value equation for each item and solve the equations for all items simultaneously. Such a solution is probably impractical, however. As a practical approach to it, inventory problems generally concentrate only on those items which appear to have a high potential of cost reduction. Another possibility for handling the crowded storeroom case is to assign a second, higher cost-of-storage to space greater than some quantity of space which represents the practical limit of available space for the item in question. This is similar to proposing that the cost W applies so long as the quantity does not exceed a stated value Q'. When $Q>Q'$, it is necessary to use another, more expensive space W'. The statements for the storage cost term become:

$$WQ \text{ for } Q \leqslant Q'$$
$$WQ + W'(Q - Q') \text{ for } Q > Q'.$$

The last and most difficult measurement problem is of the interest rate, I. This term at first glance appears clear-cut; it might be either the cost of borrowed working capital or the loss of investment oppotunity in short-term notes for the hospital which has surplus cash. Either one of these figures is commonly used. The true interest rate, as reflected in hospital management decisions, may be much higher than these rates. The result of using the lower rate would be to make the purchasing agent tie too much money in inventories. (As I increases, Q_{min} decreases.) The selection of the appropriate interest rate may be quite difficult. Further discussion of this question appears in the chapter on capital investment and cost effectiveness.

Other Uses of Total Value Analysis

Total value analysis can be applied to other problems than the inventory order quantity. In general, it is applicable whenever a model can be devised which expresses the total value or cost of the process in terms of the variable under study. The comparison of two alternative processes over a range of outputs has already been graphically illustrated in conceptual form (see figs. 6-1 through 6-5). The method can be extended to cover other decisions and to determine critical points where the preferred decision changes. It can also be extended to stochastic situations as the following example will illustrate.

Example 2. Consider as an example a department such as radiology, which has a fixed physical facility and has experienced growing demand which now begins to tax the capacity of the facility under its present 40-hour a week operations. The short-run daily demand, D, consists of scheduled and unscheduled components, and the scheduled demand is a significant part of the total. In this situation, we shall include only the emergency or unscheduled demand which occurs during the regular working hours. That is, emergencies receiving service at night are irrelevant to the problem and will be ignored. Demand has a mean $\bar{D}$, and a variance σ_D^2. The form of the demand curve is shown in figure 6-11. There is a capacity D_1 of the existing regular service which cannot be increased in the short run. We will call the present capacity state 1. There is a cost of providing service at this capacity, TC_1, and a probability p that this capacity will be exceeded on any given day. As the total demand D grows, the probability p will increase. (We are obviously ruling out the possibility of expanding the department and increasing its hourly capacity. Thus we are discussing and modeling those demands at or near $\bar{D} = D_1$.) As a final assumption, let us assume that the costs of failing to meet demand (bad public relations, medical hazards, and unnecessary delay of discharge) are very high, and we wish to avoid any such occurrence. There are two alternative solutions: (a) schedule an additional shift. This might be done in the evening or on Saturdays (state 2); and (b) arrange to operate the department on an overtime basis when necessary only (state 3).

The costs of operation can be divided into two categories: *fixed* (those which

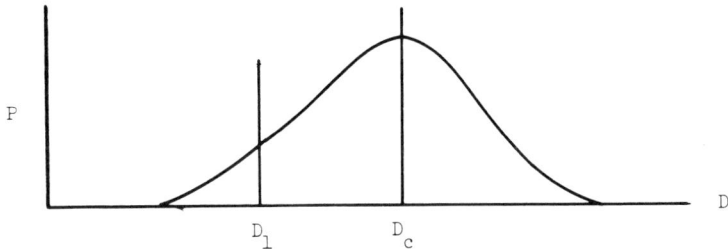

Figure 6-11. Probability Distribution of Demand for Service D.

would be incurred even if there were no demand on a particular day, such as heat, depreciation, supervision) and *variable* (those which will increase with each unit of demand, such as supplies). Labor costs will be fixed if a definite number of hours will be worked regardless of the demand. This is the case in state 1 and state 2. They will be variable if hours are worked only when the demand is present (state 3). Using the concepts of fixed and variable costs, it is possible to write algebraic models which describe the costs under each state. For state 1, where the demand on any given day is less than the capacity ($D \leq D_1$), the total costs, TC_1, are as follows:

$$TC_1 = F_1 + H_1 + K_1 D,$$

where

F_1 = cost of fixed items (equipment, overhead)
H_1 = cost of regularly scheduled man hours
K_1 = cost of variable items (supplies).

For state 2 all the fixed costs in state 1 will be incurred plus an additional fixed cost for the additional man hours scheduled and variable costs for the total demand:

$$TC_2 = F_1 + H_1 + H_2 + K_1 D,$$

where H_2 = cost of additional regularly scheduled hours. Since the decisions are made in advance, independent of the actual demand, this equation applies for any value of D.

For state 3, no additional costs are incurred unless demand is present, but the variable costs are quite high because they include both supplies and manpower. (The manpower might be at "time and one-half" as well.) Two equations are necessary to describe state 3, depending on whether or not demand exceeds the state 1 capacity.

For $D \leq D_1$:

$$TC_3 = F_1 + H_1 + K_1 D,$$

and for $D > D_1$:

$$TC_3 = F_1 + H_1 + K_1 D_1 + (K_1 + K_3)(D - D_1)$$

K_3 = variable overtime manpower

The equations for the three states are shown graphically in figure 6-12. Looking at this figure, it appears that there is some level of demand D_c where state 2 becomes cheaper than state 3. If the daily demand were a constant rather than a variable depending in part on a random process, the selection of the alternative would be simple. The total value equations could be evaluated for the expected demand and the lesser chosen. It is clear that alternative 2 is preferable for any D less than D_c, where the two lines intersect on figure 6-12. This point, D_c, can be calculated algebraically. To simplify the calculation, the equations for states 2 and 3 can be rewritten summarizing the fixed terms into single constants.

$$TC_2 = F_1 + H_1 + H_2 + K_1 D = C_2 + K_1 D$$

and, for $D > D_1$,

$$TC_3 = F_1 + H_1 + K_1 D_1 + (K_1 + K_3)(D - D_1) = C_3 + (K_1 + K_3)(D - D_1)$$

where $C_3 = F_1 + H_1 + K_1 D_1$.

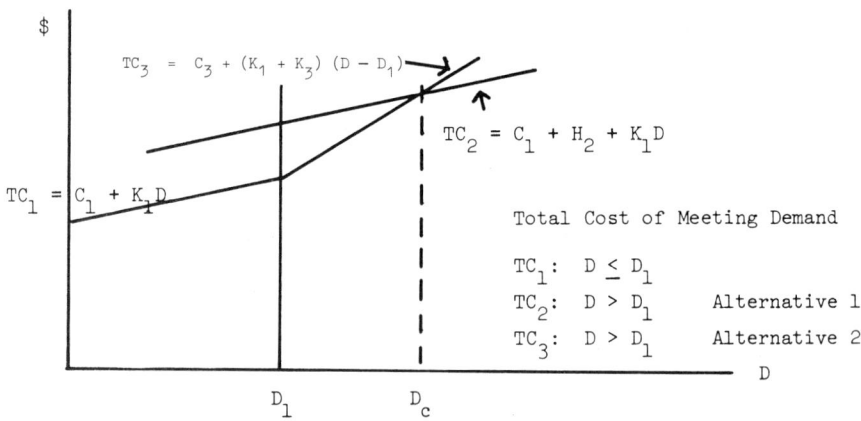

Figure 6-12. Total Cost of Meeting Demand.

(The case where $D \leqslant D_1$ is no longer relevant to the problem. It is clear that the solution will not lie in this area.)

The solution is obtained by finding the point D_c where the costs of the two states are equal:

at $D = D_c$,
$$TC_2 = TC_3$$
$$C_2 + K_1 D_c = C_3 + (K_1 + K_3)(D_c - D_1)$$
$$K_1 D_c - K_3 D_c = C_3 - C_2 - (K_1 + K_3)D_1$$
$$\frac{C_2 - C_3 + (K_1 + K_3)D_1}{(K_1 + K_3) - K_1} = D_c$$

but $C_2 - C_3 = (F_1 + H_1 + H_2) - (F_1 + H_1 + K_1 D_1) = H_2 - K_1 D_1$.

substituting $\dfrac{H_2 - K_1 D_1 + (K_1 + K_3)D_1}{(K_1 + K_3) - K_1} = D_c$ or $\dfrac{H_2 + K_3 D_1}{K_3} = D_c$

For a stochastic process the solution is not so simple, however. The total cost of each level of demand is different, and the total cost of all levels will be the sum of each level under the alternative selected, times the probability that that level will occur.

$$\sum_{D=0}^{\infty} TC_D p_D$$

For state 2, for each daily demand

$$TC_2 = C_2 + K_1 D$$
$$\sum_{D=0}^{\infty} TC_2 p_D = C_2 \sum_{D=0}^{\infty} p_D + K_1 \sum_{D=0}^{\infty} D p_D \ .$$

Since

$$\sum_{D=0}^{\infty} p_D = 1, \text{ by definition}$$
$$\sum_{D=0}^{\infty} TC_2 p_D = C_2 + K_1 \sum_{D=0}^{\infty} D p_D \ .$$

Similarly, for state 3,

$$\sum_{D=0}^{\infty} TC_3 p_D = F_1 + H_1 + K_1 \sum_{D=0}^{\infty} Dp_D + K_3 \left(\sum_{D=D_1+1}^{\infty} (D-D_1) p_D \right)$$

As before, these cost equations can be compared and the lesser value selected. (Notice that under stochastic demand there can be some levels of $D \leq D_1$ even though the mean demand $\bar{D} > D_1$. Under state 3, these are handled at the same cost as state 1; but under state 2, extra costs are incurred for staffing which remains idle.)

In order to reach a decision regarding the preferred state, the terms of this equation must be evaluated. There are two ways to do this—by approximation based upon actual demand experience, or by an analytic solution of the value of $\sum_{D=0}^{\infty} Dp_D$ which can be done under certain assumptions regarding the demand distribution. These are illustrated in the following sections.

Example 2A–Solution by Approximation. Suppose that the demand curve in figure 6-11 is for a moderate-size x-ray department, having capacity of twenty-five examinations per day. The demand distribution has been as follows for the past year, with extra demand met by overtime when necessary. The question is whether the department should continue this practice or reorganize to a six day week.

Number of Examinations	Number of Days Occurring	Number of Procedures	Cumulative Number of Procedures	Probability p_D	Cumulative Probability	Dp_D
less than 20	17	308	308	0.046	0.046	0.87
20	12	240	546	0.033	0.079	0.66
21	18	378	924	0.049	0.128	1.03
22	31	682	1606	0.085	0.213	1.87
23	48	1104	2710	0.132	0.345	3.04
24	57	1368	4078	0.156	0.501	3.74
25 (D_1)	53	1325	5403	0.145	0.646	3.62
26	55	1430	6833	0.151	0.797	3.93
27	40	1080	7913	0.110	0.907	2.97
28	19	532	8445	0.052	0.959	1.46
29	12	348	8793	0.033	0.992	0.96
30	3	30	8823	0.008	1.000	0.24
Total	365	8823				24.39

$\sum_{D=0}^{\infty} Dp_D = 24.4,$ $\sum_{D=D_1+1}^{\infty} p_D = 0.35,$ $\sum_{D=D_1+1}^{\infty} Dp_D = 9.56$

The cost under state 2 $= C_2 + K_1 \sum_{D=0}^{\infty} Dp_D = C_2 + 24.4 K_1$

and under state 3 =

$$F_1 + H_1 + K_1 \sum_{D=0}^{\infty} Dp_D + K_3 \sum_{D=D_1+1}^{\infty} Dp_D - K_3 D_1 \sum_{D=D_1+1}^{\infty} p_D$$

$$= C_3 + 24.4 K_1 + 0.8 K_3$$

These values can be easily calculated when the cost data are supplied.

For the data presented, the range of the distribution of D is only slightly more than 11 units. For a much larger demand, say in the laboratory, where the distribution of D is between 200 and 300 tests per day, or in the laundry, where D might be of order of magnitude 2,000 to 3,000 pounds per day, manual calculation of $\sum Dp_D$ would be tedious or impossible. In such a situation, one might wish to substitute grouped frequencies, using the cost value of the frequency midpoint, to reduce the amount of calculation. An interval of 100 pounds per day could be used for the frequency distribution, with the cost of the interval assumed to be that of the midpoint. Another way to arrive at a solution would be to program the calculations for a computer, although for most nonrecurring problems the time required for writing and checking the program will be greater than that required to solve the problem manually. Once the program was written the costs TC_2 and TC_3 could be evaluated for several hypothetical distributions of demand. By successive trials, one could determine the approximate demand necessary to justify state 2. This is, in effect, a simple simulation routine.

Example 2B—Analytic Solution. For certain demand distributions it may be possible to derive an analytic solution to the terms $\sum Dp_D$. For example, for a Poisson process of demand,

$$p_D = \frac{e^{-\lambda}\lambda^D}{D!},$$

where λ is the mean of demand, $\bar{D}$,

$$Dp_D = \frac{De^{-\lambda}\lambda^D}{D!} = \frac{e^{-\lambda}\lambda^D}{(D-1)!} = \left(\frac{e^{-\lambda}\lambda^{D-1}}{(D-1)!}\right) \lambda.$$

But $\dfrac{e^{-\lambda}\lambda^{D-1}}{(D-1)!}$ is a Poisson process as well

and $\displaystyle\sum_{D=D_1+1}^{\infty} \lambda \dfrac{e^{-\lambda}\lambda^{D-1}}{(D-1)!} = \lambda \sum_{D=D_1}^{\infty} \dfrac{e^{-\lambda}\lambda^{D}}{D!}$,

$$TC_2 = C_2 + K_1 \sum_{D=0}^{\infty} Dp_D$$

$$= C_2 + K_1 \overline{D} \;.$$

Taking the equation for TC_3 ,

$$TC_3 = F_1 + H_1 + K_1 \sum_{D=0}^{\infty} Dp_D + K_3 \sum_{D=D_1+1}^{\infty} Dp_D - K_3 D_1 \sum_{D=D_1+1}^{\infty} p_D$$

and using the reduction of the Poisson equations above:

$$TC_3 = F_1 + H_1 + K_1\overline{D} + K_3\overline{D} \sum_{D=D_1}^{\infty} p_D - K_3 D_1 \sum_{D=D_1+1}^{\infty} p_D$$

Solving for $\overline{D}$ at the critical point where $TC_2 = TC_3$,

$$C_2 + K_1\overline{D} = F_1 + H_1 + K_1\overline{D} + K_3\overline{D} \sum_{D=D_1}^{\infty} p_D - K_3 D_1 \sum_{D=D_1+1}^{\infty} p_D$$

substituting $\quad C_2 = F_1 + H_1 + H_2$

$$F_1 + H_1 + H_2 + K_1\overline{D} = F_1 + H_1 + K_1\overline{D} + K_3\overline{D} \sum_{D=D_1}^{\infty} p_D - K_3 D_1 \sum_{D=D_1+1}^{\infty} p_D$$

Subtracting $(F_1 + H_1 + K_1\overline{D})$ from both sides and rearranging yields

$$\overline{D} = \dfrac{H_2 + K_3 D_1 \sum_{D=D_1+1}^{\infty} p_D}{K_3 \sum_{D=D_1}^{\infty} p_D}$$

This can be evaluated with the help of a cumulative table of the Poisson distribution. For actual values of $\overline{D}$ less than the solution, state 3 (overtime) is preferred, otherwise state 2.

Summary

In this chapter, the notion of minimizing total cost has been introduced as a rule for making health and hospital decisions. The first section illustrates this conceptually in a resource allocation framework. It is pointed out that resources have a cost, so that the more resources are used, the higher their cost will be. On the other hand, there are costs or values involved in failing to provide a resource as well. These costs tend to diminish as more resources are made available. If all these costs and values could be measured, and if hospital problems were deterministic, the appropriate amount of resources for a given situation could easily be determined. Resources would be provided until the cost of providing the last unit of resources (the marginal cost) exactly equalled the cost or value of not providing the service it represents. In practice it is often very difficult to measure these costs and values. Even when they can be measured, their interaction can be quite complex. Models are used to describe the resources allocation problems so that the appropriate decisions can be made. These are abstractions of the problem which permit study of impact of various decisions, and the eventual selection of the optimal solution. They are often mathematical or graphic, and they frequently require computers for their solution.

The model for total value analysis is one of the most flexible and fundamental of these analytic tools. It is an algebraic statement of the costs which are incurred under various possible solutions to the problem. The first illustration of the total value model is an inventory problem selecting the quantity of a supply which should be ordered at one time. The usage of the item is assumed to be deterministic. Costs are stated in terms of the order quantity, and it is found that some increase as the quantity increases, while others decrease. A minimum cost solution is reached by graphic methods.

The second illustration uses total value analysis to establish the critical point at which a department should expand its regular schedule rather than rely on overtime to meet increasing demand. The solution can be formulated for the deterministic case. The model can be expanded to accommodate the stochastic variation in demand and solved by a trial and error approach. The possibility of exact solution by algebraic methods is also explored. This rests on the assumption that demand follows the Poisson distribution.

In the chapters which follow, other common forms of models will be discussed. These all rest upon the same conceptualization—seeking the minimum cost solution. Chapter 7 will describe the technique of simulation and illustrate ways in which it can be used to model decisions involving stochastic processes.

Chapter 8 will review deterministic and stochastic mathematical models which permit the analysis of complex situations involving selection from among large numbers of courses of action. These are called mathematical programming models. Chapter 9 deals with a form of analysis where both capital investment and operating costs are affected by the resource allocation decision. This important area of decision making will be explored in terms of problems where most of the elements can be reduced to monetary terms and problems where many aspects cannot be expressed in this way.

Additional Readings

Bowman, E.H. and R.B. Fetter. *Analysis for Production and Operations Management*, 3rd Ed., R.D. Irwin, Homewood, Ill., 1967, ch. 8, "Total Value Analysis," ch. 9, "Incremental Analysis."

Churchman, C. West. *The Systems Approach*, Dell Publishing Co., New York, 1968.

Sloan, A.P. *My Years with General Motors*, McFadden-Bartell, New York, 1965.

7 Queueing and Simulation Models for Resource Allocation

Resource Allocation in Stochastic Processes

Problem Description

The problem of random, or stochastic, variation is described in chapter 3, with examples of both demand fluctuations and resource (absenteeism) fluctuations. This variation obviously creates problems for resource allocation. There is a clear tradeoff between the ability to handle demand when it occurs and the cost of the resources provided. The following hypothetical example will illustrate this.

Suppose that a certain disease strikes randomly, following a Poisson distribution, and that a certain resource, such as an oxygen tent, is needed whenever it occurs. To simplify the problem, assume that one unit of the resource is needed by each patient for twenty-four hours at the start of his illness and is not needed again. If the expected number of patients demanding the resource is five, actual distribution of demand over a year will be as follows.

Number of Patients (k) (Number of resource units demanded)	Chance of Occurring[a]	No. of Days per Year Expected	No. of Days kth Resource Used
0	.01	3	—
1	.03	12	362
2	.08	29	350
3	.14	51	321
4	.18	66	270
5	.18	66	204
6	.15	55	138
7	.10	36	83
8	.06	22	47
9	.04	15	25
10	.02	7	10
11	.01	3	3
Total	1.00	365	1813

[a] A Poisson distribution with a mean of 5.0.

If seven resource units are available, 87 percent of the demand will be met, and of 7 × 365 = 2,555 unit-days available, 1,728 will be used, or 68 percent. If nine

135

are available, 97 percent of the need will be met, but only 1,800 of 3,285 available unit days, or 55 percent, of the resources will be used. If each of the units cost the same amount, the marginal cost of each unit will be constant. The marginal contribution of each additional unit will decline steadily, however. The ninth unit will contribute only 25 use-days per year to meeting demand, although it will cost as much as the first. How many units must be purchased depends on what value is assigned to meeting the patient's need, for the marginal cost of the last unit purchased is equal to the value per patient, times the marginal number of patients who will use it. Obviously, if the resource is life saving, and there are no substitutes for it, 11 or more will be purchased. This is also likely to be the case if the resource is inexpensive even if it is of limited value. On the other hand, if it is expensive and regarded as of limited value, a much smaller number, perhaps seven or eight, would be provided.

The ability to make an analysis of this kind depends upon two factors: (a) being able to measure the marginal demand for each unit of resource, and (b) being able to attach some value, at least at a subjective preference level, to meeting a unit of demand.

Most realistic problems are considerably more complex than this hypothetical example. The demand for the resource will be for a variable length of time, and it will have different values to different patients. Two modeling techniques have been developed to deal with problems of this sort. The first, queueing theory, has only limited hospital application. The second, simulation, has theoretically unlimited application in stochastic problems, although in specific situations it may prove far more costly than the contribution it can make. These techniques assist with the first condition; they make it possible to measure the ability of various combinations of resources to meet given levels of demand. In many applications, this may be the less difficult of the two conditions. The clarification of the decision which results merely brings the problem of value into sharper focus.

In order to understand the nature of this form of resource allocation problem, it may be desirable to review some of the history of how decisions were made in the past. The problem of the number of beds necessary to meet an expected patient demand has been historically documented over several decades. It is also a fundamental consideration in hospitals planning which can be approached in some cases through the use of the newer techniques.

The Bed Allocation Problem

The techniques outlined in chapters 3 and 4 result in a forecast of a mean number of patient days for each kind of service, together with some information about both the stochastic variation about the mean and the error of the estimate. The initial resource allocation problem is to reach a decision about the number of beds which will be required for each type of service. Since much of the demand for hospital beds is a stochastic process, the dilemma which was outlined above, of efficiency versus risk of failing to meet the demand, must be dealt with. It is worth noting that the problem has always been solved: decisions have been made and beds provided. The history of the decision-making process has been one of increasingly sophisticated models, but their use has been to improve decisions by improving understanding of the tradeoffs involved. The models do not add to the dimensions of the problem; they merely clarify what previously was obscure.

There has been a continuing evolution in the ways in which this problem has been solved.[1] Initially the solution was largely intuitive, or based upon unquantified experience. At this stage, demand was measured directly in bed need, or rule-of-thumb allowances were made to translate patient day demand to bed need. These estimates had little consistency and neither the occupancy (efficiency) or the chance of overcrowding was made clear. In the second stage, assumptions were made that the demand for beds varied according to relatively simple known distributions, usually to the Poisson or the normal. Still later, it was agreed that the actual demand was subject to some manipulation and that within certain limits, it could be managed to gain the desired degree of occupancy. Most recently, agreement is developing that the distribution of demand is a complex one, containing some elements which are subject to manipulation through scheduling and others which are random. These may or may not follow known distributions such as the Poisson or the normal.

The simplest solution to the problem of bed needs is to accept ratios of beds to population, assuming that demand, occupancy, and the probability of being able to meet demand when it occurs will all be handled at an acceptable level. The next simplest is to consider demand in patient days, with an occupancy factor which is either arbitrarily selected or agreed upon as a management goal. If P is the number of patient days; O is the occupancy, and B is the bed need requirement, then:

$$\frac{P}{365 \times O} = B$$

Thus, if $P = 36,500$

$O = 70\%$

$$B = \frac{36,500}{365 \times 0.70} = 141 \ .$$

This simple model identifies one element of the tradeoff, the efficiency with which the resource will be used.

In order to understand the other aspect of the tradeoff, it is necessary to know the nature of the demand distribution. The mean of the demand distribution is the hospital census C:

$$C = \frac{P}{365}.$$

If C is assumed to be normally distributed, it is necessary to have empirical knowledge about the standard deviation of C, σ_C. Efforts to measure σ_C led to the suspicion that it approximated the square root of C.[2] This value,

$$\sigma_C = \sqrt{C} \quad,$$

is characteristic of the Poisson distribution and led to the assumption that the census might in fact follow that distribution. These assumptions allowed, for the first time, an estimate of the chance of having the census exceed the available bed supply. Given a bed capacity B larger than the mean census C, the probability that the census would exceed B on any given day could be obtained by referring to tabulated values of the Poisson distribution. In the case where C was large, the assumption could be made that the Poisson is approximated by the normal distribution. In this case the probability of exceeding the capacity could be calculated using the Z statistic,

$$Z = \frac{B - C}{\sigma_C}$$

and the normal table.

Using this approach, it was common to estimate bed need for a number of years using the formula:

$$B = C + Z\sqrt{C} \quad.$$

The values of Z which were used ranged from 2.5 to 4.0, with a tendency in recent years to lower values. Clearly, these estimates gave a very low probability of exceeding capacity. At $Z = 2.5$ the probability of exceeding capacity is 0.0062, and at $Z = 4$, it is less than 0.00005. The result of this is a rather low-expected occupancy which is, of course, a low efficiency in the use of beds. At $C = 100$, $Z = 4$, the expected occupancy is only a little over 70 percent. A planned occupancy of 90 percent can be achieved only if Z is 2.5 and C is 400. The meaning of Z in probabilistic terms was only rarely considered.

These weaknesses, failing to consider the chance of overflow specifically and permitting inefficient occupancy, were partially overcome by the practice of lumping all kinds of beds and demands into a figure for the hospital as a whole.

While this aggregation of demand was probably not justified, it did act in part to counteract the very conservative, but rather inefficient result of the formula.

With the flurry of attention devoted to the problem in 1960, the weaknesses of the formula were more clearly understood, and it was generally abandoned in favor of selected levels of occupancy which were known to be practical, and not unduly risky, based upon previous experience on meeting demand.[3] These occupancies were adjusted to the individual services. Beds in the more schedulable services, such as surgery, are given high expected occupancy, such as 90 percent, while those services with large random demand are given low occupancy. Those services such as obstetrics and the intensive care unit, where the demand appears to follow a Poisson process, can still be treated as such.

Other Facility Size Questions

Unfortunately bed need is not the only question of facility size which must be answered. For example, operating rooms, recovery rooms, and x-ray treatment facilities must be related in some manner to anticipated demand. Many of these facilities serve a combination of several different demand generating processes. While assumption of a purely random process might be justified in some of these, that is rarely true of all of them. Often there are a variety of ways of manipulating or controlling the demand processes, and one of the management questions is to understand the advantages which might accrue from a manipulation.

Other areas in the hospital, such as the recovery room, present demand problems much too complex for easy analysis. Recovery room demand is generated by both scheduled and emergency surgical operations, and the exact beginning of a unit of demand for recovery room service is a stochastic phenomenon. The length of time that the patient will need the recovery room is also stochastic. The situation is further complicated by the fact that the room rarely operates in a steady state, but rather fills up during the morning to some peak and empties out after that point. The calculation of the number of beds needed to meet the peak demand and the chances of exceeding the available beds is not likely to be simple. It is doubtful that the recovery room arrivals, length of stay, or census would follow any well-known distribution. Even if they did, it would be possible to manipulate the distributions by changing the number of operating rooms, or possibly the order in which difficult cases were scheduled.

Other difficult problems lie in the area of scheduling resources once the quantity has been fixed. For example, consider an x-ray department which has four different kinds of demands for service: (a) medical emergencies; (b) high priority diagnostic requests where delay in meeting the requests will result in unnecessary additional hospitalization; (c) other inpatient x-rays; and (d) nonemergency outpatient work. The size of the emergency demand is sufficiently small that the actual physical facilities might be constructed on the expected total demand without "built-in" protection for emergencies. If this were done, however, certain limits would have to be placed on the scheduling of lower priority work to avoid the danger of being unable to meet high priority work satisfactorily. If these limits were set too high, serious costs or even dangers could be incurred. Exactly what these limits would be presents a rather difficult analytic problem, even if one assumes that the emergency demand follows a Poisson process and the second priority demand is normally distributed. Queueing theory and simulation are the techniques which have been applied to solving these resource allocation problems.

Queueing Theory Models

One of the earliest examples of models of the size of facilities was the exploration of the various aspects of the obstetrical service. This work was begun by John D. Thompson at Yale University in the late 1950s and has resulted in a series of papers by him, Robert B. Fetter, and others on the obstetrics problem and similar ones approachable by the same technique.[4] Other researchers have attempted queueing theory applications to an increasing range of hospital problems, but the relatively simple obstetrical problem provides an appropriate illustration.

Problem Description

A simplified form of the problem of obstetrical demand is relatively easy to perceive. A flow chart of this is shown in figure 7-1. The patient arrives for delivery, presumably in the early stages of labor. She then goes to a labor room for preparation and supervision, where she remains for a varying number of hours. When delivery is imminent, she is moved to the delivery room proper where she stays for a shorter, but also variable length of time. In most hospitals, it is considered good policy to keep the mother under close supervision for a period of one to two hours after delivery. This supervision is provided either in a special obstetrical recovery room, or in another part of the delivery suite. At the end of this time, the patient is ready to move to the obstetrical floor, where she will remain for several days and from which she will be discharged. It can be seen that the distribution of occurrence of each one of these phenomena is, at least in part, random. The arrival rate has been checked repeatedly. Although it seems to have minor seasonal and hourly variations, these are usually insignificant, and a Poisson distribution of arrivals is a very close approximation. The mean number of patients arriving hourly is the total number of births per year divided by 365 X

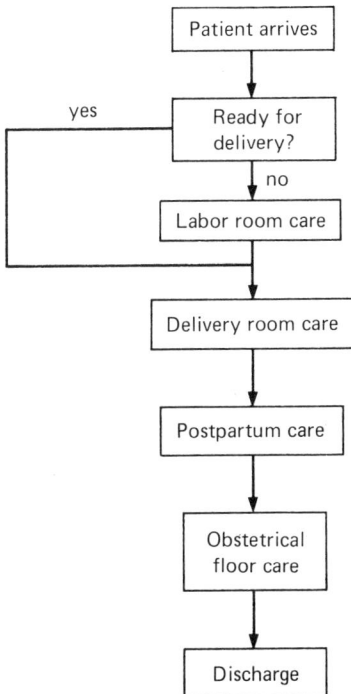

Figure 7-1. Simplified Obstetrical Care Flow Chart.

24. Within the system, it is possible to measure empirically the distribution of service times for each of the care units. Thompson did this for each of the units in the delivery suite itself, using data from Yale New Haven Hospital.[5] These distributions are shown in tables 7-1 through 7-3.

The problem is to construct a model which will allow the effect of various size-of-facility decisions to be checked. Most problems of this sort fall into a class familiar to operations researchers as *queueing problems*. These problems exist whenever service has to be provided in sequence for "customers" who arrive at the service point. Examples of queueing problems are traffic arriving at toll gates, airplanes arriving at airports, and customers arriving at supermarket checkout stations. When the problem is as concrete as these, it is easy to see that the number of service facilities or the average time spent in service has a direct effect on the length of the waiting line or queue which develops. When the arrivals are irregular, if enough facilities are supplied to service the maximum rate of arrivals, the result will be idle facilities at less active times. The dimensions of the problem which must be described are the service time, the time between arrivals, the number of service facilities, sometimes called *channels*

Table 7-1
Distribution of Length of Stay in Labor Rooms, Yale-New Haven Hospital

Hours	Number of Patients	Probability of Occurrence in a Given Patient
0-.99	89	.189
1-1.99	63	.133
2-2.99	46	.098
3-3.99	62	.131
4-4.99	42	.089
5-5.99	22	.047
6-6.99	22	.047
7-7.99	14	.030
8-8.99	14	.030
9-9.99	15	.032
10-10.99	13	.028
11-11.99	12	.025
12-12.99	7	.015
13-13.99	2	.004
14-14.99	5	.011
15-15.99	3	.006
16-16.99	7	.015
17-17.99	0	.000
18-18.99	7	.015
19-19.99	0	.000
20-20.99	1	.002
21-21.99	7	.015
22-22.99	1	.002
23-23.99	0	.000
Over 24	17	.036
Total pts.	471	1.000
Average stay	5.87	

Source: J.D. Thompson et al., "Yale Studies in Hospital Function and Design," unpublished compilation of papers in USPHS Grant W-53, 1959.

or *gates*, and the length of the queue. Although service and arrival times could be constant, in realistic problems they are usually stochastic functions and are described in terms of their mean, standard deviation, and frequency distribution. The distributions given in tables 7-1 through 7-3 are in fact the service times for the three kinds of facilities which comprise the modern labor and delivery suite. The reciprocal of the mean service times is the maximum service rate. Thus, if the mean service time in the labor area is 7.5 hours, the service rate per service

Table 7-2
Distribution of Length of Stay in Delivery Rooms, Yale-New Haven Hospital

Hours	Number of Patients	Probability of Occurrence in a Given Patient
.00-.24	0	.000
.25-.49	57	.154
.50-.74	134	.362
.75-.99	83	.224
1.00-1.24	56	.151
1.25-1.49	19	.051
1.50-1.74	15	.041
1.75-1.99	8	.022
2.00-2.24	2	.005
2.25-2.49	0	.000
2.50-2.74	1	.003
2.75-2.99	0	.000
3.00-3.24	1	.003
3.25-3.49	0	.000
3.50-3.74	1	.003
3.75-3.99	0	.000
Total pts.	377	1.000
Average stay	0.85	

Source: Thompson, "Yale Studies."

facility would be 1 per 7.5 hours, or slightly more than 3 per day at 100 percent efficiency. Similarly, the mean time between arrivals is the reciprocal of the arrival rate.

Queueing Solution

A branch of operations research called *queueing theory* has been developed, which allows theoretical solutions to queueing problems where the distributions of arrivals and service times follow certain known mathematical distributions. Thus where the arrival is Poisson distributed and the service times follow negative exponential distributions, it is possible to calculate from queueing theory formulae the number of "customers" which will be processed per hour, the queue length, and the idle time of facilities for any given set of numerical values.

Thompson and his co-workers at first attempted solutions to the obstetrical suite problem by treating it as a multichanneled, sequential queueing theory

Table 7-3
Distribution of Length of Stay in Postpartum Area, Yale-New Haven Hospital

Hours	Number of Patients	Probability of Occurrence in a Given Patient
.00-.24	3	.007
.25-.49	9	.022
.50-.74	47	.115
.75-.99	73	.179
1.00-1.24	107	.262
1.25-1.49	55	.134
1.50-1.74	46	.113
1.75-1.99	21	.051
2.00-2.24	19	.048
2.25-2.49	12	.029
2.50-2.74	2	.005
2.75-2.99	4	.010
3.00-3.24	4	.010
3.25-3.49	0	.000
Over 4	6	.015
Total pts.	408	1.000
Average stay	1.30	

Source: Thompson, "Yale Studies."

problem. The calculated results for the delivery rooms are shown in table 7-4. This table shows that once in 100 hours, three delivery rooms would be required, while five would be required only once in 10,000 hours. Slightly less than two-thirds of the time (64.13%), no delivery room is required.

Table 7-4
Predicted Usage of Delivery Rooms, Yale-New Haven Hospital, By Queueing Theory

Number of Patients Needing Delivery Room	Predicted Frequency
0	0.6413
1	0.2849
2	0.0633
3	0.0094
4	0.0010
5	0.0001

Source: Thompson, "Yale Studies."

Adopting Solution to Decision

The problem of how many rooms should be built is still unanswered; some cost of turning a patient away must be balanced against the cost of providing an additional room. Because the cost of turning a patient away is almost unmeasurable, one approach would be to allow the physicians on the obstetrical service to decide the risk that they are willing to tolerate. Such a decision would be subject to trustee review. The data in table 7-4 can be translated into more easily understood terms by noting that there are 24 hours a day and 8,760 hours in a year. The same data could be presented as follows:

Rooms Built	Need Another Room	Last Room Used
1	1.4 times a day	28%
2	every fourth day	6%
3	nine times a year	1%
4	once a year	negligible
5	negligible	negligible

It seems clear that the decision lies between three and four rooms. A compromise solution might be reached by building three full-sized rooms and a large labor room which could be converted when necessary.

Verification of Model

In order to verify the queueing theory solution, Thompson and his staff collected additional data on the actual use of delivery rooms. These data showed an error in the predicted values:[6]

Patients	Queueing Prediction	Actual
0	0.6413	0.6118
1	0.2849	0.2983
2	0.0633	0.0802
3	0.0094	0.0069
4	0.0010	0.0024
5	0.0001	0.0004

Although the difference is small, the frequency of need for four rooms is twice the predicted value. In this particular case, the error could prove troublesome, since it affects the value of both the alternatives under consideration. The cause of the error apparently lies in the assumptions of Poisson distributions for arrival and service times. Thompson noted that applicability of this solution was limited to cases where the arrival rate was a true Poisson process. One cause of deviation from the Poisson is the practice of admitting normal women on a scheduled basis for induction into labor. This practice has been common in recent years. In some hospitals, as many as 20 to 30 percent of births are induced, enough to create serious distortions in the distribution of the arrival times. Thompson also noted that in these cases the mean service time in the labor area is likely to increase substantially. Thus two distributions are affected by this practice. In order to develop a more accurate and flexible model to explore the impact of problems of this kind, Thompson and his group turned to simulation solutions to the queueing problem in the obstetrical suite. These are discussed below.

Applications of Queueing Theory

The development of theoretical solutions to queueing problems continues on a worldwide basis. "Analytic" or theoretical solutions to a wide variety of problems now exist. It is possible to handle multiple queues, with varying priorities, multiple service channels under a variety of service time distributions, and sequential servicing stations as well as combinations of these. The ability to solve these problems analytically is still dependent, however, on having situations where the actual service and arrival distributions are close to a limited number of known theoretical distributions. This restriction has limited the usefulness of queueing theory in practical hospital problems. The usefulness of these models so far has been limited to their contribution to the general understanding of the problem. In the hands of skilled operations researchers, they are of great value in formulating and understanding general problems. However, because of their lack of immediate practical value in hospitals and the mathematical difficulty of the solutions, they will not be discussed further in this text.

Simulation as a Solution to the Facility Size Problem

Another operations research technique, formally called Monte Carlo Simulation, is far less restricted to known mathematical distributions and has found more practical application in hospitals. Thompson and Fetter were among the first to demonstrate this usefulness by application to the delivery suite problem,[7] but a wide variety of other applications to areas such as admissions scheduling, patient nursing requirements, operating rooms, and outpatient clinics have been demonstrated or are being developed at the present time. In many of these areas, simulation is used for both scheduling and facility requirement analyses. Others will undoubtedly develop as familiarity with the technique and computer capability increase.

Monte Carlo Simulation is a technique of reproducing or modeling a stochastic process of interest, in such a way that the parameters of interest can be measured by relatively inexpensive artificial trials of the model. Thus a simulation of the delivery suite problem would allow the selection of a given number of each of labor rooms, delivery rooms and postpartum facilities, and the testing of various combinations of arrival rates and service times against the chosen quantities of facilities. The output of the simulation would be estimates of the amount of time the facilities were idle, and the probability of exceeding capacity of each of the various elements. As in the case with any model, certain simplifications from reality are likely to be necessary. However, the technique of simulation is sufficiently expansible that it can be refined to a high degree if the problem justifies it in terms of additional expense necessary to make the modifications.

The simplest example of simulation is the problem of estimating the area of an irregular surface. Such a surface is shown in figure 7-2. It can be seen that one method of measuring the surface would be to count the number of squares within the grid which are included in the surface and to multiply the area of a single square by that number to obtain the total area. It should also be clear, however, that the surface is entirely contained within the area of 6,300 squares—90 × 70. If one were to take a random sample of squares, one might determine the percentage of these 6,300 squares which lie within the surface. That percentage multiplied by 6,300 would yield the area within confidence limits indicated by the sample size. Using a table of random numbers, in which all digits have equal probability of occurrence, one might take four digit numbers, translate these to coordinates of the figure and locate them within or without the surface. Thus, if the first random number were 0122, one would locate this and indicate that it was outside the figure. The next random number might be 2081, which is within the figure. Random numbers such as 1691 which might appear in the table would be ignored since they are outside the 6,300 squares of interest. In a more complex problem, such a procedure might be highly desirable.

Constructing Simulation Routines

The same approach can be extended to solve the delivery suite problem. For example, consider simply the problem of the number of labor rooms which are desirable. Any suggested solution can be tested by simulation to determine the number of times a patient will be forced to wait for a labor room, and the percentage of the times that each labor room will be occupied. The procedure is as follows:

1. Specify the number of labor rooms, the frequency distribution of patients arriving per hour, and the frequency distribution of service time in the labor room

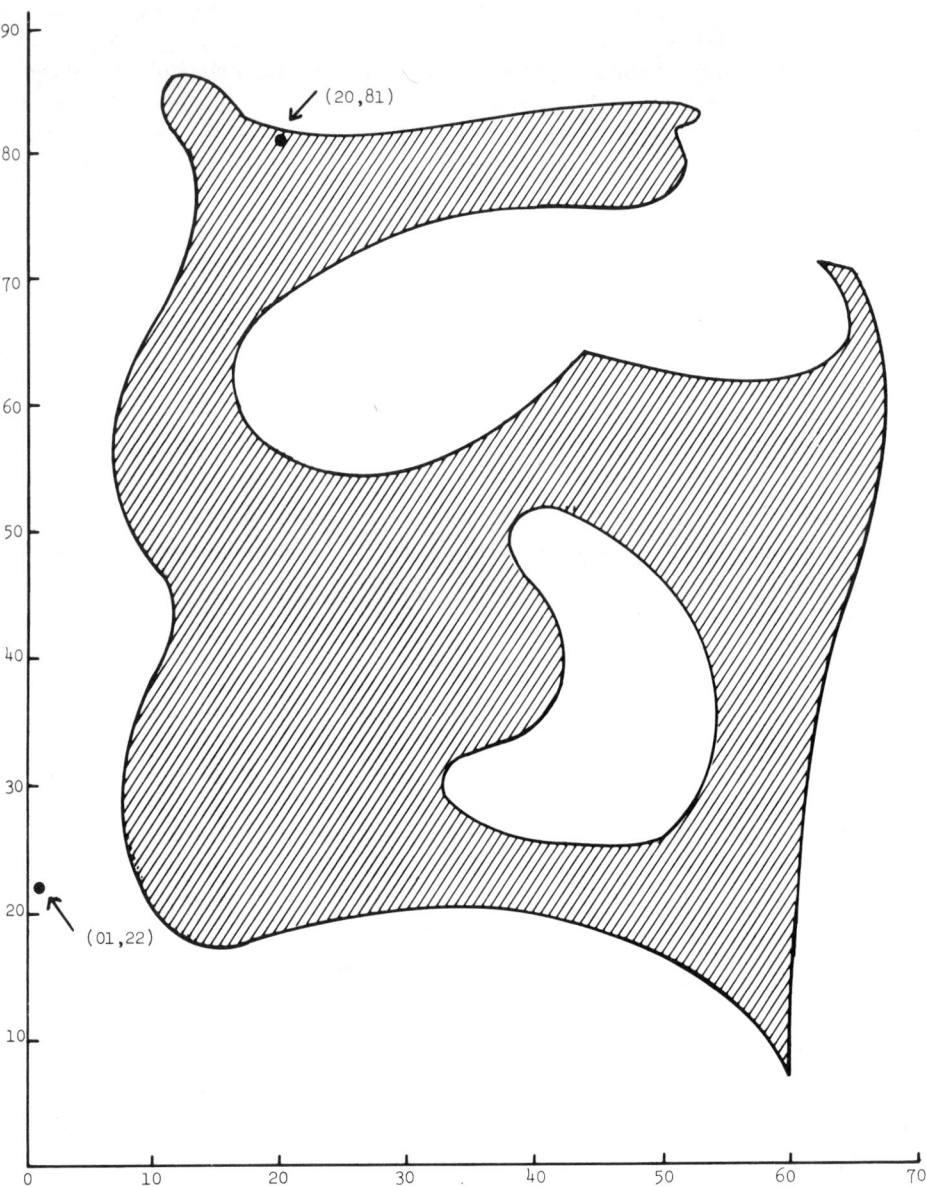

Figure 7-2. Estimating Area of an Irregular Surface. Source: Adapted from E. H. Bowman, and R. B. Fetter, *Analysis for Production and Operations Management*, 3rd Edition, p. 418.

2. Express the two frequency distributions into cumulative probability distributions. For example, the arrival distribution might be as follows, for a small delivery room service

Patients per Hour	Probability of Occurrence	Cumulative Probability
0	0.905	0.905
1	0.090	0.995
2	0.005	1.000
3 or more	neg	

Similar probability distributions for length of stay are given in tables 7-1 through 7-3.

3. Operate the facility for several hundred simulated hours in the following manner:
   A. From a random number table, select a three-digit random number. If it is less than 905 proceed to step (B). Otherwise:
      (1) Review the labor suite for available beds. If there is an unoccupied bed, change it to occupied status. If there is no bed available, place the patient in queue status
      (2) Using a second random number, assign a length of stay in the labor room to the patient using the cumulative probability of discharge shown in table 7-5. Calculate the clock hour at which the patient is to be discharged
      (3) If the first random number was greater than 995, (including 000) return at (A) (1), repeat steps (1), (2), and go to (B)
   B. Count the number of available beds, occupied beds, and patients in queue for this hour
   C. Advance the simulation clock one hour
   D. Review the hours of patients in available beds. If any are to be discharged in this hour, count them as discharges and restore their beds to available status
   E. Review the available beds and the queue. Remove patients from the queue to the available beds until either the queue is zero or the number of available beds is zero
   F. Return to step (A) and repeat the sequence until a sufficient sample has been obtained.

In a real problem, the delivery rooms, recovery rooms, and postpartum care beds usage would also be simulated. The discharges from step (D) would be delivery room arrivals.

It can be seen that in order to carry out the simulation, a number of counters are required which will keep track of various statistics of interest. The first is the clock which is simply incremented by one hour with each pass through the procedure and which serves as the measure of the number of trials of the

Table 7-5

Cumulative Probability of Discharge from Labor Rooms, Yale-New Haven Hospital

Hours	Cumulative Probability of Discharge
0–.99	.189
1 –	.322
2 –	.420
3 –	.551
4 –	.640
5 –	.687
6 –	.734
7 –	.765
8 –	.794
9 –	.825
10 –	.853
11 –	.828
12 –	.894
13 –	.897
14 –	.909
15 –	.914
16 –	.930
17 –	.930
18 –	.944
19 –	.944
20 –	.945
21 –	.960
22 –	.962

simulation. The results of the simulation generate hourly data on available and occupied beds, or facilities, number of discharges, number of arrivals, and queue lengths. After several hundred hours have been run, frequency distributions can be constructed for each of these. At the start of the simulation, the available beds are set to the desired number of beds in the unit, while all other counters, including the clock, are set at zero. There is obviously a period while the use of the unit builds up to a steady state. For a continuous operation such as the labor rooms, the unit will never again return to the starting state. In such a situation, the start-up period should be simulated, but then excluded from the data of interest. Thus, after several days of simulated operation of the delivery room, all the counters would be set back to zero except the census and the available beds, which would be left in the state in which they were found. New data on queue lengths and idle time would be collected by simulating the system from that point forward.

Computerizing Simulation Models

Clearly, there is a great deal of work involved in even a simple simulation. The device would not be a practical one without the aid of computers. A number of computer programs have been developed specifically for simulation; these simplify the problem of inputting and referencing the necessary probability distributions and arrange for the generation of the appropriate random numbers. Some of these programs are in almost identical structure to the example presented above. Others do not advance the clock by single increments as indicated in the example, but rather generate events and assign clock times to the occurrence of these events using random numbers and the available probability distributions. The events are then ordered by the machine and processed. One advantage to this approach is that it simplifies changing the arrival structure. For example, if 30 percent of the obstetrical deliveries were to be induced in a scheduled manner, the scheduled time of arrival for several hundred patients could be selected and then input into the computer program. The arrival of the remainder of patients would change to a distribution similar to the initial one, but with a mean of seven-tenths the original mean. These arrivals could be generated by the machine in the manner outlined above. In programs of this type, the events which are scheduled by the operator are called *exogenous*, and those which are generated by the machine are called *endogenous*.

Surgical Simulation Model—An Example

Rather elaborate hospital subsystems have now been successfully simulated by various researchers. Applications include outpatient services, obstetrical units, admitting systems, and other areas of the hospital. One such effort develops a simulation of a complete surgical subsystem, including preoperative beds, operating rooms, recovery rooms, postoperative beds. This simulation was done by the Yale group led by Thompson and Fetter, and is reported in detail in a master's thesis by Kavet.[8]

The central event in this simulation is the demand for operating rooms. This event is made exogenous, except for emergencies which are generated endogenously. Demands for various surgical beds—preoperative, recovery room, intensive care, postoperative—are generated endogenously depending upon the operating room demand. This arrangement, which is somewhat of a distortion of real life, was selected to allow manipulation of operating room scheduling. The model is a flexible one with broad usefulness. With appropriate data, it can provide estimates to the following questions:

1. For given numbers of operating rooms, what are the expected levels of usage and probabilities of overflow?
2. What is the impact of scheduling changes upon these measures of the operating suite?
3. Given operating room output and number of beds, what are the expected occupancy levels and probabilities of overflow in each of the following areas?: (a) recovery room, (b) intensive care units, (c) post-operative beds, (d) preoperative beds.

The simulation can be adjusted over a broad range of demand, including not only an increase in total demand, but also increases in segments of demand. For example, emergency surgery may be growing at a much faster rate than scheduled surgery. The impact of this on the above questions could be simulated.

Some of these questions could be approached individually by much smaller simulation models, or simply by inference from demand distributions. The question of bed requirements in the case where the preoperative and postoperative beds are the same (the conventional situation), could be simulated with a model similar to the example of the labor rooms. All that would be necessary would be descriptions of emergency and scheduled admission demands, and a description of the service time, or average length of stay. The case of a special preoperative preparation unit could be similarly explored with a sequential model. In this case, it would be necessary to have two demand distributions as before, but at least three service time distributions: emergency preoperative, scheduled preoperative, and postoperative. Presumably, the postoperative stay is independent of whether or not the procedure was an emergency. If this proves untrue, the distribution must be separated.

Sensitivity Analysis of Simulations

The amount of data necessary to establish the frequency distributions on which a simulation is based depends more on the process itself than on the simulation. Samples are used to provide the information, and the usual sampling inferences are possible. The simulation itself can be used to explore the impact of shifts in the input data. Small changes in certain distributions may result in large changes in the result. These distributions must be measured to narrow tolerances. Others will not affect the result significantly and can be estimated by small samples. In most applications, it is wise to collect a small amount of data on which to test the model. Extensive data collection and high precision are deferred until after the sensitivity of the model has been explored. Then attention can be devoted to the more important inputs.

Confidence Limits of Simulations

Bowman and Fetter offer three guidelines to understanding the results of simulation.[9] Assuming that the input data are sufficiently accurate, the confidence limits are related to the number of "trials" of the simulation in the same manner as the confidence limits of a sample statistic are related to the sample size.

1. The accuracy of the simulation only improves as the square root of the number of trials
2. It is best not to rely on simulation results when the distribution of the trials is very different from the expected distribution (e.g., if 100 trials of the surgical simulation showed five emergencies, but the expected percentage of emergencies was 20 percent of the total surgery, additional trials are indicated)
3. The statistics generated by the simulation can be treated as random sample statistics. If 100 hours trial of the labor room simulation, above, showed a mean occupancy of 60 percent, the standard deviation of the occupancy would be:

$$\sigma_P = \sqrt{\frac{P(1-P)}{n}} = \sqrt{\frac{0.6 \times 0.4}{100}} \cong 0.05$$

Applications of Simulation

Simulation appears temptingly simple as a way to solve allocation problems. It does not require great facility with mathematics or mastery of complex theory, as most other resource allocation techniques do. It is often easy to visualize a system and to assume that a simple simulation model can be constructed. *In fact, however, simulation is expensive and tedious for most hospital problems.*

Often the simple model which is originally conceived turns out to be too inflexible to solve the really interesting problem, and further refinement must be built on. Data collection becomes a serious consideration. For the surgical system simulation developed by Kavet, the following information is necessary: (a) frequency of emergency surgery (by service), (b) demand for scheduled surgery (by service), (c) scheduling policies, and (d) distribution of the following service times—preoperative stay (by emergency and scheduled, by service), operation times (by emergency and scheduled, by service), recovery room stay (by service), intensive care stay (by service), and postoperative stay (by service). "Service" in this case is one of four different classes of seriousness of surgery. If this factor is included, 36 different distributions are required. If it is excluded, only ten are needed, but such questions as, "What would be the bed demand generated by an additional orthopedic operating room?" cannot be answered. The problem of programming the model for the computer should not be overlooked. Although the programs, like the models, are straightforward, their length and complexity offer countless chances for error. The program for the surgical subsystem has 68 variables and more than 400 statements. Its development, debugging, and application took well over a thousand hours of the time of at least a half dozen people.

The long-range future of simulation in hospitals is bright. Once a program such as the surgical subsystem has been developed, its application can be extended to a variety of specific situations with only a fraction of the effort necessary for its original development. (This is still likely to be several hundred hours.) With further improvements in data collection, the day will probably come when simulations are used routinely to establish scheduling rules and to size facilities to meet demand.

Use of Simulation in Scheduling Policies

Simulation permits the implication of certain decisions to be explored at relatively low cost, and as such it has wider application than simply in sizing facilities. It is presently feasible to simulate the impact of selected policies over a period of time and thus evaluate the policies. It may be possible some day to simulate alternative immediate decisions on a daily basis and select the best, but this is currently not practical. What can be done is to use the simulation to establish scheduling rules which have known probabilities of overcrowding and inefficiency. Simulation has been used to improve scheduling policies for hospital admissions in at least two cases, which are reviewed here as examples.

The hospital bed with its associated services is a high cost resource subject to fluctuating demand. Even though the cost of leaving a bed empty can be partially reduced by varying nurse staff to meet census, there remains a fixed cost for facilities and overhead expenses which cannot be avoided when the bed is empty, and also costs which are involved in varying staffing. Hospitals, therefore, are interested in minimizing both the mean and variation of the number of empty beds they have. This is done primarily by adjusting the advance scheduling of nonemergency admissions.

Young's Admission Scheduling Model

Formulation. Young has formulated this problem as one of selecting an optimum number of scheduled admissions related to the census level.[10] In essence, his procedure was to establish a number of beds to be left vacant for emergency admissions, and to define a number B, the beds available for patients in the hospital and nonemergency admissions.

$$B = (\text{Capacity}) - (\text{number of beds allowed for emergencies})$$

Assuming that the admitting officer has a current report on the census, she admits previously scheduled patients plus a number from a standby waiting line so that the total number of patients in the hospital is equal to B: Number to be admitted = $B -$ (Census).

Young first developed an analytic solution to this problem using queueing theory, and later verified the results in a small 30-bed unit by simulation. His analytic results permit calculation of the average occupancy, the average overflow, and the variances of these statistics for B's varying values.[a] When these equations are solved, the chances of overflow and the gain in occupancy are known for each possible value of B. The second problem, attaching values to these levels, must also be solved to reach a decision. The B level to be used can

---

[a]The calculations involve ratios of cumulative terms of the Poisson distribution, where each term takes the form:

$$\sum_{B}^{\infty} \frac{\rho^B e^{-\rho}}{B!}$$

where ρ is the mean census of emergency patients. Estimates of these terms are possible where B and ρ are relatively small, or where $B < 2\rho$, but they become mechanically difficult in other cases. The condition $B < 2\rho$ is met when more than half the census is generated by emergencies. Unfortunately, the practical applications lie mainly in the areas where computation is difficult. The full set of Young's calculations appears in his "A Queueing Theory Approach to the Control of Hospital Inpatient Census," p. 62. Document available from University Microfilms, Inc., Ann Arbor, Michigan, Hospital Management Series 61AM 20, vol. 1.

be selected by balancing the desirability of a given mean census against the probability for overflow for the mean. Young suggests that this be done by minimizing the cost equation:

$$C_T = C_1 I + C_2 O ,$$

where I = average number of idle beds (I = capacity − average census)
O = average daily overflow
C_1 = cost associated with an idle bed
C_2 = cost associated with a one patient overflow.

I and O are provided by the simulation. C_1 and C_2 must be estimated in some manner. While C_1 might be related to the loss of revenue, C_2 must be evaluated subjectively.

Dividing by C_1:

$$C_T/C_1 = T = I + (C_2/C_1) O$$

if $C_2/C_1 = R$, then:

$$T = I + RO ,$$

R values must be selected subjectively because of the difficulty of measuring C_2. Once this has been done, T can be calculated for several values of B, and the B associated with T_{min} selected.

Using the Model for Decision Making. Young's data apply only to the single case of a 30-bed unit, over the range of emergency demand which he studied, and with the distributions of service times (length of stay) which he found at the Johns Hopkins Hospital. His specific results are not directly applicable to other situations. However, his results can be used to illustrate the nature of simulation output, and how it must be combined with other information on the value of alternatives to reach a decision.

The results of Young's analysis, applied to a 30-bed medical unit at the Johns Hopkins Hospital, show the average census and the probabilities of overflow at various B levels. These are reproduced in figures 7-3 and 7-4. Figure 7-3 shows both the theoretical results (dotted lines) and the simulation results, for varying levels of ρ, where ρ is equal to the average census of emergency patients. (λ is the arrival rate of emergency patients, and $\bar{t}$ is their length of stay). The simulation, using actual distributions, shows a rather significant difference from the queueing model, which apparently reflects deviations from the Poisson assumptions.

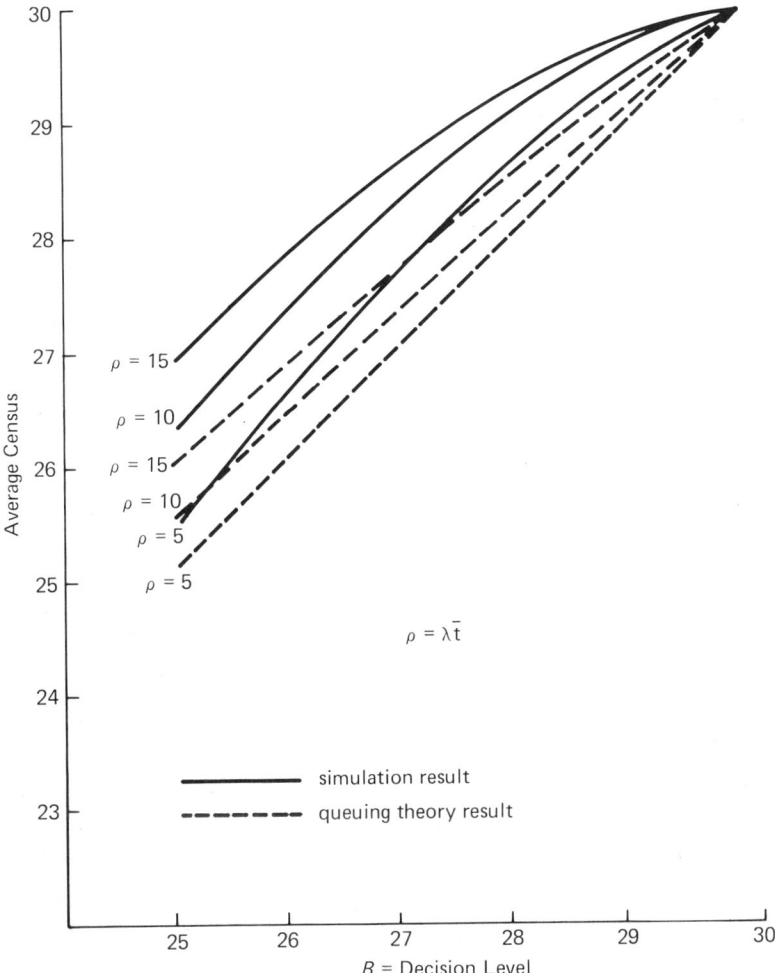

Figure 7-3. Average Census as a Function of Decision Level ($\bar{t}$ = 10 days). Source: Young, "A Queuing Theory Approach to the Control of Hospital Inpatient Census," Johns Hopkins Hospital Operations Research Division, Baltimore, 1962, p. 96.

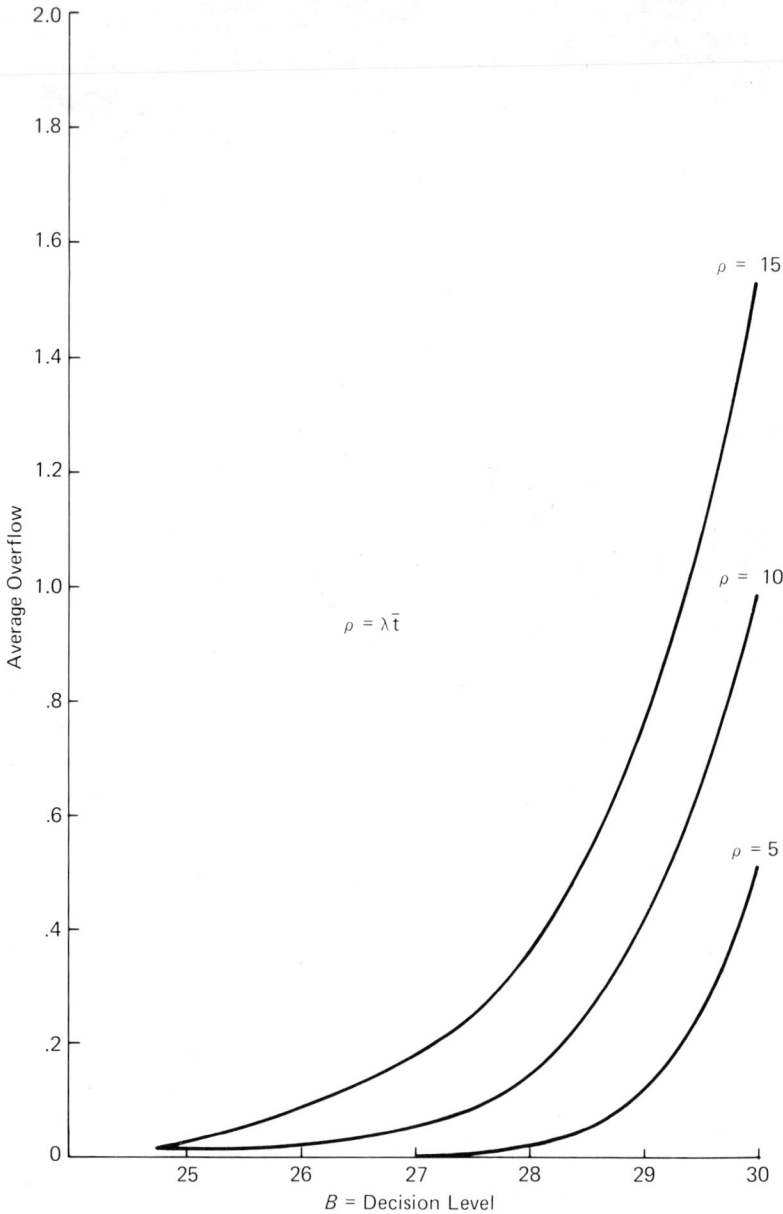

Figure 7-4. Average Overflow as a Function of Decision Level ($\bar{t} = 10$ days). Source: Young, "Inpatient Census", p. 102.

In order to reach a decision as to the appropriate B level, the first step is to select the ρ value most closely representing the hospital's expectations about the number of emergencies. When this is done, the results of each B decision are described in terms of their impact on census and overflow on the appropriate line of the figures. The second condition can be met by selecting a value of R. Medical and nursing advice would probably be helpful. To get realistic advice it may be necessary to reformulate the meaning of R. This can be phrased in terms of preference, as follows:

- If R is less than one, I would rather turn one patient away each day than have one empty bed
- If R is one, I do not care whether I turn one patient away or have one empty bed
- If R is two, I would rather, on the average have two empty beds than turn one patient away.

Of course, the patient may not always be "turned away." The proper phrase may be "placed in the corridor until a bed is available" or "placed in another part of the hospital." The disposition of the overflow determines the cost, and also where the cost appears. Patients in the corridor are costly to nursing. They must do the extra work (and listen to the complaints). Patients turned away are costly to the patient and the doctor.

Once R has been selected, B can be calculated by using the equation

$$T = I + R\ O$$

and selecting T_{min}. For $R = 3; \rho = 10$:

B	I (from fig. 7-3)	O (from fig. 7-4)	T
25	3.3	.025	3.4
26	2.8	.04	2.9
27	1.6	.07	1.8
28	1.1	.16	1.6
29	0.4	.45	1.7

using the simulation results from Young's data. (These values were read from the charts, but would normally be available in tabulated form. The actual output values are more accurate, of course.) The minimum is 28, and this should be the policy level. On any given day, the admitting officer will take the census, adjusted for today's discharges, subtract it from 28, and admit that number of patients from the waiting list. In the long run, if the simulation is correct, the average census will be 28.9, and an average of 0.16 patients will be "turned away," or "placed in the corridor" or whatever arrangement is agreed upon. This result follows directly from the selection of "R," the ratio of costs of overflow to costs of idle facilities. It is equally true in reverse. That is, if one selects a B level, one automatically and inevitably establishes R. Thus some value of R is implicitly set in the normal operation of the admitting office.

There is another way to approach the B level decision, using the probability that any patient will be turned away on a given day. These probabilities also result from the simulation, and are shown in figure 7-5. The probabilities can easily be translated to the number of times a year, or a month, the overflow condition will occur. For instance, for $\rho = 10$, $B = 28$, the probability of any overflow is 0.1, or one day in ten.

Using this chart, the tradeoff between census and overflow can be evaluated directly. For $\rho = 10$, the increase in probability per change in B is as follows:

B	Probability of Turning Patients Away (from fig. 7-5)	Census (from fig. 7-3)
26	0.02	27.4
27	0.04	28.3
28	0.10	29.0
29	0.31	29.7

It may be agreed that the gain in census of 0.5, in going from $B = 27$ to $B = 28$, is not worth increasing the occurrence of overflow from four days per hundred (once every twenty-five days) to once every ten days. As noted, this decision establishes the value of R automatically. All that is necessary is to find the R which yields T_{min} at $B = 27$.

Young used the data from the simulation output to calculate the relationship between R and B for various ρ. His results are shown in figure 7-6. This figure shows a value of $R = 21$ for $\rho = 10$, $B = 27$. The cost of "overflow" has been established at 21 times the cost of an empty bed.

Both approaches to reaching the final decision are probably desirable. The doctors and nurses reaching the decision can check their two intuitive feelings—about the chance of overflow and about the relative cost of overflow—against each other, and in this way reach a fuller understanding of the B level they recommend.

Dunn's Admission Scheduling Model

Young's simulation has a number of oversimplifications. One of these is that most hospitals work from a system of fixed advance scheduling, rather than

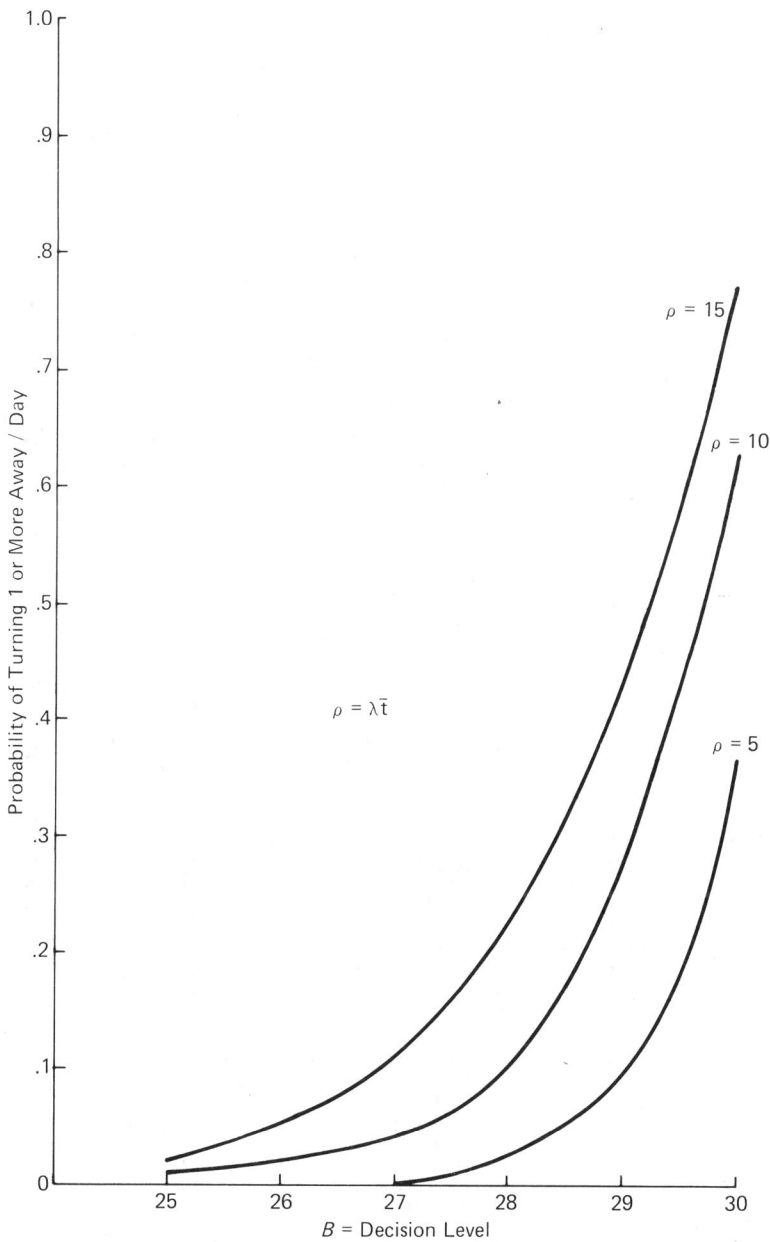

Figure 7-5. Probability of Turning One or More Patients Away per Day vs. B ($\bar{t}$ = 10 days). Source: Young, "Inpatient Census", p. 99.

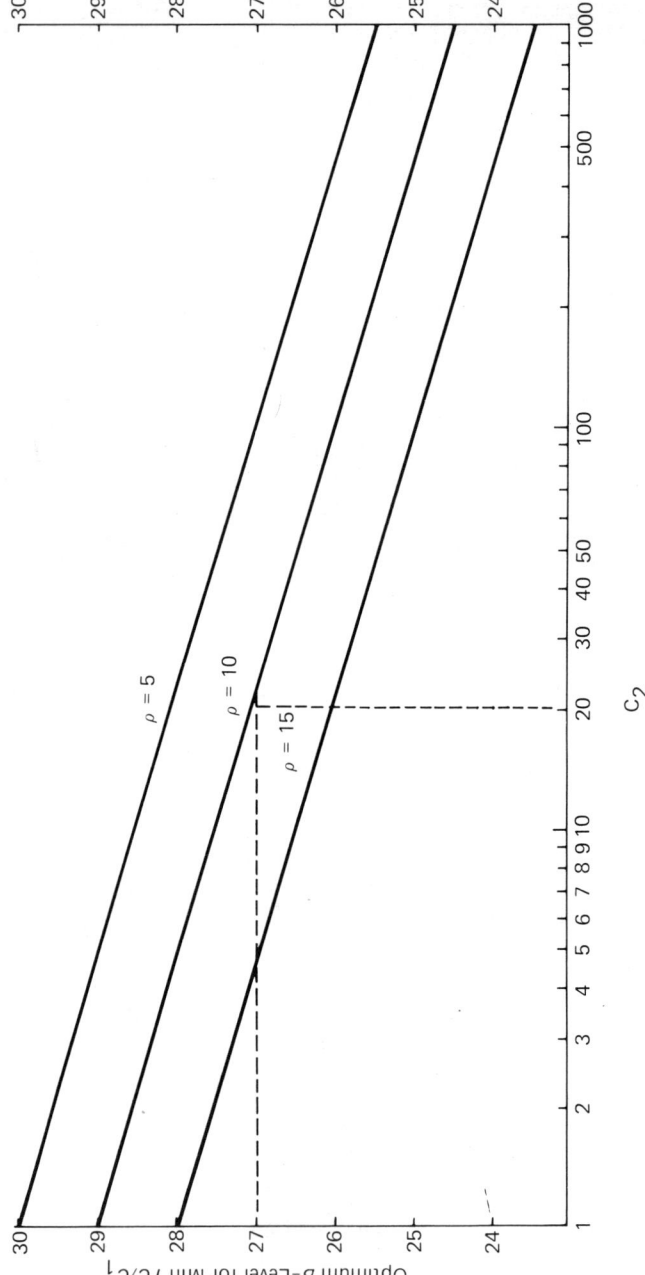

Figure 7-6. Optimum B-Level as a Function of Cost Ratios. Source: Young, "Inpatient Census," p. 129.

having a list of patients waiting and ready to come on a few hours notice. Admitting scheduling rules for this situation are more complex, and have at least the following components:

1. A rule for the maximum number of patients who can be scheduled for a given day in the future
2. A rule for the number of nonemergency patients who can be accepted from a waiting list for admission on the current day, after previously scheduled patients have been accommodated. (These patients are usually "urgent")

Dunn later worked on the admission scheduling problem in purely empirical terms, using a more complicated formulation of policies, and relying on simulation alone to provide decision-making information. He classified admission into three categories.[11] (a) scheduled: fixed date in future; (b) urgent: no fixed date, to be admitted from a waiting list as soon as service is available; and (c) emergency: admit immediately. On any given day, the admissions are the sum of these three. For a distant future day i, a limit of K scheduled admissions could be set, based upon the expected number of discharges adjusted for the day of the week ($\overline{D}_i$) and reduced by a relatively conservative allowance E for emergencies and urgent admissions:

$$K_i = \overline{D}_i - E \quad .$$

As the i day approaches, the number of scheduled admissions can be increased, by changing urgent admissions to scheduled patients for day i. (This gives both the patient and the doctor more advance notice.)

$$S_i = K_i + U_i$$

Dunn wished to establish the term U_i three days in advance of the ith day, by comparing the current census, scheduled admissions, predicted discharges and the B level which had been set by policy. The equation for estimating U_i for three days in advance is:

$$\sum_{i=1}^{3} U_i = B - C_1 + \sum_{i=1}^{3} \overline{D}_i - \sum_{i=1}^{3} K_i + 3\lambda$$

$$= B - C_1 + \sum_{i=1}^{3} (\overline{D}_i - K_i) + 3\lambda$$

The simulation requires distributions for emergency arrivals, urgent arrivals, and length of stay (subclassified as necessary). These items are treated as endogenous events. Scheduled patients are treated as exogenous events, but the number of these events is established based upon past experience. Both the scheduled and the urgent arrivals are likely to be nonstationary. Dunn discovered significant seasonal variations in his application at the Henry Ford Hospital. There will obviously be day of the week variations. The various services should be handled independently, according to the way beds are assigned. Thus obstetrical and pediatric patients would be simulated separately. So would adult medical and adult surgical, if beds were segregated in this way.

The decision making proceeds in two stages. A B level must be set in a manner similar to Young's analysis. Then for a given B level, various values of K can be evaluated, subject to the constraint that

$$\overline{K} + \overline{U} + \lambda = \overline{D} = \overline{C}/\overline{t}$$

(The sum of the averages of all forms of admissions, scheduled, urgent, and emergency is equal to the average number of discharges, or the average census divided by the grand mean length of stay.)

The parameters of interest in the second level of the decision are: the average delay to schedule a nonemergency patient, the average delay to admit an urgent patient, and the number of scheduled patients cancelled or treated as "overflow." (This will usually be zero in the range of K and U of interest. It should be checked, however, to avoid an unrealistic decision.) The lower K, the more beds will be available for urgent patients, and the shorter their delay. At the same time, the lower K, the longer the interval between the decision to schedule an admission and the actual date which it occurs. The simulation can be run for several values of K, and the tradeoff most acceptable to the medical staff selected. The possibilities of assigning relative values to U and K directly are not promising. Among other factors, the mean delay to schedule in the real situation may influence the doctors' decision to class a patient as urgent. Within acceptable occupancy ranges, the selection of the appropriate level of K is best left to the doctors themselves, who presumably can include the medical aspects of delay in both situations. Administrative input to the decision is also required, however. A low value for the sum of K and U leads to low occupancy; a high sum leads to overflow.

This application illustrates the expansibility of simulation techniques to increasingly complex and realistic situations. Work by Briggs expanded the Dunn model, taking estimates of future discharges and day of the week variation into account.[12] With this flexibility, any real situation could be studied. Beds can be allocated to several different subspecialties, with K and B levels tested for each example. The impact of doing this on the total census of the hospital can be demonstrated by comparing simulations with and without such allocations. The possibility that too long a delay would cause a scheduled patient to become urgent, or an urgent patient to become an emergency, could be incorporated into the model and tested for its impact on census and overflow. (For instance, the simulation could be established so that any urgent patient on the list more than five days became an emergency. The result of this would be an increased probability of overflow, which could be measured by the simulation.) The opportunities to handle overflow by early discharges rather than turning patients away might also be incorporated. The latter two possibilities would require substantial empirical study if the conditions postulated were to be meaningful. Evaluations of the possibilities for early discharge or the necessity to reclassify urgent patients would be required. These might be highly speculative at best. The cost of gaining the information would be several times the cost of determining the original distributions. Finally, once so many possibilities had been taken into account, the very limited ability to place meaningful values on the alternatives would be strained to the point of breaking. Thus while simulation models themselves can be expanded almost indefinitely, the practicalities of data gathering and decision making form a definite limit on the technique.

Additional Readings

Elementary discussions of queueing theory appear in:

Flagle, C.D., Huggins, W.H., Roy, R.H. *Operations Research and Systems Engineering*, The Johns Hopkins Press, Baltimore, Maryland, 1960, p. 132.

Churchman, C.W., Ackoff, R.L., Arnoff, E.L. *Introduction to Operations Research*, John Wiley and Sons, Inc., New York, 1957, chapter 14.

Discussions of simulation can be found in works such as those above, and in:

Bowman, E.H., and R.B. Fetter. *Analysis for Production and Operations Management*, 3rd Ed., R.D. Irwin, Homewood, Ill., 1967, chapter 11.

Kiviat, P.J. "Digital Computer Simulation: Modeling Concepts," RAND Corp. Memorandum RM5378-P.R., Santa Monica, Calif., 1967.

8 PERT and Mathematical Programming Models

Introduction

There is an important class of resource allocation problems dealing with the optimum arrangement of a set of resources which can be distributed in a variety of ways. The assignment of patients to beds, nurses to nursing stations, and demand to facilities such as operating rooms are examples of problems in the class. These problems recur constantly in hospitals and are solved routinely by supervisory personnel, using established policies and criteria for guidance. The goal is usually to gain maximum benefit from the available resources, but alternatively it may be to minimize the resources required for a given level of demand. The problem is generally deterministic. Both the demands to which distribution should be made and the quantity of resources available for distribution are fixed, and the distribution should optimize the achievement of the goal.

Highly sophisticated, computer-oriented models exist to aid in the solution of the class of problem. They have been used successfully in a number of industrial applications. Hospital applications have so far been limited, but the promise of eventual success is encouraging. The models generally are called *mathematical programming* models. Linear programming models are the most common examples. These models rest upon the formulation of a quantitative statement of the relationship between resource allocation and goal achievement called an *objective function*. They proceed by seeking the mathematical optimum solution to the objective function, using the computer as a substitute for (or in some cases an aide to) the human decision-making process. This chapter will describe the general mechanism by which these problems are solved, but the emphasis will be on examples of hospital application and the way in which hospital problems must be formulated to use the models.

The concept of an objective function is not unique to mathematical programming. Total value analysis, described in chapter 6, is one common way of formulating an objective function. The statement of costs related to order quantity in the inventory model is an objective function which is minimized with respect to total cost in the solution. Similarly the formula developed by Young in the admission scheduling simulation is an objective function which is minimized by selecting the desired bed level. Young's original equation (from chapter 7) is a total value equation:

$$C_T = C_1 I + C_2 O$$

where

C_T = total cost
C_1 = cost of idle beds
C_2 = cost of overflow
T = expected number of idle beds
O = expected overflow

PERT and CPM

One straight-forward and easily applied technique which resembles mathematical programming, but is much simpler in concept is called Program Evaluation Review Technique (PERT) or Critical Path Method (CPM). It was developed in nonhospital applications but it has also been applied to hospitals. In addition to its immediate practical value, it is useful in demonstrating the basic process of seeking the optimum solution from among an array of alternatives. Its application is in sequential scheduling problems, where certain activities cannot be begun until others have been completed. Building construction and massive development projects for military and aerospace applications are the most common examples, but it may be applied to other forms of planning and development activity. The numerous publications about its application range from marketing programs to preparing annual corporate reports.[1,2]

Illustration

The technique can be most clearly illustrated by a construction and program development example. Consider the following hypothetical illustration: the problem is to build a small building, install a computer, and prepare for certain production data processing activities. The project termination comes when the computer replaces the present manual processing of payroll and employee work records. The situation can be described by a series of *tasks* which must be performed, and *events*, points in time at which one or more tasks must be completed before other tasks can be begun. It is important to define events and tasks so that the events follow in logical sequence; no successor event can precede any earlier event. Events also should be clearly definable and if possible related to the normal management records. The tasks are defined in large part by the selection of events. It should be possible to estimate the amount of time necessary for each task.

For the illustration the tasks are:

Task	Time (weeks)	Predecessor Tasks
a. Contract negotiation for construction	4	None
b. Computer delivery delay	17	None
c. Support equipment selection and ordering	4	None
d. Forms delivery delay	3	None
e. Construction	26	a
f. Computer installation	4	b,e
g. Support equipment delivery delay	12	c
h. Forms distribution	1	d
i. Employee recruitment	2	f,g
j. Training	4	i
k. Computer trials and debugging	6	f,g
l. Dummy runs	2	j,k

There is clearly a sequence to these tasks, and a minimum time in which they can be performed. There is also the possibility of lost time, if certain events are not started at the appropriate time. For instance, the new reporting forms must be distributed to users before the change-over day. Since delivery will require three weeks and distribution one, the order must be placed at least four weeks prior to the expected date of completion of "dummy runs," task l. The goal of PERT charting is to avoid such delays and to identify the critical components where any delay will increase the total time in the project. The objective function is the total project time, which is to be minimized by identifying the critical components and making sure they are properly scheduled.

The sequencing of the tasks can best be charted by working backwards. Starting with the change-over event, there are two tasks, l and h, which immediately precede the event. This can be represented graphically, with arrows for tasks and circles for events:

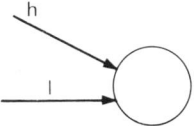

Task l cannot be begun, however, until tasks j and k are complete. This defines another event:

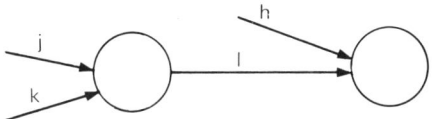

But j is preceded by i, k is preceded by f, and i is preceded by both f and g. This defines two more events, requiring the completion of these tasks.

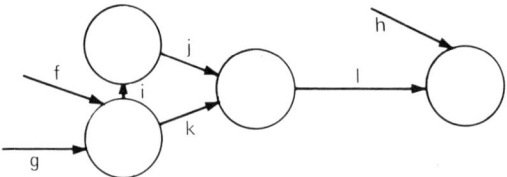

When this process has been completed, there is a network describing the relation of tasks and events. This is shown in figure 8-1. The estimated times for completion of each task are shown. (The lengths of the arrows do not represent the time estimates.)

The events, and the tasks which they conclude are as follows.

	Event	Completed Task Letter
1	Start	—
2	Contract signed	a
3	Construction complete	e
4	Computer delivery	b
5	Support equipment ordered	c
6	Support equipment delivered, computer installed	f,g
7	Hiring complete	i
8	Debugging, training complete	j,k
9	Forms delivery	d
10	Change-over	h,l

By using figure 8-1 and calculating the longest time to reach each event, this indicates the critical path (shown as figure 8-2):

Task	Time
a	4
e	26
o	0
f	4
k (or i,j)	6
l	2
Total	42

and the minimum time (the sum of the critical path times), 42 weeks. There is one "dummy task" shown as a dotted line, on the critical path, with zero time to complete. This indicates that task b cannot be completed until task

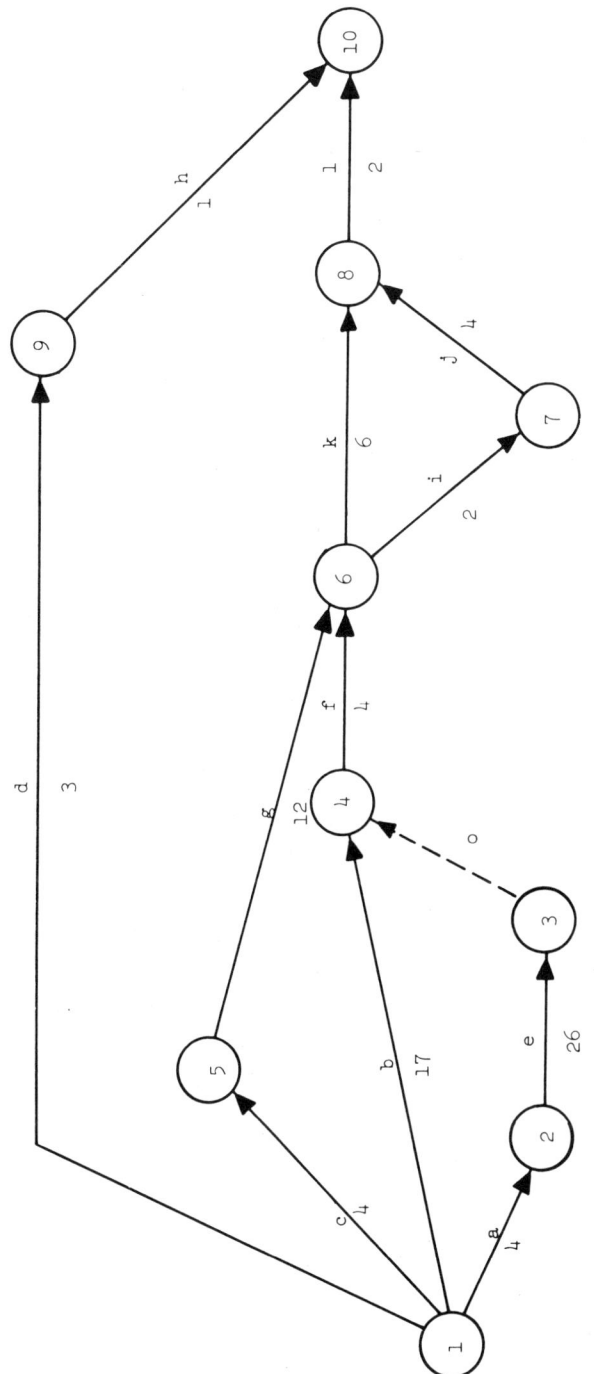

Figure 8-1. PERT Chart of a Hypothetical Program.

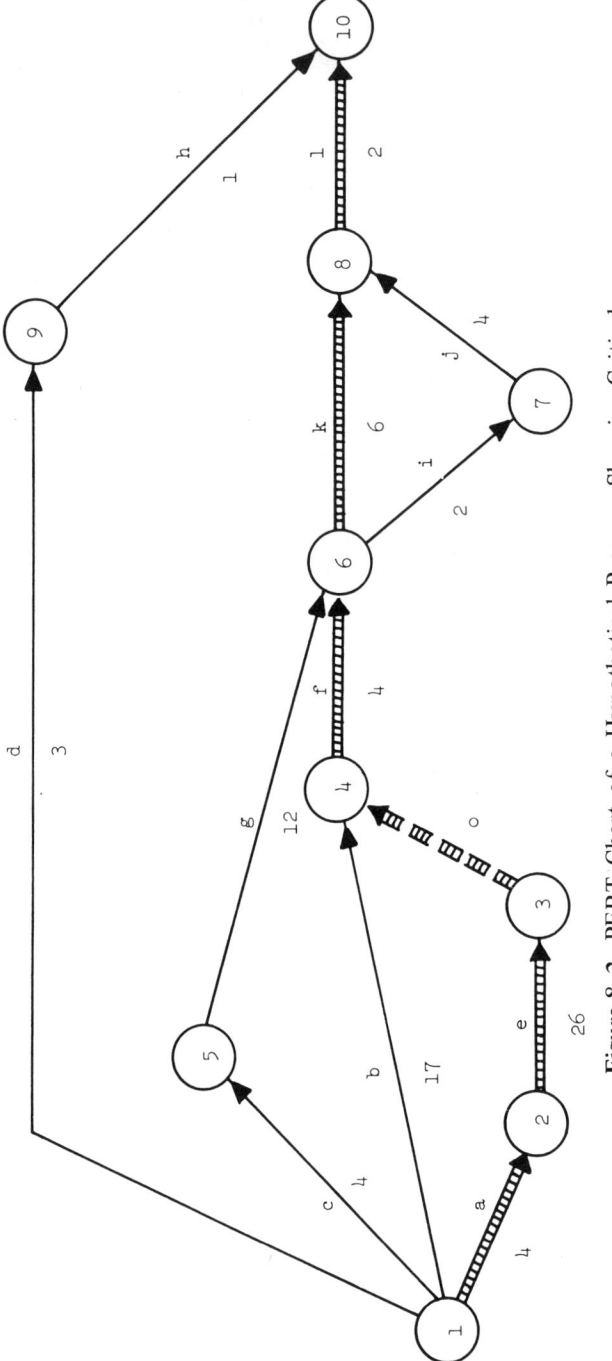

Figure 8-2. PERT Chart of a Hypothetical Program Showing Critical Path.

e is complete, but can be done immediately once event 3 occurs. Task k is on the critical path, but the time to complete the other tasks in the section is the same.

Savings in total project times will result only from reduction in times for critical path tasks. Even for these, the amount of savings is limited. It can be calculated by looking at the slack time for other paths.

Path	Slack
b	13
c,g	18
i,j	0
d,h	38

The latest possible starting times for noncritical tasks can also be calculated from these data. If the critical path is begun at week zero:

Week	Tasks Started
0	a
4	e
13	b
18	c
22	g
30	f
34	k,i
36	j
38	d
40	l
41	h

Delays become immediately recognizable from this list.

Handling Variation in Estimates

Additional refinements can be made to PERT. One of the most useful is to handle variation which can be expected about the estimates of task times. Obviously no future event can be predicted with certainty. It is common to make estimates on the basis of *optimistic, most likely,* and *pessimistic,* based upon the subjective judgments of the persons responsible for the work. These terms are self-defining, but one authority suggests:[3]

Optimistic—An estimate of the *minimum* time an activity will take, if unusual good luck is experienced and everything "goes right the first time."

Most likely—An estimate of the normal time an activity will take, a result which would occur most often if the activity could be repeated a number of times under similar circumstances.

Pessimistic—An estimate of the maximum time an activity will take, if unusually bad luck is experienced. It should reflect the possibility of initial failure and fresh start, but should not be influenced by such factors as "catastrophic events"—strikes, fires, power failures, and so on—unless these hazards are inherent risks in the activity.

Formulae have been developed which allow probability estimates for the overall project time, and the probabilities of completing sections on schedule.[4] If a is optimistic; b, pessimistic; m, most likely; the expected time, t_e, will be:

$$t_e = \frac{a + 4m + b}{6}$$

These expected times can be used instead of single point estimates indicated in the illustration. Given a reasonable number of tasks, the overall minimum expected completion time T_e will be the sum of the t_e values for the critical path[a]:

$$T_e = \sum_{i=1}^{n} t_{e_i},$$

if there are n tasks on the critical path.

The calculations become quite tedious, but a variety of computer programs

---

[a]Estimation of standard deviations of individual tasks can also be made:

$$\sigma_i = \frac{b-a}{6}$$

While individual estimates of σ_i will have little validity, the standard deviation of the total (or a reasonably large segment) can also be estimated. If there are n tasks on the critical path:

$$T_e = \sum_{i=1}^{n} (t_e)_i$$

$$\sigma_{T_e}^2 = \sum_{i=1}^{n} \sigma_i^2 (t_e)_i \div T_e$$

or $(\sigma_1^2 t_{e1} + \sigma_2^2 t_{e2} + \ldots + \sigma_n^2 t_{e_n}) \div T_e$

This value is treated as though T_e followed the normal distribution. (Heyel, *Encyclopedia of Management*, appendix) are available. These identify the critical path, calculate slack times, and chart latest possible starting times. They also handle probability calculations.

PERT/cost

Another modification of PERT attaches costs to the time estimates of the various segments. This changes the objective function to a cost basis. Often task times can be reduced by increasing costs (using overtime, more expensive machinery, prefabricated materials, or other means). If a value can be assigned to reducing the time, then the tasks on the critical path can be speeded up until the cost of further speed-up is equal to the value of the time gained. In the hypothetical illustration shown in figure 8-1, if the firm lost $1,000 per week for each week change-over was delayed, but the construction time (task e) could be cut 5 percent for each additional $1,000 expended, the additional charges would be paid up to the point where the savings was no longer greater than the expenditure. For each $1,000 expenditure:

Increment	Expenditure	Savings	Value
1	$1,000	.05 × 26 = 1.3 weeks	$1,300
2	1,000	.05 × 24.7 = 1.25 weeks	1,250
3	1,000	.05 × 23.4 = 1.17 weeks	1,170
4	1,000	.05 × 22.2 = 1.11 weeks	1,110
5	1,000	.05 × 21.1 = 1.05 weeks	1,050
6	1,000	.05 × 20.05 = 1.00 weeks	1,000

The firm would be willing to increase the contract cost by $6,000, anticipating a reduction of nearly seven weeks, saving $6,900. The total cost will be reduced $900. The seventh $1,000 would save only $950, however, and would not be justified. Of course the savings would be obtained only while the construction task was on the critical path. No expenditure would be made for speeding tasks not on the critical path, nor would the construction time be shortened beyond 13 weeks. (This is the slack in the alternative process b.) Computer programs called PERT/cost programs exist for analyzing a variety of cost tradeoff situations like this.

Modeling for Mathematical Programming

There is a class of decisions which occurs frequently in hospitals and other industries, but which none of the models discussed so far—total value, queueing, simulation, PERT—will solve. This class of problem involves the optimal relationship between a set of desired outcomes and a set of available resources.

The traditional example is in menu planning (so much protein, so much fat, so much iron, etc.) and a variety of foods (steak, sweet potatoes, milk, etc.) used to gain the outcome. Similar problems are not hard to find. We can specify such problems in terms of the resources to be utilized and the outputs to be delivered.

Resource Set	Outputs
1. Foods	1. Nutrition
2. Intensive, intermediate, self-care beds	2. Patient needs for care
3. R.N.s, L.P.N.s, aides	3. Nursing needs of patients
4. Operating rooms—general, urological neurological, orthopedic	4. Patient demands for operating rooms
5. Medical services—x-ray, laboratory physical therapy, etc.	5. Patient demands for medical services

The output set and the resource set do not match on a one-to-one basis. That is a food, like "steak," generally fills part of several nutritional needs. No specific food supplies one and only one nutrient and conversely, no nutrient is supplied by only one food. The same condition applies to the other resources and outputs on the list, to varying degrees. A registered nurse can fulfill both needs for her services and needs for less skilled services. General surgery can be done in rooms equipped for nuerosurgery, etc. This condition makes the problem of determining the optimal allocation of resources more difficult to solve. If it did not exist, the problem would be trivial.

As a matter of fact, problems within this class are among the most difficult, because of the many possible interrelationships among the variables. Methods of solving them are lengthy and demanding. Generally speaking, problems in this class are solved by using the computer to seek the most desirable solution from among the large number of theoretical possibilities. The technique which is used is called in its most general form *mathematical programming*. Linear programming, nonlinear programming, dynamic programming, integer programming, and other specific techniques of mathematical programming have been developed. Of these, the most widely applied is linear programming, primarily because it is simpler than the other types of programming and because many problems can be closely approximated by linear functions. In the following sections, simplified examples will be used to illustrate the approach used in solving mathematical programming models. Linear and integer formats will be used to demonstrate how problems can be solved by graphic and algebraic methods and to show the meaning of the solution and the information usually provided. The technology of linear programming is demanding and best left to experienced analysts,[5] but administrators and other hospital personnel have roles in helping formulate the approach and in appraising the appropriateness of the assumptions involved, as well as in application of the results.

A Simplified Hospital Production Problem

Consider that a hospital offers a variety of services (nursing care, operating rooms, laboratory, physical therapy, radiology, etc.) and that each of these has some capacity under normal operating circumstances. Only so many operations, lab tests, x-rays, etc., can be performed in a given time period such as a month. The amounts of these services required, however, depend upon the kinds of patients coming to the hospital. Some patients require much laboratory work and no operating room time, others, such as elective surgery patients, require almost the opposite. Then for a given set of operating policies and physical plant arrangements, there must be some ideal "mix" of kinds of patients which will optimize the use of the various capacities. Perhaps this mix will use the capacity of each service. However, it may use less than the capacity of some services, because the hospital treats no kinds of patients whose needs involve only those services which are at less than capacity. The problem is of some practical interest: if a hospital already exists, so that its capacities are fixed, it will be able to treat this mix of patients with minimum idle capacity. Any other mix will result in greater idle capacity and therefore higher costs. Through regional planning, the hospital might be aided in getting its optimum mix of patients.

The general problem has been modeled in a linear programming format and solved in a representative hospital by William Dowling.[6] The following illustration is a greatly simplified version of the problem developed by Dowling to illustrate the application of linear programming. The illustration includes both graphic and algebraic solutions and shows the way in which the real world is reduced to a model, the assumptions which must be made in modeling, the conceptual approach to solution, and the meaning of the information supplied with the solution. The following elements which are common to all programming problems will be defined and discussed: (a) production coefficients, (b) production or capacity constraint, (c) assumption of linearity, (d) solution space and boundary conditions, (e) the objective function, and (f) the dual problem and shadow prices.

Problem Formulation. In formulating the problem, it is necessary to specify all the resources or services which are supplied by the hospital, the amount of each service required to treat patients of different types, the total amount of the service which is available, and the number of patients of each type which must be treated over a given time period. Many of these pieces of information are random variables from stochastic processes, but it will not be possible for us to treat them as such. We must make an assumption that a "typical" month exists and that we may use the expected value of the stochastic distributions of such factors as number of each type of patient and the amount of each service required. Programming models are deterministic, with rare exceptions.

Most hospitals can identify more than twenty services, and the number of types of patients can be subdivided almost infinitely if desired. For illustrative purposes, we will reduce the number of services to five—nursing, surgery, laboratory, physical therapy, and x-ray. To make it possible to show the solution graphically we will reduce the number of patient types to two—medical and surgical. These restrictions, unlike the ones in the preceding paragraph, are solely for convenience. Computerized solutions are commonly reached to problems with several hundred resources and similarly large numbers of outputs (in this problem, the output of the hospital is measured in terms of the number of patients of each type treated per time period).

Production Coefficients and Capacities. We may now collect the information in a convenient form, called a *technology matrix*, shown in table 8-1, which displays the services in the rows and the patient types in the columns. For each service and patient type combination there is a value; for example, the expected number of days of nursing care for a medical patient is nine, and each medical patient will receive no operations, fifteen laboratory tests, one physical-therapy treatment, and four x-ray procedures. These values are called *production coefficients*, or *input-output coefficients*.

The hospital has policies regarding the amounts of each service which can be made available, based upon the time required to perform each service and the number of man-hours or facility hours which are available. These are the *capacities* of each service, shown in table 8-2. Another way to express these capacities is in terms of hospital output (i.e., the number of medical or surgical patients they will permit the hospital to treat). These values are shown in table 8-3. If there are 73,000 nursing days available, and each medical patient requires nine days, 73,000 ÷ 9 equals 8,111 medical patients can be treated, and so forth.

Linearity Assumptions. If we assume that each patient requires nine days of nursing care if medical or seven if surgical, and the other values shown in the technology matrix, we are assuming that the production coefficients are

Table 8-1
Hospital Technology Matrix

Inputs	Diagnostic Categories	
	Medical	Surgical
Nursing Days	9	7
Operations	–	1
Laboratory tests	15	12
P T treatments	1	2
X-ray procedures	4	2

Table 8-2
Facility Constraints

Facility	Capacity Per Day	Capacity Per Year
200 nursing beds	200 nursing days (1/bed/day)	73,000 nursing days
4 operating rooms	20 operations (5/room/day)	6,000 operations
Laboratory	350 tests	105,000 tests
Physical therapy	45 treatments	13,500 treatments
3 x-ray rooms	78 procedures (26/room/day)	23,400 procedures

Table 8-3
Maximum Patient Capacity per Year by Case Type

	Case Type	
Facility	Medical	Surgical
Nursing beds	8,111	10,429
Operating rooms	–	6,000
Laboratory	7,000	8,750
Physical therapy	13,500	6,750
X-ray	5,850	11,700

constant, so that the relationship between the variables is linear, that is there are no economies in treating greater numbers of patients. If one medical patient requires 9 days to treat, two consume 18 days of patient care, and ten consume 90 days. This is the most important *linearity* assumption, and the one which permits the application of linear programming. It also permits us to represent the problem on a graph with straight lines. (*Nonlinear programming* permits the analyst to deal with nonlinear relationships between the variables. The technology is much more difficult and less fully developed. Practical applications, therefore, remain rare.) A second, less critical linearity assumption is made in specifying the objective function (below), but the need for this assumption can often be eliminated or reduced.

Solution Space and Boundary Conditions. It is now possible to represent the problem graphically, and this is done in figure 8-3. If the two types of patients, medical and surgical, are shown on the axes of a graph, the capacities of the various services can be shown as lines representing all possible combinations of medical and surgical patients which can be treated. For example, from table 8-3, the x-ray capacity permits treating either 5,850 medical patients or 11,700 surgical patients or any combination of medical (M) and surgical patients (S) such that

$$4M + 2S \leqslant 23{,}400 \quad \text{(from Tables 8-1 and 8-2)}$$

The capacity line for x-ray, $4M + 2S = 23{,}400$ is shown on figure 8-3 as line AA'. So long as the policies and facilities of the hospital remain the same, no combination of medical and surgical patients lying outside the triangle formed by line AA' and the axes can be treated. The other services can be represented by similar lines, and these have been shown on figure 8-3. It is worth noting that the equation for surgery

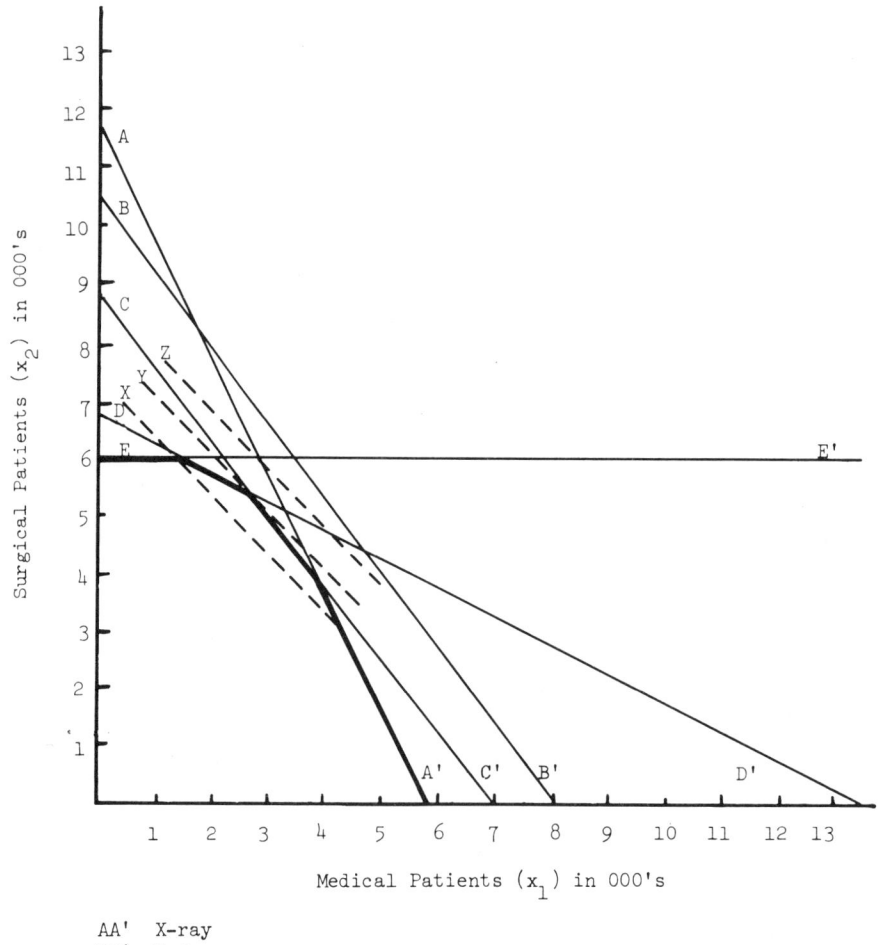

AA'	X-ray
BB'	Beds
CC'	Laboratory
DD'	Physical Therapy
EE'	Operating Rooms

Figure 8-3. Graphic Solution: Hospital Production Model.

$$0\,M + 1\,S = 6{,}000$$

yields a horizontal line at $S = 6{,}000$. Any number of medical patients can be treated without exceeding the capacity of the operating room since in our simplified example they do not require surgery. Remembering that any possible (or "feasible") solution to our problem must lie on or within the capacity lines, then the possible combination of medical and surgical patients lies within the polygon shown in the heavy line of figure 8-3. This polygon is called the *solution space*, and represents the set of all feasible solutions within the capacity constraints. Assuming the hospital seeks to treat as many patients as possible, any move in a northeasternly direction from the origin is desirable. Thus the *optimal* solution will lie somewhere on the polygon away from the x and y axes. This set of lines is called the *production possibility frontier*. Assuming that increasing production is desirable, no point short of the frontier will be optimum. It will always be possible to increase production by moving out to the frontier, where the capacity of at least one service is reached. By extension of this argument, it can be shown that in fact, for most problems, the optimum will lie at an intersection of two lines of the polygon. In most of these cases the capacity of two services is fully consumed.

Objective Function. In order to select which of the points on the production possibility frontier is most desirable, we must now specify an *objective function*, a statement of the relative desirability of our various outcomes. In industrial applications of programming, this is usually the "profit," or contribution to revenue made from the sale of each unit of production. Thus, if medical patients earned a profit of $150 each and surgical $100, the objective function would be:

$$Z = 150\,M + 100\,S.$$

This function would be maximized by taking medical patients rather than surgical so long as not more than 1½ (150/100) of a surgical patient was sacrificed for each additional medical patient.

The use of "profits" is somewhat pointless, if not impossible, for hospitals. Markets do not exist which fix profits on various kinds of patients. What alternatives are there? Some methods must be found to assign relative weights to each kind of output, if the objective function is to be specified. There are arguments to support the use of the relative average costs of treating each type of patient as the weights, but these are subject to dispute. This argument is based on the assumption that the long-run cost of treatment of a given type patient is the average cost as reflected by past experience. If medical patients cost $1,000 each to treat, and a patient is left untreated, an additional $1,000 will have to be spent to treat that patient. Conceivably, a panel of "experts" might be convened to assign weights to the various types of patients. Most simply, we might assign them equal value,

$$Z = M + S$$

and attempt to find the point on the production possibility frontier which maximizes this objective function. This can be done by noting that any given value of Z generates one of a set of parallel lines called "isomers." Three isomers of $Z = M + S$ are shown in figure 8-3, as the dotted lines X, Y and Z. It appears that Y, which is at $8,084 = M + S$, is the highest which touches the frontier, and therefore represents the optimum solution.

At this solution, the optimum output will be 5,418 surgical patients and 2,666 medical patients. The laboratory and physical therapy services will be fully utilized, but the operating rooms, nursing, and x-ray departments will not. There is no point in the solution space where a larger total number of patients can be produced, however. The unused resources are said to be *slack* resources, and a measure of their slack can be introduced as a *slack variable*. S_N, the quantity necessary to make the inequality, $(9M + 7S \leqslant 73,000)$ an equality, $(9M + 7S + S_N = 73,000)$ is the slack variable for the nursing resources, and at the solution it will be greater than zero.

The original problem has now been solved, but there are a number of other aspects to linear programming which are important.

Other Constraints. Often it will be desirable to constrain the desired solution of a programming problem to a limited portion of the solution space. This may be done by writing *constraints* or limitations into the problem, in addition to the capacity constraints which have been discussed. Figure 8-4 shows two additional constraints upon our example:

and $\qquad$ $S \geqslant 4,000$, shown by the line II'
$\qquad\qquad$ $M \geqslant 3,000$, shown by the line JJ'

These constraints, combined with the capacity constraints, restrict the solution space to the polygon KLM, and exclude the previous optimum solution G. The new solution will be at L where the isomer W touches the new production possibility frontier LM.

Other constraints, called *nonnegativity constraints*, are implicit in the problem, but must be stated to solve the problem algebraically. It is clear that only nonnegative numbers of patients can be treated. Thus any feasible solution lies in the realm

$$M \geqslant 0,$$
$$S \geqslant 0$$

Simplex Method. Graphic solutions, while useful for illustration, are impractical with three outputs and impossible with more than three. Algebraically however, our problem is stated as follows:

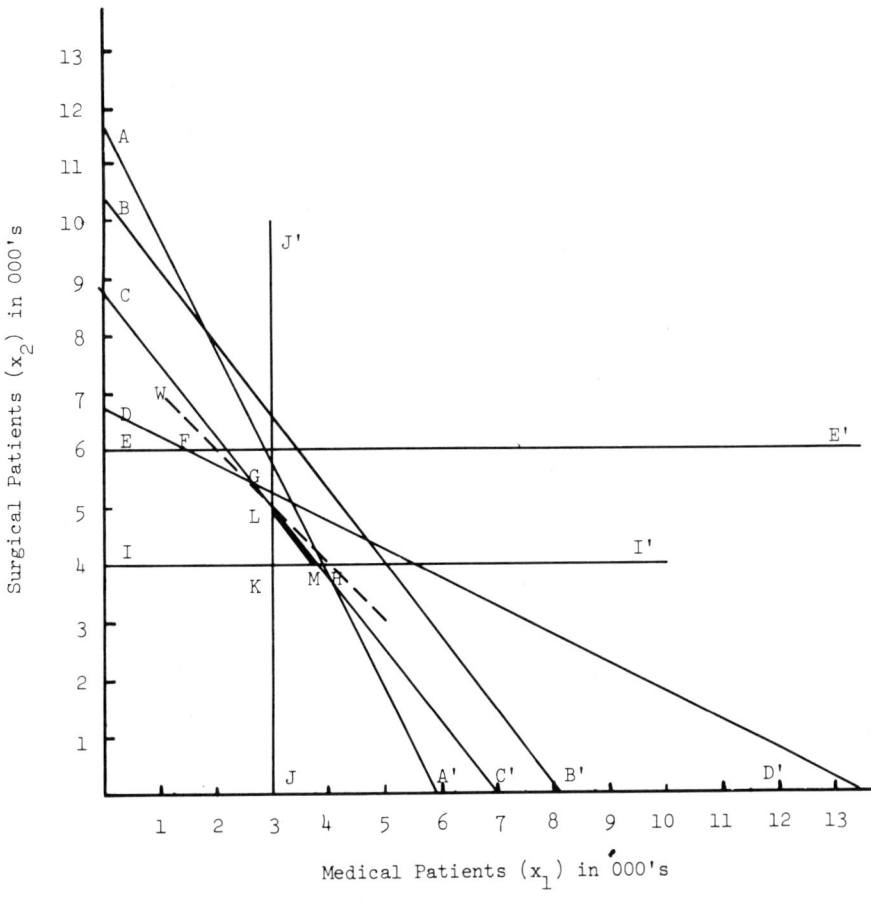

AA'	X-ray
BB'	Beds
CC'	Laboratory
DD'	Physical Therapy
EE'	Operating Rooms

Figure 8-4. Graphic Solution: Hospital Production Model.

Maximize:

$$Z = M + S$$

Subject to:

(Nursing)	$9M + 7S$	$\leq$	73,000
(Surgery)	S	$\leq$	6,000
(Laboratory)	$15M + 12S$	$\leq$	105,000

and

(Physical Therapy)	M	$+ \; 2S$	$\leq$	13,500
(X-ray)	$4M$	$+ \; 2S$	$\leq$	23,400
		M	$\geq$	3,000
		S	$\geq$	4,000

or

$$M, S \geq 0$$

(The last statement, $M, S \geq 0$ becomes redundant with the addition of the preceding constraint statements.)

This problem can be solved algebraically by a procedure known as the *simplex method* which determines the precise optimum solution. (The method will not be described here but can be studied in any basic programming text.)

The Dual and the Shadow Price. To each linear programming problem there exists a mathematical opposite, or *dual*. In the commonest form of linear programming, the original problem or *primal* is to maximize profit or some proxy for profit subject to a series of capacity constraints upon the quantities of outputs produced. Algebraically, if the outputs are Y's; the profit contributions, P's; the capacities, K's; and the slack variables S's, for two outputs and three resources:

Maximize: $Z = P_1 Y_1 + P_2 Y_2$

Subject to: $a_{11} Y_1 + a_{21} Y_2 + S_1 = K_1$

$a_{12} Y_1 + a_{22} Y_2 + S_2 = K_2$

$a_{13} Y_1 + a_{23} Y_2 + S_3 = K_3$

where: $Y_1, Y_2, S_1, S_2, S_3 \geq 0$

The dual will be framed in terms of the *value* or contribution of the resources, V_1, V_2, V_3, consumed per unit of output, rather than the quantity units, Y's. The dual problem is to minimize these values, whereas the original problem was to maximize output. Certain other algebraic rearrangements are necessary as well, and the dual to the original problem becomes:

Minimize: $Z' = K_1 V_1 + K_2 V_2 + K_3 V_3$

Subject to: $a_{11} V_1 + a_{12} V_2 + a_{13} V_3 - L_1 = P_1$

$a_{21} V_1 + a_{22} V_2 + a_{23} V_3 - L_2 = P_2$

where: $V_1, V_2, V_3, L_1, L_2 \geq 0$

The new slack variables, L_1 and L^2, are called the *dual* slack variables and represent the losses (which may be zero) associated with the two products at the solution.

For the illustrative example shown in figure 8-3 the primal was:

Maximize: $Z = M + S$

Subject to:
$$9M + 7S \leq 73{,}000$$
$$S \leq 6{,}000$$
$$15M + 12S \leq 105{,}000$$
$$M + 2S \leq 13{,}500$$
$$4M + 2S \leq 23{,}400$$

The dual is:

Minimize:

$$Z = 73{,}000\, V_1 + 6{,}000\, V_2 + 105{,}000\, V_3 + 13{,}500\, V_4 + 23{,}400\, V_5$$

Subject to:

$$9 V_1 + 0 V_2 + 15 V_3 + V_4 + 4 V_5 \geq 1$$
$$7 V_1 + V_2 + 12 V_3 + 2 V_4 + 2 V_5 \geq 1$$

The dual formulation has a number of properties of interest to the operations researcher. These are described in the texts on linear programming. For the hospital administrator, two of these are worthy of special note.

1. If the problem can be solved, the solution for its dual and primal specification is the same.
2. At the solution, the values of V represent the *marginal value* (or profit) *contribution* of the various resources.

Thus the value of additional units of any resource not fully utilized will be zero, and the value of additional units of any resource fully used at the solution will be given by the V value for that resource. This value, which represents the change in the objective function obtained for a change of one unit of the resource is called the *shadow price*. Because the primal and the dual have one and only one point in common, the shadow price is obtained directly from the algebraic, or simplex, solution.

For the illustration, the shadow prices of the resources are:

Laboratory = 0.06 patients/test per year

Physical therapy = 0.17 patients/test per year

That is to say, if the capacity of the laboratory were increased by one test per year, the optimum value of the objective function would increase by 0.06 patients (i.e., the hospital could treat 0.06 more patients for each one test increase in the capacity of the laboratory). If the capacity of physical therapy were increased by one treatment per year, the objective function would increase by 0.17 patients. The shadow price of all other resources is zero. They are not fully utilized at the solution, and enlarging them will not change the objective function value.

Opportunity Costs. One final inference can be made from the solution to a linear programming problem, and that is the opportunity cost of deviating from the solution (i.e., moving along the production possibility frontier from the optimum solution point). For the illustration, at the solution G, the number of patients treated is 2,667 medical and 5,417 surgical. The opportunity cost of treating one more medical patient is a loss of 1.25 surgical patients, occasioned by the constraint on laboratory capacity. Thus the opportunity cost is -0.25 patients. The cost of treating one more surgical patient is -2.0 medical patients. The opportunity cost is thus -1.00 patients.

A "Transportation Model" Example

In order to further demonstrate the practical utility of programming models and to discuss further the selection of realistic objective functions, consider the following assignment problem. It is taken from the x-ray department, and it is presented in an integer format as a daily scheduling problem. In this case, two objective functions, both related to cost, will be explored. The first assumes that costs are proportional to time spent. The second uses judgmentally assigned costs to adjust for danger and inconvenience. The problem, which is generically the same as many other assignment problems in hospitals, including that of the optimum assignment of nurses, is solved by a specialized method called the transportation method. In this problem there are four resources or rooms, X_1, X_2, X_3, and X_4. The services needed can be designated $1, 2, 3, \ldots, n$, where there are n different kinds of x-ray procedures. The total quantity of each procedure demanded (say to provide x-ray services to a given number of patients) can be designated $Y_1, \ldots, Y_j, \ldots, Y_n$. For simplicity in the illustration, let $n = 3$, and as an aid in understanding the problem, let:

Service 1: upper and lower G.I. exams

Service 2: special dye studies
Service 3: skeletal and chest x-rays.

The assignment of demand to rooms can be specified in the form of an *assignment matrix*:

Service	Rooms X_1	X_2	X_3	X_4	Demand
1	x_{11}	x_{21}	x_{31}	x_{41}	Y_1
2	x_{12}	x_{22}	x_{32}	x_{42}	Y_2
3	x_{13}	x_{23}	x_{33}	x_{43}	Y_3

where the x's represent the number of cases of each type assigned to each room. Certain constraints appear immediately. First any x value must be zero or greater.

$$x_{ij} \geq 0 \text{ for all } i, j$$

Next, the total service produced in all rooms must equal the demand:

$$\sum_{i=1}^{4} x_{i1} = Y_1$$

$$\sum_{i=1}^{4} x_{i2} = Y_2$$

$$\sum_{i=1}^{4} x_{i3} = Y_3$$

This will only be true, however, if we do not exceed the capacity of the rooms. That suggests another constraint, but to specify it we need actual values for the input-output (production) coefficients. These indicate the quantity of resources (rooms) required to fill a single unit of each kind of demand. Let us assume that studies of actual performance in room X_1 show that each G.I. study requires 45 minutes, each special dye study requires 120 minutes, and each skeletal or chest exam requires 15 minutes. (Of course, these values would have to be carefully checked. The actual times may be a stochastic function, with a measurable variation, but we will assume these problems away for the present.) Let us designate these values as P_{ij} (for production coefficient). For our illustration:

Production Coefficients (Minutes/Exam)

Service	Rooms			
	X_1	X_2	X_3	X_4
1	45	45	90	90
2	120	90	180	180
3	15	15	10	10

Assuming that we wish to complete our work in eight hours, or 480 minutes, another set of constraints can be formulated: The capacity of X_1 is 480. The total use of X_1 must be less or equal to that:

$$45x_{11} + 120x_{12} + 15x_{13} \leq 480$$

or

$$P_{11}x_{11} + P_{12}x_{12} + P_{13}x_{13} \leq 480$$

or

$$\sum_{j=1}^{3} P_{1j}x_{1j} \leq 480$$

$$\sum_{j=1}^{3} P_{2j}x_{2j} \leq 480$$

$$\sum_{j=1}^{3} P_{3j}x_{3j} \leq 480$$

$$\sum_{j=1}^{3} P_{4j}x_{4j} \leq 480$$

There is one other constraint in this problem, that all the x_{ij} are integers. That is, we cannot do half an exam, or split an exam between rooms.

The problem is now fully constrained. It is clear that there are some levels of demand where no solution exists, such as $Y_2 = 14$. It is impossible to do fourteen dye studies in eight hours in these four rooms. But for lower levels of demand, the problem can be solved, and usually there are several possibilities.

In order to find the optimum solution, it is necessary to specify what is to be optimized. This is the objective function, designated by the letter Z. The simplest objective function for this problem is time. If we attempt to minimize the total time the rooms are in use, the objective function is the measure of the total time consumed by any particular schedule. This is:

$$Z = \sum_{j=1}^{3} P_{1j}x_{1j} + \sum_{j=1}^{3} P_{2j}x_{2j} + \sum_{j=1}^{3} P_{3j}x_{3j} + \sum_{j=1}^{3} P_{4j}x_{4j} ,$$

or in a shorter notation;

$$Z = \sum_{i=1}^{4} \sum_{j=1}^{3} P_{ij}x_{ij} .$$

The objective function coefficients here are the same as the production function coefficients.

Trial Solution

We should be able to test our model, and find an optimum (minimum) of the objective function Z. Let us take a specimen demand

$$Y_1 = 10$$
$$Y_2 = 8$$
$$Y_3 = 25$$

We can pick any starting point, but since we can save at least 30 minutes any time we do a dye study in room 2, let us start there. To assist in an orderly computation, we will temporarily add a "slack" measure, S_j, equal to the services which are as yet unassigned. Our constraints imply that these must be zero when we are finished. We will also display our problem in the form of a matrix showing resources (rooms) in columns, and demands (services) in rows. Such a matrix is called a *tableau*. Column totals may never exceed capacity constraints, while row totals never exceed demand. By the insertion of slack variables (S_j), the row totals may be kept equal to the demand.

Trial Schedule # 1

Service	Room				S_j	Y_j
	1	2	3	4		
1					10	10
2	3	5	0	0	0	8
3					25	25
$\sum_{j=1}^{3} P_{ij}x_{ij}$ (≤ 480)	360	450	0	0		

It will be helpful to have another "slack" measure, for available (unscheduled) room time equal to $480 - \sum_{j=1}^{3} P_{ij} x_{ij}$

At this stage,

Slack   120   30   480   480.

Continuing with the G.I. examinations:

Trial Schedule #2

Service	Rooms				S_j	Y_j
	1	2	3	4		
1	2	0	5	3	0	10
2	3	5	0	0	0	8
3					25	25
$\sum_{j=1}^{3} P_{ij} x_{ij}$ (≤ 480)	450	450	450	270		
Slack ($480 - \sum_{j=1}^{3} P_{ij} x_{ij}$)	30	30	30	210		

And last the skeletal exams:

Trial Schedule #3

Service	Rooms				S_j	Y_j
	1	2	3	4		
1	2	0	5	3	0	10
2	3	5	0	0	0	8
3	0	1	3	21	0	25
$\sum_{j=1}^{3} P_{ij} x_{ij}$ (≤ 480)	450	465	480	480		
Slack ($480 - \sum_{j=1}^{3} P_{ij} x_{ij}$)	30	15	0	0		

Trial 3 yields a solution, since all demand has been met. The value of the objective function is:

$$Z = 450 + 465 + 480 + 480 = 1875$$

This may not be the minimum, however. Some improvement might be possible if some G.I. studies were moved out of room 3, and dye studies moved in.

Trial Schedule #4

Service	Rooms				Y_j
	1	2	3	4	
1	4	0	3	3	10
2	2	5	1	0	8
3	0	1	3	21	25
$\sum_{j=1}^{3} P_{ij}x_{ij} (\leq 480)$	420	465	480	480	
Slack $(480 - \sum_{j=1}^{3} P_{ij}x_{ij})$	60	15	0	0	

This decreases the objective function to 1845. The same maneuver can be repeated:

Trial Schedule #5

Service	Rooms				Y_j
	1	2	3	4	
1	10	0	0	0	10
2	0	5	2	1	8
3	0	2	3	20	25
$\sum_{j=1}^{3} P_{ij}x_{ij} (\leq 480)$	450	480	390	380	
Slack $(480 - \sum_{j=1}^{3} P_{ij}x_{ij})$	30	0	90	100	

This decreases the objection function to 1700. A systematic trial can be run for each element to check the minimum. Inspection reveals that only one skeletal exam is scheduled at greater than minimum time, so that no significant improvement appears possible.

Improving the Model Precision

The procedure followed so far with the hypothetical illustration is not unlike that which might be followed in a real problem. A much restricted, oversimplified version of the problem might be formulated, modeled, and tested with crude or even imaginary data. If an encouraging result is obtained, as it has been in this case, the major components of the model can be reviewed to improve the practical usefulness of the result. One element which will clearly require expansion is the list of services. Most modern radiology departments offer a wide variety of services. These elements can be expanded easily. Each additional service requires a specification of the demand, the input-output coefficients, and the contribution, in each alternative, to the objective function. The number of resources (rooms) can also be expanded as necessary. The problem will soon become unwieldy for manual solution. The method of solution is relatively simple, and computer programs are available to solve problems of this type, even for a large number of services and resources. Other elements may present more problems, however.

Input-Output Coefficients. These relate each service to the quantity of each alternative resource which may be used. They must usually be derived from empirical studies of the department, although it is occasionally possible to get the information from various existing records. Collection and preparation of the data are often the most costly part of the project. While accuracy and detail are important to make the model useful, it is possible to extend the specificity of the model unnecessarily. Three elements eventually limit the usefulness of additional precision in the coefficients. They are the cost of additional data collection, the reliability of more precise subdivision of services, and size limits on computer capability. In the illustration, there are dozens of specific x-ray examinations which could be considered. However, the length of each procedure is actually stochastic, not deterministic. It is only useful to treat the individual coefficients separately so long as there is a significant and nontrivial difference between mean values of coefficients and there are sufficient quantities of demand for each service to make the model useful. It will clearly be desirable to group services which are similar in their input-output characteristics, even though they are quite different in all other respects.

Sensitivity Analysis. Sensitivity analysis, the technique described in the preceding chapter, can be used to evaluate needs for additional data. Trial solutions can be generated for specific changes in the service parameters, including constraints, input-output coefficients, and modifications of the objective function. If these result in small changes in the optimum result, the value of additional data refinement is low. On the other hand, if testing shows that the model is highly sensitive to a specific parameter, specifications and data in that area must be developed to a high degree of accuracy.

Such an analysis can be performed for the illustration by postulating a relatively large error in the input-output coefficients for the dye study exams. For a 17 percent decrease, the revised production coefficients will be:

Sensitivity Analysis

Revised Production Coefficients
(17% decrease, service 2)

Service	Rooms			
	X_1	X_2	X_3	X_4
1	45	45	90	90
2	100	75	150	150
3	15	15	10	10

These yield a minimum time schedule with an objective function of 1,450 minutes.

Trial Schedule #S 1

Service	Rooms				Y_j
	1	2	3	4	
1	10	0	0	0	10
2	0	6	2	0	8
3	0	0	11	14	25
$\sum_{j=1}^{3} P_{ij} x_{ij} \;(\leqslant 480)$	450	450	410	140	
Slack $(480 - \sum_{j=1}^{3} P_{ij} x_{ij})$	30	30	70	340	

$Z = 1{,}450$

Since the previous minimum was at 1700, a change of −17 percent in this input parameter produces a change of 15 percent in the objective function. An increase of a similar magnitude will exceed capacity constraints on the demand, but assuming these are removed, it will result in an increase of 10 percent in the objective function:

Sensitivity Analysis

Revised Production Coefficients
(17% increase, service 2)

Service	Rooms			
	X_1	X_2	X_3	X_4
1	45	45	90	90
2	140	105	210	210
3	15	15	10	10

Trial Schedule #S 2

Service	Rooms				Y_j
	1	2	3	4	
1	10	0	0	0	10
2	0	5	2	1	8
3	2	0	6	17	25
$\sum_{j=1}^{3} P_{ij} x_{ij}\ (\leqslant 480)$	480	525	480	380	
Slack $(480 - \sum_{j=1}^{3} P_{ij} x_{ij}) $	0	−45	0	100	

Z = 1,865

In this case, errors in the measurement of the coefficients change the value of the objective function on approximately a one-for-one basis. This information would indicate the need for careful study of the true values within the service. A fourth service might be created composed of those kinds of dye studies which took less time than others, in addition to efforts to measure the service 2 coefficients more accurately.

It is possible to test models over multiple trials covering the range of normal operating experience by combining them with simulation routines. In the illustration, data might be collected on the distribution of demand for each of the x-ray services, and the actual impact of using the model could be compared against historical performance. By adjusting the input data, the simulation could also estimate the sensitivity of the solution to changes in the accuracy of measurement of the production coefficients. While possibilities of this kind are almost unlimited, they are also costly. As a general rule, no such involved project should be undertaken unless there is convincing evidence of an appropriately large return.

Selecting the Objective Function

If the objective function is incorrectly related to the true objectives of the organization, all results from the model are at best irrelevant and at worst impede attainment of the true goals. In the illustration, the objective function which was selected, total time, may or may not be realistic. A number of other possibilities exist for objective functions. Outside the hospital situation, in for-profit business, the contribution to profit or overhead is a common objective function. This might be appropriate in the illustration if the department were operated as the radiologist's private business. The profit objective function is developed by taking the revenue earned by each service and subtracting from it the direct cost (excluding overhead) of performing each type of examination in each room. Using the same notation as before (i: rooms; j: services) the value of the objective function for any cell in the matrix is:

$$(R_j - C_{ij})x_{ij}$$

if R_j = revenue for the jth service

C_{ij} = direct costs for the jth service in the ith room.

The total for the objective function is:

$$Z = \sum_{i=1}^{4} \sum_{j=1}^{3} (R_j - C_{ij})x_{ij} .$$

This can be expanded and restated algebraically as:

$$Z = \sum_{j=1}^{3} R_j (\sum_{i=1}^{4} x_{ij}) - \sum_{i=1}^{4} \sum_{j=1}^{3} C_{ij}x_{ij} ,$$

but since $\sum_{i=1}^{4} x_{ij} = Y_j$ (where the Y_j's are the demands)

$$Z = \sum_{j=1}^{3} R_j Y_j - \sum_{i=1}^{4} \sum_{j=1}^{3} C_{ij} x_{ij} ,$$

(The logic of the above algebra is easy to follow. It simply states that since the revenue is constant on each row j, the revenue can be calculated by looking only at the row totals. The costs vary by both row and column and must be summed individually by cell.)

In the illustration as we have considered it so far,

$$\sum_{j=1}^{3} R_j Y_j$$

is a constant. It thus does not affect the location of the optimum, and it could be ignored, if desired. Another form of the objective function results:

$$Z = \sum_{i=1}^{4} \sum_{j=1}^{3} C_{ij} x_{ij} .$$

This is a direct cost objective function which is to be *minimized* in the solution. (Minimized if the minus sign is dropped.) Since time for personnel and equipment is an important component of direct costs, this objective function is conceptually very similar to the original one. Other substitutes or "proxies" for direct cost might be used instead of time. The time spent by the radiologist is one possibility since it represents a scarce and expensive element in the overall cost.

Still another concept for the objective function might be explored. This involves a subjective notion of values of the various exams. An entire subjective value system for the worth of each service (analogous to revenue) and its negative values, such as patient safety and discomfort (analogous to direct cost) could be constructed for each room. The radiologist and the chief technician might recommend that certain exams are safer, or more convenient, or more likely to yield accurate results in some rooms than in others. While these opinions are less tangible than accounting data on direct costs, it would be foolish to ignore them in a scheduling model. There are ways of incorporating these judgments into an objective function if they can be reduced to quantitative terms.

To continue the illustration, suppose that cost accounting studies indicate the following direct costs per test:

| | Rooms | | | |
Service	1	2	3	4
1	$32.50	$32.50	$ 55.00	$ 55.00
2	85.00	70.00	115.00	115.00
3	2.25	2.25	2.25	2.25

However, in discussing the matter with the chief radiologist, he points out that there are distinct safety factors involved. Considering radiation exposure, patient comfort and diagnostic accuracy, he feels that certain exams should never be scheduled in some rooms. Room 4, he feels, should never be used for dye studies. Room 3 should be used only as a last resort for this purpose. Room 1 is preferable to room 2 for G.I. studies because of patient comfort. Rooms 1, 2, and 3 are better than room 4 for all studies. After considerable thought and the trial of various alternatives, he agrees that the following table of penalty factors correctly represents his views.

| | Rooms | | | |
Service	1	2	3	4
1	1	2	2	3
2	1	1	3	∞
3	1	1	1	2

This conclusion could be used directly as an objective function. It is the same as saying it is twice as desirable to do a G.I. study in room 1 than room 2 or 3, three times as desirable as room 4, etc. It also implies that G.I. studies in room 4 are about as undesirable as dye studies in room 3. The ∞ (infinity) symbol has the effect of ruling out the possibility of a dye study in room 4. If these values are used by themselves as an objective function, however, the opportunity to minimize accounting costs is lost. (There is no preference between several options carrying different dollar costs.) It is possible to combine the two estimates, by taking the element-by-element product of the cost matrix and the preference matrix. This yields an objective function in "adjusted cost dollars":

| | Rooms | | | |
Service	1	2	3	4
1	$32.50	$65.00	$110.00	$165.00
2	85.00	70.00	345.00	∞
3	2.25	2.25	2.25	4.50

Any solution to the scheduling problem yields a value of the adjusted cost objective function, and at least one solution yields a minimum. For example, the minimum solution for total time (section 3):

Trial Schedule #5

Service	Rooms				Y_j
	1	2	3	4	
1	10	0	0	0	10
2	0	5	2	1	8
3	0	2	3	21	25
Slack (min)	90	15	0	0	

yields the objective function value:

Service	Rooms			
	1	2	3	4
1	$325.	$ 0	0	0
2	0	350.	690.	∞
3	0	4.50	6.75	94.5
$\sum_{j=1}^{3} C_{ij}x_{ij}$	$325.	$354.50	$696.75	$ ∞

$$Z = \sum_{i=1}^{4} \sum_{j=1}^{3} C_{ij}x_{ij} = \infty$$

This clearly is not the minimum of the new objective function. To improve it, the dye study in room 4 must be rescheduled, and then the other rows reviewed to find the minimum. Costs could be reduced if the exams done in rooms 3 and 4 were transferred to room 1, and two G.I. exams were moved to room 3:

Trial Schedule #5A

Service	Rooms				Y_j
	1	2	3	4	
1	2	0	5	3	10
2	3	5	0	0	8
3	0	1	3	21	25
$\sum_{j=1}^{3} P_{ij}x_{ij}$ ($\leq$ 480)	450	465	480	480	

Slack $(480 - \sum_{j=1}^{3} P_{ij} x_{ij})$ 30   15   0   0

Objective Function Trial #5A

Service	Rooms			
	1	2	3	4
1	$ 65.00	$ 0	$550.00	$495.00
2	255.00	350.00	0	0
3	0	2.25	6.75	94.50
$\sum_{j=1}^{3} C_{ij} x_{ij}$	$320.00	$352.25	$556.75	$589.50

$$Z = \sum_{i=1}^{4} \sum_{j=1}^{3} C_{ij} x_{ij} = 1,818.5$$

A few additional possibilities exist, and the minimum objective function value is $1,702. (The interested student can derive the schedule or schedules which yield the minimum.)

Summary

In this section, a form of mathematical programming model has been described by means of a hypothetical problem. The problem, scheduling of x-ray facilities, was one of allocating a fixed set of resources to meet a known, deterministic demand. The problem was described in terms of *constraints*, governing the demand which must be met and the resources available, *input-output coefficients*, or *production coefficients*, which relate each unit of demand to the resources it consumes in each possible allocation, and an *objective function* which relates the contribution of each possible combination of demand and resources to the goals of the operation. A simplified version of the problem was stated, and formulated in a *matrix* or *tableau*. A solution was reached in an iterative process which made a number of trials aimed at optimizing the objective function.

Next the model was studied for possible refinements. The value of more precise information for the production coefficients was tested by sensitivity analysis. Alternative objective functions were explored, including contribution to profit or overhead, direct costs alone, and various proxies for accounting costs. Subjective estimates combining accounting costs with weighting factors for intangibles were selected for a new "adjusted cost" objective function, and the problem was solved again.

Programming Models

Extensive work has been done on the computer solution of certain forms of mathematical programming models. The form of programming which has been most completely worked out is the linear form, where the input-output coefficients and the objective function can be stated in linear equations. A number of specific programs have been published with varying capabilities in terms of the number of elements, the kinds of constraints, and the form of the coefficients and objective functions they can accommodate. These programs are in daily use in industrial settings, solving such problems as the appropriate patterns of shipment between several plants and several warehouses, scheduling of several products among several plants, and similar uses. Not all the applications are of a scheduling nature. The oil industry uses linear programming to assist in selecting the optimum quantities of the several products which can be made from crude oil and selecting the proper combination of antiknock chemicals for high octane gasoline.

Limitations

The major limitation of linear programming is the need for a linear relation between the quantity of demand met and the quantity of resources required. This means that the resource requirement X for any given demand met, Y can be calculated from an equation of the form:

$$X = aY + K,$$

where K is a constant. This is the same as saying that the amount of resource consumed by any unit of Y is a constant, independent of the total number of units produced by that resource. The $Y + 1$ unit will require an additional amount of resource a, regardless of whether Y is very small or very large. The amount a is the input-output coefficient which is necessary to formulate the problem. If the relationship between X and Y cannot be stated in this form, it is nonlinear. When this occurs, nonlinear rather than linear programming must be used, and the problem becomes much more difficult to solve.

The objective function must also be a linear function of the demand met. That is, objective functions of the type: $Z = aY + b$ can be solved, while those of the type $Z = aY^2 + bY + c$ or $Z = e^{ax} + b$ cannot. Often a linear approximation can be used if the true relationship is not linear. This is particularly true of the objective function requirement, where several linear functions can be used to approximate a single nonlinear function. Linear approximations can also be used for nonlinear production relationships. The critical question is the same as with other considerations of the accuracy of models: "Does the introduction of the approximation result in a serious distortion of the solution?" In the illustration used previously it is quite possible that the production relationship is not truly linear. Doing ten G.I. exams in room 1 will not require exactly 10 times as long as doing one. The question is whether the error which is introduced by assuming linearity is important. In the illustration, where the difference between room 1 and room 3 is a change of 100 percent, from 45 to 90 minutes, it is hardly likely that the deviation from linearity would be important.

Linear programming also assumes continuity of both the production coefficients and the objective function. That is, any value for the solution is acceptable, even if it is not an integer. Here the second illustration seriously violates the linear programming assumptions. The linear programming solution to the problem with the initial objective function would schedule an additional one-third of a dye study in room two and show 5.3 dye studies in the solution. This solution would be unacceptable because the fractions result in a serious departure from the optimal schedule. Again the question is not whether the assumption introduces an error, but whether the error was important. If the illustration had used laboratory tests, with ten times the service volume, we would probably assume that a solution of 53.3 was only trivially different from 53 and ignore the restriction. Otherwise we would be limited to transportation models and other solution techniques identified as *integer programming*.

Simplex Solution

The basic method of solving a linear programming model is the *simplex* method which approaches, and ultimately reaches, the optimum solution, by a series of algebraic solutions to the constraints. After each solution, the program calculates the shadow price of each possible adjustment to the solution. The one making the greatest contribution to the objective function is adopted, and the process is repeated. When no adjustment will make a contribution to the objective function without violating the constraints, the optimum has been reached. The remaining shadow prices represent the values of additional resources or additional demand.

Other Solution Techniques

There are other forms of linear programming techniques which fit limited cases. The transportation solution is the most common, and resembles the method used in the x-ray scheduling illustration. The simplex method can be used in any linear programming problem, while degenerate solution techniques are applicable only to restricted sets of problems.

A number of texts detail the process of the simplex technique, various special techniques, and modifications to accommodate special problems such as non-linearity of the objective function. The interested student is referred to these works, which are listed in the Additional Readings. There are in addition to linear models a variety of nonlinear models, models covering integer requirements, models dealing with stochastic instead of deterministic relationships, and others. Little application of these has been made in hospitals, and they will not be discussed here.

Hospital Applications of Mathematical Programming

There have been a number of fruitful efforts to apply mathematical programming to hospitals. These have been principally in the areas of hospital location,[7] nurse staffing,[8] nursing unit design,[9] and menu planning.[10] Of these, only the menu planning problem has so far reached practical application. It is used routinely by a number of hospitals and services offering menus for hospital use, and has been proven to reduce the dollar cost of raw food.

Balintfy's Menu Planning Model

These problems are easy to formulate in mathematical programming models, although the models are usually difficult to solve. Balintfy's menu-planning model considers the cost of food as the objective function to be minimized, nutritional requirements as the demand, and various food items as the resources. The input-output coefficients are the amounts of each nutritional requirements supplied by a serving of food. For example:

Menu Item	Protein per Serving	Vitamin C per Serving
Beef Stew	16 gms.	20 mg.
Cherry Cobbler	21 gms.	8 mg.

The constraints quickly become very complicated. Foods must be grouped, so that the program picks traditional meals with entrees, vegetables, desserts, etc. Servings must be integers of 1 from each group. The noninteger solution turns out to be unsatisfactory—it does not yeild a solution similar to the integer solution for a single meal. Either meals must be planned in cycles, or integer solutions must be found. Balintfy chose the former course, using the noninteger solution and planning several meals at a time. The model was still not realistic, however. Constraints were needed for color, flavor, texture, and repetition of the same item within the cycle. These problems were all overcome, but at the expense of a complex, two-stage model which reached far beyond the elementary simplex solution. The final result is a program which improves significantly upon the dietician's unaided judgment but does not mathematically guarantee an optimum. The computer solution is reviewed by a skilled dietician, who can alter it to take care of factors not included in the model by making substitutions referring to the shadow prices.

Wolfe's Nurse Staffing Model

Wolfe studied the problem of the optimal mix of nursing staff on a patient unit. Most patient units are staffed with several levels of personnel skill, including head nurses, staff nurses, practical nurses, and aides. These personnel must perform a variety of tasks: bed-making, administering medication, giving personal care to patients, etc. It is clear that not all classes of personnel can do all jobs equally well. There are penalties both ways. An untrained aide cannot give medications because she may make serious errors, but if a head nurse makes beds, her time is much more expensive to the hospital than an aide's.

In this problem, the hours of personnel time are the resources, and the tasks which must be done are the demands. The input-output coefficients are the times required for each class of personnel to perform each task. The objective function, which must be minimized, is some measure of cost. It cannot be simply payroll dollars, however. (If this were used all tasks would be assigned to the lowest paid employees.) Wolfe solved this problem by calculating the dollar cost for each task—the number of man minutes required times the wage per minute for each class of personnel. He then asked a panel of nurses to establish subjective values for intangible costs. The coefficients for the objective function were the sum of the two costs. (This is the same problem and the same solution as was shown earlier in the daily x-ray scheduling with a cost objective function.)

In order to establish intangible costs realistically, it was necessary to sort the patients by level of care required. The cost for a practical nurse to give personal care to a critically ill patient was different from the cost for a registered nurse, but the difference was less important if the patient was not critically ill. This distinction was built into the model, but the result was a large increase in the number of possible tasks demanded.

After considerable effort, Wolfe and his nursing panel divided the demand for nursing care into nine task groups, as shown below:

1. Technical tasks 1: bedside nursing procedures which can be performed after on-the-job training
2. Technical tasks 2: bedside nursing procedures requiring "advanced" (i.e., academic) training

3. Preparatory care 1 and 2: patient related activities away from the bedside associated with Technical tasks 1 and 2
4. Clerical tasks, 1, 2, and 3: record keeping and related tasks in order of increasing clinical significance
5. Housekeeping
6. Escorting and emergency errands
7. Maintenance, checking and ordering supplies
8. Supervising and teaching
9. Evaluation of patient care needs and assignment

The first three groups are subdivided by severity of patient illness or importance of work, making a total of sixteen tasks. The relationships between each of these were established by work measurement. (To reduce the cost of data collection, it was assumed that the unit times were the same for all levels of personnel.) The objective function value for the ith task and the jth personnel level becomes

$$Z_{ij} = x_{ij}w_j + V_{ij} ,$$

or the time required (the variable x_{ij}) times the wage per minute (w_j), plus the intangible costs assigned by the panel V_{ij}. A sample of these values is shown in table 8-4.

The constraints for the problem proved to be more difficult to handle than the objective function. Since personnel were to be assigned only for a full eight-hour shift, it was necessary to create a "dummy" task for idle time. The eight hour constraint also created an integer problem, requiring more advanced programming techniques. As in the case of Balintfy's problem, considerable technical manipulation was required to reach a solution. The method finally chosen was a noninteger technique, followed by trials of the noninteger optimum to approximate an integer optimum.

Other Approaches to the Nurse Staffing Problem

Hospitals must assign nursing staff to nursing units. These are sometimes called "nursing stations" or "floors," but in general they are geographically identified collections of patient facilities. The demand for service on each unit varies stochastically because of variation in both the number and degree of illness of patients. One solution to this problem is simply to treat the needs of a given station as a fixed, deterministic value, and establish a constant staff requirement for each unit. Alternatively, an effort can be made to accommodate to the variation by transferring staff, or using a pool of "float" staff which can be assigned to the units of greatest need. The latter method has advantages in

Table 8-4
Nursing Care Task Values

Task Complex	Head Nurse	Assistant Head Nurse	General Staff Nurse	Licensed Practical Nurse	Nursing Aide	Ward Clerk
Technical Task 1						
Class I	$ 8.52	$ 7.92	$ 7.56	$ 5.28	$ 4.32	$∞
Class II	14.10	13.10	12.50	8.80	8.50	∞
Class III	9.87	9.17	8.75	7.49	9.24	∞
Technical Task 2						
Class I	1.41	1.31	1.25	1.01	∞	∞
Class II	5.64	5.24	5.00	4.28	∞	∞
Class III	5.64	5.24	5.00	5.36	∞	∞
Preparatory Care 1	33.84	31.44	30.00	21.12	17.76	43.92
Preparatory Care 2	14.30	13.30	12.50	12.30	∞	∞
Clerical Task 1	8.46	7.86	7.50	5.28	4.32	8.88
Clerical Task 2	20.86	19.46	18.62	13.44	20.72	9.80
Clerical Task 3	5.64	5.68	6.24	6.76	∞	∞
Housekeeping Duties	12.69	11.79	11.25	7.92	6.39	14.94
Escort and Errand	14.10	13.10	12.50	9.10	8.40	13.40
Supervising and Teaching	4.23	4.35	4.68	5.13	∞	∞
Evaluation and Assignment	32.43	34.50	39.79	44.26	∞	∞
Maintenance Checking & Ordering supplies	4.23	3.93	3.75	2.64	4.17	2.10

Source: Wolfe and Young "Staffing the Nursing Unit," *Nursing Research* 14, no. 4, (1965) p. 301.
Note: Infinite costs were assigned where performance of a task by a given skill level was considered to be impossible or unsafe.

optimizing the use of a scarce resource or in reducing the cost of nursing.[11] When a variable staff approach is used, the nursing department faces a daily resource allocation problem. The available personnel in each class of nursing employee must be assigned to the several floors. This assignment can be done manually, relying solely upon the supervisor's judgment, but it is time consuming and different supervisors have different abilities to do well with it.[12] The combination of the possibility of a rewarding solution and difficulty with unaided manual solution strongly encourage the development of more specific, less subjective criteria for the solution. These will at least speed the manual solution and reduce the variation between supervisors. They may also permit use of the computer in reaching a solution and the eventual application of mathematical programming techniques.

The following example establishes the necessary information to describe the nurse staffing problem in a specific hospital. The example chosen is a *progressive patient care* hospital where patients are assigned to units according to their degree of illness. The same approach could be applied to a conventional hospital by treating all adult medical-surgical floor censuses as being composed of subgroups with varying degree of illness. One possible procedure to follow in formulating the problem is as follows:

- The nursing units are specified by size and function
- The nursing needs of each of the three shifts are separated, under the assumption that short-term intershift transfer is not a practical solution
- Standard assignments are prescribed for the evening and night shifts based upon average total census. Guidelines are established for the shift supervisor to use in transferring personnel between units. (These shifts present less flexibility, and therefore are handled more arbitrarily)
- Standards are established for the hours per patient day of care required by the typical patient on each unit during the day shift
- A policy of a staffing increment is established for the day shift, (i.e., no person will be assigned to a unit for less than four hours or less than eight hours). Minimum staffing standards for each census on each unit are calculated. These are some specified fraction of the standard, and include the staffing increment constraint
- Each day, from input information of census and available staff, the supervisor (or the computer) assigns minimum staff and checks availability of personnel to make sure minima are met
- If minima are not met, shift supervisor must decide on appropriate action. (Floor closed, LPN substituted for RN, etc.)
- The balance of the available staff are assigned beginning with the greatest shortage in terms of hours of care below standard. Personnel are assigned to the units up to some agreed upon maximum. When no further assignments can be made, either because all personnel are assigned or because any further assignment would be over maximum, the assignment is complete
- Supervisor reviews assignment, changes it if she feels it necessary, acts on staff remaining for assignment, and issues the result

The standards relate the hours of care believed to be needed by each patient on each floor to the demand, which is the total census on each floor. These standards can be developed in several ways. Traditionally they are a consensus of nursing judgment, carefully and formally compiled.[13] This consensus may be augmented, however, by reference to staffing patterns in nearby hospitals, reported for members of Hospital Administrative Services, or to published research,[14] or by use of consultants and specialized studies such as the CASH program in California.[15] At the present time, the standards must remain subjective.

The length of the staffing increment and the minima and maxima are constraints. Generally an eight-hour increment is probably necessary, although it reduces the flexibility of the result. In some situations, however, as with a "float" pool of part-time nurses, four-hour increments may be feasible. Minima represent relatively undesirable situations which should be identified for control purposes, as well as a practical initial solution. They are calculated in terms of assignment patterns following the increment constraint, for each possible level of census and for each class of nursing personnel. This speeds the solution, since presumably the majority of personnel are assigned automatically in the process of meeting the minima. The minima include constraints such as "at least one R.N." wherever appropriate. In many hospitals, the evening and night shift are staffed at or near the minimum levels. Since little flexibility remains on these shifts, they receive little additional attention.

The objective function in this model is the deviation from standard in hours per patient day. It differs substantially from the Wolfe approach in not taking the cost of individual tasks into account. It could be expanded by subjective weighting of skill levels and also by weighting of the deviation according to its magnitude. Additional assignments are made to each floor, according to the increment constraint, until the objective function is minimized, or until all personnel are assigned. The problem as formulated is actually a degenerate integer programming problem which apparently could be programmed for computer solution without difficulty. Similar programs exist, and are commercially available.[16] A closely related formulation using the square of deviation was made and solved by Warner.[17]

Summary

The works of Balintfy and Wolfe are examples of pioneering efforts at mathematical programming applications. They show the same pattern of problem identification, major difficulties, and eventual success. The difficulties come when the theoretical models are tailored to realistic conditions, and they appear in the form of numerous (and often troublesome) constraints as well as difficulties in formulating objective functions and problems in accurate specification of demands and production coefficients. Overcoming the difficulties increased the scope and complexity of the programming, and individually tailored programs had to be devised. Thus the procedure for developing mathematical programming models is expensive and requires strong technical skills. It may also require large, high-speed computers. The eventual promise is quite high, however, because of the number of costly problems which the method can solve. There is already voluminous technical literature and a growing supply of computer capability. It seems certain, therefore, that the number of practical applications will mount rapidly in the 1970s.

One of the major jobs which must be done to facilitate programming solutions is the reduction of subjective, nonquantitative policies and criteria to specific quantitative statements. This task will fall on the hospital personnel for they have the professional knowledge necessary to specify constraints, coefficients, and objectives in a realistic way. While doctors, nurses, and other clinical professions must be included in this process, so must representatives of hospital administration. They can play major roles both in representing consumer interests in cost and convenience and in coordinating and stimulating the work of others.

Additional Readings

Baumol, W.J. *Economic Theory and Operations Analysis*. 2nd Ed., Prentice-Hall, Englewood Cliffs, N.J., 1965.

Bowman, E.H. and R.B. Fetter. *Analysis for Production and Operations Management*. 3rd Ed., R.D. Irwin, Inc., Homewood, Ill., 1967.

Hillier, E.F. and Lieberman. *Introduction to Operations Research*. Holden-Day, San Francisco, 1967.

9 Evaluating Capital Investment Opportunities

Introduction

A large class of management decisions deal with alternatives differing in both the amount of capital and of operating expenses. Some of these involve the substitution of capital for labor, such as the installation of an automated cart delivery system. Others involve exactly the opposite, such as the purchase of laundry service with corresponding savings of capital investments in laundry equipment. Some involve lease of equipment, resulting in a recurring operating expense, rather than a purchase, which results in a one-time capital expense. The most complicated decisions in this class are those relating to expansion of services. In these, commitments are made to both capital and operating expenses in expectation of some level of goal achievement. The offering of a new service, such as a mental health clinic, is an example.

Decisions in this class are obviously important. They are all planning decisions which often involve large sums of money and long lead times between decision and implementation. They interact importantly with each other. For example, the decision to build a laundry rather than purchase services will consume significant amounts of capital and force commitments of building space. As a result, management's willingness to support a mental health clinic may be substantially reduced. These decisions are unique, which means that there is little opportunity for learning. Operators can make errors in recurring decisions such as daily staffing levels. They learn from these and avoid the errors in the future. The same is not true of investment decisions, except in limited degree. Finally, unlike many operating decisions, they are difficult and costly to reverse. Once capital has been put in place as buildings and equipment it becomes impossible to return to exactly the original condition.

The goal in decisions of this class is the same as in other management decisions—to gain the maximum benefit from a given level of expenditures. There is a systematic pattern of analysis which will aid in achieving this goal. This begins with careful estimates of the level of future demand, including an understanding of the uncertainty of the forecast and the stochastic variation. Techniques described in chapters 1 to 5 are useful in preparing these forecasts and analyses. Second, it is necessary to establish careful cost estimates for both capital and operating expenses under each alternative. The models discussed in chapters 6 through 8 are useful for doing this, together with conventional accounting and budgeting techniques. Third, in order to compare alternatives, capital and operating expenditures must be reduced to equivalency. The techniques for doing this, discounting cash flow and finding the internal rate of return, will be explained in this chapter. Fourth, the alternative offering the greatest achievement for a given expenditure, or the necessary achievement for a minimal expenditure, must be selected. Since achievement in health services is not always measured by any single measure, like profit or dollar savings, this determination is sometimes quite difficult. Techniques for improving the quality of this decision, called cost-benefit analysis, will also be discussed in this chapter. This topic will be developed in stages, beginning with decisions involving the substitution of capital for labor, and vice versa. In these cases, the measure of achievement is usually minimizing dollars expended. Nonmonetary considerations, while always present, are generally minor. After exploration of these cases, the more difficult evaluations will be explored. These involve investment alternatives with differing expenditures of both capital and operating dollars and with differing achievements of a nonmonetary nature.

Decisions Involving Principally Monetary Costs

There are a relatively large number of subsidiary processes in hospitals where the goal of management is cost minimization within a framework of achievement of a given quantity and quality of output. Most production processes fit this condition as well in hospitals as they do in industry. Examples include food production, laundry, housekeeping, and payroll processing. While some of these activities have a direct impact on patient care, they are generally performed to a fairly clear level of quality of service or product. The principal management goal is to achieve that level of performance with minimum expenditure. In various subprocesses, or sometimes in whole processes, there are alternatives which involve adjustment of the relative levels of capital and operating expenditures. The decisions evaluating these alternatives are called *make-or-buy decisions*, reflecting one common form of the problem. Make-or-buy decisions occur when the hospital has the alternative of performing the process itself (make) or purchasing the completed service (buy). Usually, although not always, the make alternative involves heavier capital investment and lower operating investment, and the buy alternative little or no capital investment. The problem is to evaluate the various capital and operating expense combinations to determine whether they are desirable and to rank order them by their desirability.

The problem is approached in the following steps.

  – The demand for the item or service in question is estimated
  – The operating expenses to meet the possible levels of demand are budgeted in detail for each alternative
  – A complete budget of capital requirements is prepared for each alternative

- The savings in operating expenses (cash flow) each year is expressed as a return on capital expenditures
- The return on capital investment becomes the measure by which the decision is made

Operating Costs

There is a framework for analyzing operating costs which is suitable for any alternative, either "make" or "buy." This approach assumes that there is a *cash flow*, certain out-of-pocket expenditures associated with the alternative, and that the major elements of this cash flow will lie in easily measured expenses connected directly with the alternative. Under these assumptions, the total operating cost can be measured by taking the sum of the elements:

1. Labor cost—the cost of direct labor used in the alternative
2. Materials cost—the cost of direct supplies used in the alternative
3. Identifiable indirect cost—the costs of indirect labor and supplies involved in preparing for production, cleaning up, direct supervision spoilage, equipment maintenance, and other activities which do not result directly in production, but which are incurred if the alternative is adopted.

There are other elements of the total cost of the alternative which are excluded from the elements above. These are the cost of capital consumed in production and the cost of indirect items, usually called *overhead*, which cannot be related to any specific alternative.

Exact measurement and differentiation of identifiable indirect cost and overhead is usually difficult and estimates must be made. Overhead costs are general costs of business which are assumed to be the same under both alternatives. Therefore they are not relevant to the decision and are ignored in the cash flow. If a cost item can be assigned to an alternative, it is generally better to do so and classify it as an "identifiable" cost rather than "overhead." A typical example is the cost of first line supervision for small production processes. If it is estimated that in-hospital production will require two new employees under a foreman who now supervises eight other persons, it is usually wiser to assign 20 percent of the foreman's time to the cost of production than to assign the foreman's time to overhead. Omitting a cost for foreman's services is the same as assuming that the foreman previously did nothing productive with 20 percent of his time. If this error is repeated five times, supervision will have to be increased by one person to restore the original workloads. Then overhead costs will rise and the total costs of some of the five items may exceed their costs of purchased instead of manufactured.

Direct labor cost measurement is straightforward. The work force required to meet the manufacturing demand is estimated and priced at current or projected wage rates. Both fringe and cash benefits are included. The estimate may be prepared on a variable cost basis of man hours per unit of each level of employee required. In small volume production, however, this is often inaccurate, since a fixed total number of employees must be added to carry out the job. It is best to view the project from the aspect of total annual new payroll, even if a variable cost in man hours per unit is also prepared.

Materials costs can be estimated very closely on a per unit basis. Prices should be based upon current or projected purchase prices, plus shipping and handling costs. Small supply costs can be estimated on an annual basis.

Identifiable indirect costs can be estimated by careful study of the process requirements. In addition to direct supervision, these may include personnel costs on additional personnel (insurance, hiring, etc.), additional housekeeping and equipment maintenance costs, routine spoilage costs, and inventory costs on the finished product. Personnel services costs may be calculated in terms of costs per employee or cost per hour for the new direct labor. This is particularly justified when the change in the work force is relatively large or where there is a large efficient personnel department. In small institutions there are likely to be only a few persons performing these services. Total expenditures are not likely to change for a small change in the work force. If direct labor costs have been calculated on a total hours per year basis, the estimate may already include sufficient time to perform some of these tasks such as make-ready and clean-up. They should not be counted twice, of course. Warehousing and interest costs on the inventory will also be a part of indirect costs. These will depend on the average inventory, in the manner described in the inventory analysis model.

Measurement of direct labor, materials, and indirect costs, while demanding careful analysis and study of the process itself, is a straightforward task. Ways of measuring the actual costs and of preparing the data are presented in textbooks of engineering economics. Some hospital applications are shown in Smalley and Freeman.[1] It is possible to summarize the cost measurement discussion to this point in algebraic terms. For convenience, we will identify the alternative with the greater capital requirement as the "make" or "manufacture" alternative.

If OC_m is the total operating cost if the product is manufactured for an annual demand U:[2]

$$OC_m = F + U\left(\sum_i h_i + \sum_j m_j\right)$$

where F = the sum of all identifiable indirect costs incurred by undertaking manufacture (supervision, labor, etc.)

$\sum_i h_i$ = sum of all variable direct labor costs per unit of product

$$\sum_j m_j = \text{sum of all direct material costs per unit product}$$

The same procedure can be used to establish the operating cost under the "buy" alternative. This can be designated OC_p. The difference between the two will be the total annual cash flow, c:

$$OC_p - OC_m = c \quad .$$

If the capital costs of the "make" alternative are greater, OC_m must be less than OC_p. Otherwise, there would be no reason to make the capital investment. If both capital and operating costs are greater for a given alternative it is obviously rejected.

The future trend of the cash flow is clearly important. Purchase prices can vary substantially, often falling in the case of newly introduced items. If such reductions are anticipated, it is best to calculate the cash flow for each future year. To do this, a separate estimate must be prepared for both terms for each year throughout the anticipated life of the investment. For example, consider an investment for a "make" alternative, with an initial year cash flow savings of $3,000. If the purchase price is expected to drop $1,000 per year, the savings will be:

Year	Cash Flow Savings
1	$3,000
2	2,000
3	1,000
4 and after	0 or less

The project will have a life of only three years. After that time, it will obviously be cheaper to purchase.

Capital Costs

The amount of the additional investment (or where both methods require investment, the amount of each, and difference between the two) must now be calculated. It includes all items of space and equipment which must be purchased or evaluated if they are diverted from other uses. Obviously, any renovation and equipment installation costs must be included. Certain "sunk" costs involved in starting up the manufacturing process can also be included. Costs of special training for personnel, spoilage in initial production, costs of permits or licenses needed, and similar items are among these. For many projects, the cost of additional facilities and equipment will depend on the local situation. Idle space may be available, or equipment may be already in the hospital which will reduce the capital requirement substantially and will greatly increase the rate of return. Thus two hospitals may quite justifiably reach widely different conclusions with regard to capital requirements. Also, once a hospital has made a given investment, it will continue to use its equipment so long as the present value of cash flow exceeds the dollars which could be obtained if the equipment were sold and the space devoted to other uses. A hospital which had already made the investment necessary to manufacture would continue to do so until the value of reversing its investment exceeded its cash flow at present value. This condition would clearly require a much lower purchase price for the "buy" alternative than that which a similar hospital, without the investment, would be willing to pay.

The net investment required will be designated as C. For two alternatives, each requiring investment, C will be the marginal investment $C = C_m - C_p$ where the subscripts m and p designate the alternatives as before. (The order, however, has been reversed. Thus when both c and C have the same sign, the cash flows are in the opposite direction.) The capital investment is a form of cash flow as well. It is a large, lump sum payment, which is returned to the hospital by the savings in cash flow in future years. The decision which must be made has to do with whether these expected future savings justify the investment which is required.

Present Value of Cash Flow

Even if the cash flow return is expected to remain stable over the life of the investment, the value of future earnings is not the same as that of cash actually in hand. The value of $100 a year from now is not $100, but $100 less the amount this money could earn over a year. This amount is, of course, the interest rate on investments, I, which was introduced in the inventory model.

The value of c dollars one year in the future is[a]

$$\frac{c}{(1+I)}$$

and at two years in the future is

$$\frac{c}{(1+I)} \div (1+I) = \frac{c}{(1+I)^2}$$

---

[a]This assumes that the money will be received in a lump sum t periods in the future. The actual earning stream from manufacture is continuous throughout the time periods, but the assumption of discrete intervals is usually acceptable. The continuous income stream formula is ce^{-It} and can be used if desired. Its derivation is beyond the scope of this text.

or at a future time t

$$\frac{c}{(1+I)^t}$$

If the cash flow from the investment is discounted for each year of the life of the investment, and the sum of these years is taken, the total present value is obtained. Under the case of where the expected cash flow is constant, $I = 5$ percent, and the life expected is five years, the current value can be calculated as follows:

Year	Expected Cash Flow	Discount at 5%	Present Value
1	$3,000	$\frac{1}{(1+0.05)} = 0.952$	$ 2,860
2	3,000	$\frac{1}{(1+0.05)^2} = 0.909$	2,730
3	3,000	$\frac{1}{(1+0.05)^3} = 0.862$	2,590
4	3,000	$\frac{1}{(1+0.05)^4} = 0.826$	2,360
5	3,000	$\frac{1}{(1+0.05)^5} = 0.787$	2,480
		Total Present Value	$13,010

In the situation where a variable cash flow is projected, perhaps due to declining market price or to varying annual volumes of use, the present value can be calculated in the same manner:

Year	Expected Cash Flow	Discount at 5%	Present Value
1	$5,000	0.952	$ 4,760
2	4,000	0.909	3,640
3	3,000	0.862	2,590
4	2,000	0.826	1,650
5	1,000	0.787	787
		Total Present Value	$13,427

Although the average annual cash flow for the two projects is the same, ($3,000 per year over the five-year life) the present value of the second project is slightly higher.

The value of the capital investment at the end of the life of the project must also be considered and discounted as indicated above. For example, if the equipment purchased for the project were estimated to have a resale value of $2,000 at the end of the five years, the present value of this would be

$$2{,}000 \times \frac{1}{(1.05)^5} = \$1{,}570$$

at 5 percent interest.

It should be noted that present value of an income stream is affected by the interest rate. At higher interests, dollars to be received in the future are discounted more heavily. Thus at a ten percent interest rate, the difference between the first and second projects is greater; the advantage goes more obviously to the second. Considering the salvage value to be the same in each case, $2,000 after five years, and the interest rate to be 15 percent, the projects can be compared as follows:

	Project 1		Project 2	
Year	Expected Cash Flow	Present Value (I = 15%)	Expected Cash Flow	Present Value (I = 15%)
1	$3,000	$ 2,610	$5,000	$ 4,350
2	3,000	2,268	4,000	3,024
3	3,000	1,974	3,000	1,974
4	3,000	1,716	2,000	1,144
5	3,000	1,494	1,000	497
Salvage	2,000	996	2,000	996
Total present value		$11,058		$11,585

The difference continues to widen. At 5 percent it was $420; at 15 percent $530.

The estimation of the present value of an income stream can be expressed algebraically as:

$$V = \sum_{t=1}^{T} \frac{c_t}{(1+I)^t} + \frac{S}{(1+I)^T},$$

where

V = present value of the cash flow stream
t = time period (usually a year)
T = life of investment
c_t = cash flow in period t
I = interest rate
S = salvage value.

Where c_t is constant (that is cash flow is expected to be the same throughout the project life), these equations reduce to:

$$V = c_t \sum_{t=1}^{T} \frac{1}{(1+I)^t} + \frac{S}{(1+I)^T} .$$

Calculation of the present value is not as difficult as it appears because both the individual terms $1/(1+I)^t$ and the cumulative term

$$\sum_{t=1}^{T} \frac{1}{(1+I)^t}$$

have been tabulated over a wide range of I and T. These tables are appended to this chapter.

Estimating Project Life

Clearly one does not expect the forecasted cash flow to continue forever. Prices change; work volumes change; equipment wears out; processes and equipment are made obsolete. In addition, present values of distant future expenditures are quite small. Discounted at 6 percent, one dollar fifty years from now is worth only five cents now. The life of the investment, which enters the present value calculation as T, is an estimate of how long it will be until the changes in each of these factors have seriously affected the estimates of cash flow.

The selection of the project life, T, is arbitrary at best, but there are some helpful guidelines.

1. For simple, relatively self-contained projects where technology is changing relatively slowly, the accounting (depreciation) life of the shortest-lived major piece of equipment can be used. Examples are power boilers, buildings, laundry and kitchen equipment, etc.
2. In rapidly changing situations where investments in equipment are likely to be outmoded or purchase prices are subject to large changes, a conservative estimate of useful life, usually much less than the accounting life, is appropriate. Examples are computers and medical equipment such as cardiac monitors and dialysis equipment
3. For complex projects involving several major investments of different life, or situations where the capital investment is not a critical feature for the plan, an estimate of reasonable life before one would normally expect to reconsider the decision is in order. In making the estimate it should be remembered that a shorter project life is more conservative; that is, it anticipates recovery of an initial investment in a shorter period of time
4. Particularly in case 3, it may be necessary to allow for the replacement of minor and shorter-lived equipment. Thus, if one alternative were a whole hospital or a major component, a project life of twenty-five to fifty years

would be reasonable. The equipment might have to be replaced every ten years, however, at a significant present value of expenditure.

Using the Net Present Value

A hospital would consider an investment only if it returned at least the original capital. Thus the net present value of the project must equal the investment at some interest rate (greater than zero). To restate this in algebraic terms, where C equals the marginal investment, there must be some interest rate at which $C = V$ if an investment is to be made. But this is the same as

$$C = \sum_{t=1}^{T} \frac{c_t}{(1+I)^t} + \frac{S}{(1+I)^T}.$$

At this point C, c_t, S, and T have been estimated. Despite the formidable difficulties which appear to be involved algebraically, it must be possible to solve this equation for I because I is the only remaining unknown. We shall do this by trial and error, picking a series of interest rates producing values for V both greater and less than C, and finally selecting the value of I which reduces the cash flow stream to a net present value of C. This value is the *internal rate of return* for the project. The tables will clearly be helpful in finding the internal rate of return. It is also a rather simple matter to program a computer to solve the problem.

The meaning of the internal rate of return is easiest to understand in terms of an investment in a mortgage with a fixed maturity date and interest rate. To invest capital in a project with a life T and an interest rate I is equivalent to purchasing a mortgage for the same amount, with the same interest I and a life to maturity of T. If all other factors are equal, the mortgage and the investment are equally desirable. Another analogy is in terms of stock purchase rather than mortgages. This is more realistic because stock purchases, like investments in projects, involve substantial risk. To say that a given project has an investment of $5,000, and an internal rate of return of 10 percent over a five-year life, is the same as saying that it is equal to an opportunity to purchase $5,000 worth of common stocks which will pay $500 per year dividends and which can be sold in five years for $5,000. We can use the present value equation to show that this is exactly so:

where

$c_t = 500$ $S = 5,000$ $T = 5$ $I = 10\%$

then

$$V = 500 \sum_{t=1}^{5} \frac{1}{(1+0.1)^t} + 5{,}000 \frac{1}{(1+0.1)^5}$$

$$\sum_{t=1}^{5} \frac{1}{(1+0.1)^t} = 3.79$$

$$\frac{1}{(1+0.1)^5} = 0.621$$

$$V = 1{,}890 + 3{,}110 = \$5{,}000 \quad .$$

It is now possible to select between any two alternatives. If the interest rate, or the internal rate of return is higher on one, then that is the one we prefer (all other things being equal). If the two rates are the same, we are indifferent. To the extent that we can rely on the assumptions involved, our decision is made for us. The assumptions, to reiterate, are: (a) assumptions in forecasting—stability of process, linearity or nonlinearity, etc. (uncertainty and risk); (b) assumptions in cost estimating—These have to do with reliability of estimates of resource requirements, forecasts of price trends and forecasts of project life (uncertainty and risk); and (c) assumption of monetary values of project—Projects which have nonmonetary values cannot be judged upon their rate of return alone (quality, satisfaction, and intangibles). These factors and one other—the possibility that we should save our money for something better (liquidity)—may lead us to decide that all other factors are *not* equal.

Many of the critical assumptions are elements of risk. That is, there is no quantitative estimating technique other than Bayesian, or subjective, estimates of probability which can be applied. The decision—which may be made by a board of trustees or an administrator—to invest in an opportunity which has a lower rate of return is the same as saying that the risk involved in the assumptions for the higher rate exceeds the gain in expected return. The sensitivity of the rate of return can be tested by systematically revising the assumptions and recalculating the rate. This process is called *sensitivity analysis*, and it is desirable for all major investments which cannot be easily reversed. An example can be found by looking at the demand forecast. Many manufacturing processes are highly sensitive to demand changes. While the cost of purchase usually increases nearly linearly with quantity, the cost of manufacture may be an erratic, discontinuous function reflecting manpower and equipment limits. If there is uncertainty about the demand forecast, several possibilities can be tried, and the impact upon the rate of return measured. In this way, the sensitivity of the rate to the assumption can be determined. If the rate is insensitive, there is little risk attributable to this factor, even though the forecast may be very crude. Perhaps the crudeness of the forecast, however, would not deter a rational investor from making the investment.

Example

The following example will serve to review the analysis of present value and rate of return.[b]

A hospital of 200 beds purchases steam from its local power company. It has no power plant of its own, although land is available for constructing one. This land was set aside at the time the hospital was built and has since been unused. Currently, about 2,000,000 pounds of steam are purchased monthly, at $3.475 per 1000 pounds. However, because of air pollution control measures, the power company has announced an increase of $0.25 per 1000 pounds. At this price, the question is raised as to whether the hospital should produce its own heat.

After considerable discussion with architects and engineers the following proposal is developed for building and operating a power plant:

I. Capital investment
   A. Building
       2500 square foot building with stack, 75-year life $37,500
   B. Equipment
       1. 3 boilers and associated equipment   51,000
       2. Repiping and installation costs   32,500
       3. Total, 25-year life $83,500
   C. Salvage
       1. Building and stack will have no value at end of life
       2. Scrap metal value of the boilers will equal the cost of removing them

II. Operating Costs
   A. Labor and Supervision
      State law requires 24-hour coverage by licensed stationary engineers. An assistant chief hospital engineer will cover absences when necessary and will supervise the operators
      1. 4 Lic. St. Engrs. $31,200 p.a.
         $650/mth × 4 × 12

---

[b]Costs for this and all subsequent projects are hypothetical.

2. Supervision
   520 hrs/yr × $4.25/hr   2,200 p.a.
3. Fringe benefits @ 12%   4,000 p.a.
B. Supplies
   1. Fuel—natural gas
      6.5 million cubic ft./mth at $460/million cubic ft.
      6.5 × $460 × 12 $36,000 p.a.
   2. Other supplies   2,500 p.a.
C. Total annual operating costs $75,900 p.a.

The costs of the current system are found to be the cost of steam purchased, $84,200 from invoices for the last 12 months, plus supervision of the contract, including review of volume and pressure metering. This is estimated to take one-tenth of the time of the assistant chief engineer, or $900 per year. There is no inventory, of course, and production is continuous rather than batch.

$$OC_P = 84,200 + 900 = \$85,100$$
$$OC_M = \$75,900$$

under present conditions. If an increase of $.25/1000 pounds is imposed, at 24,000,000 pounds per year:

$$OC_P' = 85,100 + 6,000 = \$91,100$$
$$c = OC_P' - OC_M = \$15,200$$

Future cost increases in steam are expected to parallel those in stationary engineer wages, so that the revised value of c will remain approximately constant. The life of the major portion of the investment is twenty-five years. At the end of this period, the salvage value of the boiler room building will be two-thirds its construction cost, or $25,000.

Using the formula

$$C = V = \sum_{t=1}^{T} \left(\frac{c_t}{(1+I)^t} \right) + \frac{S}{(1+I)^T} \quad ,$$

$S = \$25,000$

$T = 25$ years

$C = \$121,000$

or

$$121{,}000 = 15{,}200 \sum_{t=1}^{25}\left(\frac{1}{(1+I)^t}\right) + 25{,}000 \left(\frac{1}{(1+I)^{25}}\right).$$

Evaluating the terms for several different interest rates, I:

I	$\sum_{t=1}^{25}\left(\frac{1}{(1+I)^t}\right)$	$\frac{1}{(1+I)^{25}}$	V
6	12.78	0.233	$200,081
10	9.08	0.092	140,316
15	6.46	0.030	98,942

shows that the rate lies between 10% and 15%.

Continuing the trial and error solution shows that the rate is 12 percent:

12	7.84	0.059	120,643
14	6.87	0.038	105,374

This rate of return is relatively high compared to most securities investments. One would rarely find a bond paying 12 percent over twenty-five years unless the risk associated with it were quite high. Similarly even a portfolio of common stocks managed for maximum gain would not be likely to do this well over a twenty-five-year span. Compared to other investment opportunities within the hospital, the investment may not be so desirable. Other capital opportunities—new equipment or facilities—may have a higher rate of return in dollars.

The risk of the boiler room investment appears relatively low. Changes in fuel prices and labor are likely to reflect equally in both opportunities, since the power company must also buy fuel and hire stationary engineers. The only element which it seems necessary to investigate in terms of sensitivity is the capital requirement. Possibly a small increase in usage will require a fourth boiler. Including a larger boiler house and necessary additional equipment, this may increase the original investment as much as one-third. Such a condition seems to be the worst revision likely to occur in the project. It would increase capital costs to $160,000. Reviewing the present value of savings, this investment would have a rate of return slightly more than 8 percent:

$$I = 8\%$$

$$\sum_{t=1}^{25}\left(\frac{1}{1+I}\right)^t = 10.67$$

$$\frac{1}{(1 + I)^{25}} = 0.146$$

$$V = \$165,800$$

Making the Investment Decision

If the cost estimates and calculations above were complete and perfectly accurate, the final decision on any investment opportunity would be clear. The opportunities would be ranked according to their internal rate of return, the highest rate being the most desirable. One alternative use which should be considered for the capital is an investment in securities. Such an investment has a well understood rate of return. Brokers, trust companies, or other financial advisors can generally make an accurate estimate of expected earnings. Suppose that several opportunities have been evaluated, including the example of the power plant, and that the investment portfolio has been estimated at 7 percent. There is a rank ordered list as follows:

>Project A—17%
>Project B—12% (power plant example)
>Project C—8%
>Securities—7%
>Project D—3%

Project D is clearly undesirable; it would be preferable to invest in securities. Under the assumptions of complete and accurate information, projects A, B, and C are desirable, and available funds should be invested in them, beginning with A.

To carry the example further, presume that the available funds are insufficient. The opportunities are not foreclosed, however. It may still be possible to borrow capital for the project. Loans from banks, insurance companies, bonding through governmental agencies, and other borrowing sources are available to hospitals. These agencies are willing to quote a price and terms to lend money. Their quotation is based upon the financial condition of the institution as a whole, in addition to the specific projects for which the money will be used and other factors. The interest rate which they quote can be compared to the remaining opportunities:

>Project A—17%
>Project B—12% (power plant example)
>Interest on Loan—9%
>Project C—8%
>Securities—7%

Project C now becomes undesirable. The cost of borrowing money to complete it would exceed its value. Projects A and B are desirable however and could be funded. Securities would be sold first, foregoing a revenue of 7 percent. Then loans would be arranged for the balance.

Evaluating Intangible Factors

The assumptions of complete and accurate estimates on the projects are not often met. If nothing else, the assumptions of forecasting are involved. Often the degree of risk associated with these is quite high. There are factors which are difficult to reduce to dollar terms for including in the equations for cost. The impact on employee morale, improvements in quality of service or product, better service to patients and other elements may be involved in some projects even though their primary benefit lies in dollar savings. Finally, there is a third group of intangible elements in the decision. Is the amount of funds borrowed excessive, in view of the hospitals overall financial situation? Are there other potential opportunities which may be foreclosed before they are fully investigated by using borrowing ability and assets for these projects? These considerations can be summarized under the term liquidity. *Liquidity* is measured by the availability of cash to finance new opportunities. The more projects which are adapted at any given time, the greater the loss of liquidity will be.

The combination of these factors—risk, elements which are difficult to evaluate monetarily, and liquidity—must be weighed by the board in its decision. There are techniques for improving the understanding of these elements and even for reducing many of them to quantitative terms. These techniques, however, are beyond the scope of this text; also, as a practical matter, many small capital investments will not justify such elaborate analysis. In any case, the board will inevitably place a value on these factors. Continuing the example, assume that board has authorized project A, at 17 percent but has declined to authorize project B at 12 percent, even though the interest rate to borrow money is only 9 percent. This decision is the same as saying that the value of all the intangible factors—risk that a fourth boiler may be needed, possible loss of reliability which may come from having small boilers on the site as opposed to purchasing from a larger, more flexible supply, loss of the ability to use the land on which the power house will stand, and the reduction of liquidity by $121,000—is equal to 3 percent or greater. The net internal rate of return, after adjustment for these factors, is equal to or less than the borrowing rate of 9 percent. Alternatively, if the board decides to authorize the power plant expenditure, their judgment implies that the net rate of return is still greater than 9 percent. The intangibles, therefore, are evaluated at less than 3 percent.

The fact that either decision inevitably assigns a value to the intangible elements permits a different viewpoint toward the alternative in question.

Instead of considering simply the decision to accept or reject the project, the value implicitly assigned to the intangibles can be considered in itself. Since many people have some personal notions of the worth of these items, they can compare the implicit value against those notions and thereby gain more consistent and rational decisions. This opens the opportunity to consider projects which consist largely or entirely of intangibles. Methods of doing this will be explored in the next section, on cost-benefit analysis.

Cost-Benefit Analysis

The preceding section develops techniques for evaluating decisions which require both capital and operating funds, and which can be evaluated primarily on the basis of their monetary return. For hospitals, there are many investment opportunities which do not fit this model. Their principal benefit may come in their contribution to health itself. The exact value of this contribution is very difficult to measure directly in dollar terms. Yet these opportunities compete for the scarce resources of the institution, and decisions must inevitably be made between both types. Techniques for clarifying the implications of primarily nonmonetary decisions are called *cost-benefit analysis*, and will be reviewed here.[c]

Need for Cost-Benefit Analysis

The notion of the internal rate of return of an investment has a great deal more usefulness for a firm operating for profit in a partially competitive market than it does for hospitals. One possibility lies in evaluating a new product. This product will have a predictable sales, depending on its price and other factors, and it will require a predictable capital investment and operating costs. The revenue generated by sales minus the operating costs will constitute a cash flow stream which can be equated to the capital requirements to calculate a rate of return. On that basis, various opportunities can be ranked and selected.

When hospitals wish to add a new health service, two factors prevent their using the internal rate of return on investment directly. First, they are rarely interested in cash-flow maximization alone. They wish instead to gain some return in terms of patient service. Second and related to the first, there is usually no market place in which the price can be set and the demand tested. This comes about from a number of causes, but the most striking is the widespread use of cost-based reimbursement contracts. These are designed to reimburse hospitals for their actual cash expenditures, with various arrangements for additional

---

[c]The term "cost-effectiveness" is used by some authors for the same or a closely related process.

payment for the capital costs and other items. Where the payment is accurately calculated to cover exactly cash-flow costs and straight-line depreciation, the capitalization of the difference between revenue and expenses over the life of the project will yield the initial capital cost at zero interest. Thus use of the formula for internal rate of return will lead to no investment in new services. If some form of overpayment above this level is included, the result is a completely arbitrary rate of return which depends on the basis for the overpayment calculation rather than the nature of the product at hand.[d] The charge which hospitals attach to a service is no better as an investment guideline. It is usually set quite arbitrarily, and often related neither to the cost of the service nor the value which customers might be willing to pay for it.

Many other organizations than hospitals share this condition. Nonprofit organizations such as churches and social service agencies clearly attempt to maximize other returns than monetary ones in their efforts. Governmental agencies often must decide between alternatives which do not generate any revenues. It is sometimes suggested that the services offered by agencies such as these do have monetary value and that with effort, the dollar value can be measured. In practice, however, efforts to measure the value of health lead to disputable results. So many assumptions reflecting basic social attitudes are required and so many possibilities of action and reaction exist that the estimates become simply arbitrary reflections of the viewpoint of the estimator. A more practical way to assess the results of a given investment is necessary. Cost-benefit analysis permits the institution to substitute for dollar value estimates of achievement in direct measures: lives saved, persons restored to health, or educated, or similar measures.

The problem to be aided by cost-benefit analysis can be summarized by saying that the management of an institution must have means for deciding the relative worth of several opportunities for investment which vary in: (a) the operating costs they will incur, (b) the capital investments they will require, and (c) the kind of benefit they will give. The following sections will develop the cost-benefit approach, beginning with the data collection and analysis necessary for a single project, moving to the comparison of alternatives within a single hospital showing the relationship between monetary benefit and nonmonetary benefit projects and finally considering comparisons of opportunities for several hospitals serving a community.

Cost Evaluation

As in the case of cash-flow investment opportunities, it is necessary to develop schedules of:

---

[d]The formula used for many years by Michigan Blue Cross, repayment of 102 percent of costs, results in an automatic rank ordering of projects by the ratio of operating to capital expense, which is absurdly irrelevant.

1. The annual operating expenses of the program, year by year if significant yearly variation is expected
2. The capital requirement for the program, also in the yearly form, if capital expenditures extend over several years
3. The expected life of the program or the capital investment

These budgets require a careful estimate of the demand for the service in question. Definitions and measurement of the various elements are exactly as described for cash-flow analysis. The project life or the life of the capital investment is sometimes more difficult to define. In general, the shorter life is the one which should be used unless the project is expected to be continued indefinitely. In this case, the life of the major element of the capital investment (often the building) should be selected.

Table 9-1 shows an example of a project at this stage. Annual cash flow expenditures as forecast for each year of the expected life (forty years) are shown for a proposed ambulatory care facility. Unlike the powerhouse proposal, the expenditures are not viewed as constant. This is frequently the case with large projects, whether their benefits are principally monetary or not. While this may complicate the calculations involved, it does not alter the approach to the problem. In this proposal the operating costs remain relatively constant once construction is finished. Capital must be added periodically throughout the project life. A variety of equipment is necessary, which is expected to require replacement at intervals of five to ten years. Extensive renovation is expected to be required at about ten year intervals. All expenses connected with the building will be capital for the first two years, while the building is under construction, and less than the full operating expense is anticipated during the third year. Thereafter: $270,000 per year except in the years 21, 22, 31 and 32, when $320,000 expenses will be incurred due to renovations.

In order to compare two different proposals, it is necessary to reduce the time distributions of expenditures such as the one shown in table 9-1 to a common basis. This can be done using the discounting formula previously noted, with minor adjustments.

$$V = \sum_{t=1}^{T} \frac{c_t}{(1+I)^t} - \frac{S}{(1+I)^T}$$

In this case, c_t will be the annual cash expenditure, shown in the right hand column of table 9-1. The salvage value, S, will be a return of cash. The formula has been adjusted for this by making the sign of any cash return negative. If V is positive, it will measure a net cash out flow.

Interest Rate. In order to apply this formula, it is necessary to make some assumption regarding the interest rate. Although this decision remains arbitrary

Table 9-1
Schedule of Expenses for Ambulatory Patient Facility

Year	Building	Equipment	Operating	Total
1	10,000	–	–	10,000
2	600,000	20,000	–	620,000
3	400,000	80,000	75,000	555,000
4	–	–	250,000	250,000
5	–	–	250,000	250,000
6	–	–	250,000	250,000
7	–	10,000	250,000	260,000
8	–	20,000	250,000	270,000
9	–	20,000	250,000	270,000
10	–	20,000	250,000	270,000
11	50,000	20,000	250,000	320,000
12	50,000	20,000	250,000	320,000

to some extent, it can be improved by reviewing the meaning of the interest rate and the implications of the selection. Interest is a measure of the alternative earning of capital, the amount which could be gained if it were invested in other projects than the one under study. As such it permits management to compare expenditures in two different years. For example, the $320,000 expenditure necessary in the eleventh year is less important than the same amount would be at the start of the project. A much smaller amount of money, if invested at the start of the project, would earn a large share of the $320,000 by the eleventh year. The discount formula allows this fact to be taken into account. The degree to which it is taken into account is adjusted by the interest rate I.

Although most economists agree that there should be some value of interest, there is little agreement on exactly what it should be in nonprofit applications. For profit-oriented firms where a cash flow can be capitalized, the rate should be the rate of earnings available to the firm. It can be shown that any other rate is inconsistent and leads to illogical conclusions. For hospitals and similar ventures, the best equivalent may be the earnings of investments in securities. Rates from 2 to 10 percent have been used for similar purposes.[3] Some approaches to the cost-benefit problem propose or imply a zero rate, as well.

The zero interest case simplifies the calculations and also permits a demonstration of the impact of the rate on the decision process. When $I = O$, the equation reduces to

$$V = \sum_{t=1}^{T} c_t - S ,$$

which is simply the total expected expense over the life of the project less any return from the salvage of capital. No allowance is made for differing years of expenditures. If the total cost obtained in this way is divided by the project life, the resulting average cost is the same as the accounting cost including depreciation under the straight-line method, assuming that no funds are borrowed for the project.

The possibility of borrowing funds suggests the difficulty inherent in the zero interest assumption. Clearly the borrowed money will not be obtained at zero interest. Costs which previously have not been accounted for will be incurred and must be included in the decision in some way. They might be put into the expected operating costs of the project. This creates an inequity, however. In most situations, whether or not the project is financed on borrowed funds depends not on the project itself but on the financial position of the hospital as a whole. Borrowing depends upon the total capital needs of the institution and not upon the single project. Thus if one project is weighted with the cost of borrowed money and another not, an inaccurate and misleading presentation results. Clearly, all projects should bear their share of the cost of funds. This can be done quite quickly and equitably by adopting an interest rate greater than zero.

An individual hospital considering its capital investment opportunities might select either of two rates: (a) the historic earning rate on its own investments, or (b) its own borrowing rate, which it would expect to pay for capital. These rates vary depending upon national economic conditions as well as the financial strength of the institution. The borrowing rates for leading firms and governments have been as low as 2.6 percent (in 1947)[4] and as high as 8 percent in 1969. There is some feeling that the "normal" rate is about 4 or 5 percent. Upward fluctuations are caused by inflation and downward ones by recessions. Rates of four or five percent are frequently selected for generalized cases. They are not applicable for any specific situation, however. The hospital must seek financial advice on its own rate.

It is desirable for the discount rate on all long-term projects to be consistent. *Ad hoc* rates for particular projects and differing rates reflecting short-run market conditions should be avoided. The hospital's credit position as a whole should be considered in determining the rate, and rates averaged over one to three years should generally be used for purposes of analysis, rather than unusual peak or bargain rates caused by market variation. It is not necessary for the long-term borrowing rate to be the same as the short-term rate which the hospital would pay to obtain working capital in a temporary situation. Short-run rates will often be higher than long-term situations.

Project Life. As noted above, it is often difficult to select a project life. This is particularly true for large, long-term health service projects. The life is often indeterminate. A building, for example, will last from thirty to fifty years, and the exact life is unknown. The future cost of maintenance or renovation is also unknown. It is possible that a sound structure will still have economic value for the original purpose or for some entirely different purpose at the end of the project life, yet attempting to estimate this value is highly speculative. In addition, many hospital investments are in programs which are expected to last indefinitely, or until the benefit of a given mode of treatment disappears. However, the formula requires a specific estimate of the project life.

The result of discounting is such that the total present cost of a project is relatively insensitive to small errors in the project life and in budgeting in distant periods. The discounted values of the project described in table 9-1 are shown in table 9-2 at 4 and 6 percent interest. In either case the present value of a single

Table 9-2
Discounted Values of Expenses for Ambulatory Patient Facility ($T = 40$ Years, $I = 4\%, 6\%$)

		At 4%		At 6%	
Year	Expense (000)	Discount	Present Value (000)	Discount	Present Value (000)
1	$ 10.0	.9615	$ 9.6	.9434	$ 9.4
2	620.0	.9246	573.2	.8900	551.8
3	555.0	.8890	493.4	.8396	466.0
4	250.0	.8548	213.7	.7921	198.0
5	250.0	.8219	205.5	.7473	186.8
6	250.0	.7903	197.6	.7050	176.2
7	260.0	.7599	197.6	.6651	172.9
8	270.0	.7307	197.3	.6274	169.4
9	270.0	.7026	189.7	.5919	159.8
10	270.0	.6756	182.4	.5584	150.8
11	320.0	.6496	207.9	.5268	168.6
12	320.0	.6246	199.9	.4970	159.0
13	270.0	.6006	162.2	.4688	126.6
14	270.0	.5775	155.9	.4423	119.4
15	270.0	.5553	149.9	.4173	112.7
16	270.0	.5339	144.2	.3936	106.3
17	270.0	.5134	138.6	.3714	100.3
18	270.0	.4936	133.3	.3503	94.6
19	270.0	.4746	128.2	.3305	89.2
20	270.0	.4564	123.2	.3118	84.2
21	320.0	.4388	140.4	.2942	94.1
22	320.0	.4220	135.0	.2775	88.8
23	270.0	.4057	109.5	.2618	70.7
24	270.0	.3901	105.3	.2470	66.7
25	270.0	.3751	101.3	.2330	62.9
26	270.0	.3607	97.4	.2198	59.3
27	270.0	.3468	93.6	.2074	56.0
28	270.0	.3335	90.0	.1956	52.8
29	270.0	.3207	86.6	.1846	49.8
30	270.0	.3083	83.2	.1741	47.0

Table 9-2 (Cont.)

Year	Expense (000)	At 4% Discount	At 4% Present Value (000)	At 6% Discount	At 6% Present Value (000)
31	320.0	.2965	94.9	.1643	52.6
32	320.0	.2851	91.2	.1550	49.6
33	270.0	.2741	74.0	.1462	39.5
34	270.0	.2636	71.2	.1379	37.2
35	270.0	.2534	68.4	.1301	35.1
36	270.0	.2437	65.8	.1227	33.1
37	270.0	.2343	63.3	.1158	31.3
38	270.0	.2253	60.8	.1092	29.5
39	270.0	.2166	58.5	.1031	27.8
40	270.0	.2083	56.2	.0972	26.3
Total	$11,405.0		$5,749.8		$4,412.2

year in the building life falls to less than 1 percent of the total by the fortieth year. For the ambulatory care project, a sensitivity analysis of five and ten-year errors in T reveals the following.

At = 4%

Percentage of Error Relative to $T = 40$

T	V	$\Delta V/V$
40	5750	—
35	5446	5.6%
30	5046	14.0%

At = 6%

Percentage of Error Relative to $T = 40$

T	V	$\Delta V/V$
40	4412	—
35	4264	3.5%
30	4050	8.9%

Errors in the other direction (that is, if the project actually lasts longer than forty years) will be smaller. For long projects at usual interest rates, the estimated life is a relatively insensitive element. In order to be conservative in estimating the average cost at present value, it is desirable to set T at the lower end of the reasonable life of the longest-lived major capital investment.

Benefit Evaluation

Savings of Alternative Means of Care. Occasionally it will be possible to measure dollar benefits from a new hospital service directly. Usually this occurs when the proposed service is in part a substitute for another and more expensive method of treatment. Home care programs are one example of this type. Nursing home or extended care facility beds could be another, in certain situations. In these cases, it is possible to revert to evaluating the cash-flow stream in the manner suggested for monetary projects. The results are often impressive. For example, studies of home care indicate that capital outlays are modest, and that well-managed programs can keep operating expenses at a reasonable level. It is also reasonably well substantiated that about one-fourth of the patients on home care would require hospitalization if the program were not available. In a 400 bed hospital, demand might be present for a home care program of 250 admissions per year and 32 patients average census. Such a program might require a capital investment as low as $10,000 to refurnish a small office. Operating expenses could be expected to average $46,000 per year, after the first year when referral rates are low.

The savings from the program are more difficult to estimate. The program would reduce the present average census of the hospital by eight patients. If demand is present for additional hospital services, the eight available beds will permit about 300 new admissions per year through the combined system. Since the hospital census stays the same, the operating cost should remain the same. The total savings is the value of treating 300 additional admissions under the previous system, minus the costs of the home care program. If the previous cost per admission had been $500, the value of home care in an average year would be:

$$OC_1 - OC_2 = \$500 \times 300 - \$46,000$$
$$= \$150,000 - \$46,000 = \$104,000,$$

where OC_1 is the cost necessary to process 300 patients through the acute facility. Capitalized at 4 percent over ten years, this savings is

$$V = \sum_{t=1}^{10} \frac{104,000}{(1 + 0.04)^t} = \$843,544$$

Alternatively, looking at the internal rate of return for $10,000 yields

$$10,000 = 104,000 \sum_{t=1}^{10} \frac{1}{(1 + I)^t}$$

$$\frac{10{,}000}{104{,}000} = 0.096 = \sum_{t=1}^{10} \frac{1}{(1+I)^t} \quad ,$$

indicating a rate of return greater than 50 percent.

It should be noted that the problems of evaluating revenues have been avoided. The costs have been compared to the savings in alternative expenditures which were avoided. In this case, the home care expenditure was compared to the alternative cost of caring for the additional patients, conservatively estimated at present average cost per admission. This estimation effectively reduced the problem to monetary terms.

Other Cases. In many cases, dollar savings from the substitution of a new program for other means of care cannot be measured or will not be sufficient in themselves to equal the present value of costs. The benefits which are expected must then be quantified in some other way. Generally speaking, the benefits lie in improved health, reduced suffering, and the prolongation of life. It is not possible to assign economic value to these benefits in the context of hospital care in modern nations. The clearest illustration of this point lies in the economic value of life-saving among retired persons. Economically, a life saved among the retired has a negative value.[5] It permits further expenditures of Social Security funds for both pensions and health care, and creates the possibility of a long period of severe economic dependency. On economic grounds, no project which resulted in life saving among this group of people would be financed. This conclusion is morally unacceptable. Obviously other criteria will have to be determined.

The criteria should attempt to reflect values other than monetary contributions or earnings and should be sufficiently flexible to allow for other results than simply extra years of life. Individuals and societies are likely to disagree on the exact criteria and specific applications, but it would appear that the benefits of a given project can be estimated on three major scales: (a) the number of people who will benefit, (b) the degree to which they will benefit, and (c) the characteristics of the people who will benefit. To illustrate, almost everyone would agree that if everything else were equal:

1. If two projects both prevented a fatal illness, the one which reached the larger number of people at the same cost would be better
2. If two projects reached the same number of people at the same cost, but one prevented a disease while the other simply made the disease nonfatal, the former would be preferred
3. If two projects both prevented fatal illness as in the same number of persons at the same cost, but one prevented a disease in children and young adults while the other prevented a disease occurring only among the aged, the former would be preferred

It is also clear that at a given cost, the best possibility is in disease prevention in large numbers of the young, while the worst is in temporary relief of fatal conditions in a few of the very old. Beyond that, little can be said. Decision must be made on the basis of individual proposals. Estimates relative to these three factors can easily be made, at least on a subjective basis, and they form a worthwhile part of a long-term investment proposal.

The number of patients who are likely to benefit from a proposal are closely related to the estimated demand. In many cases, such as the ambulatory facility discussed above, it is reasonable to assume that all who come will benefit. The total demand will be a measure of those benefitting. For example, if the ambulatory facility described in table 9-1 were constructed, it might accommodate 12,000 patients per year. For some the facility may be of no benefit; for others it may be life-saving. For most it will result in some intermediate degree of relief of disease. On the other hand, a proposal for facilities for specialized surgery such as organ transplants might be valueless in half the cases attempted although it is life-saving in the other half. In such cases only half the demand should be counted as benefitting.

The characteristics of patients are more difficult to conceptualize. Income and status are sometimes important, and economic value shows a distinct variation by education. Most people would agree that extreme efforts are desirable to preserve the life of the president of the United States, but few would support more general distinctions in this direction. Only age seems acceptable, and that within very broad limits. The young adult has the highest economic value, reflecting substantial investments which have been made in his rearing. Most societies also place high values on the life of young children.

The kind of benefit can be crudely characterized according to the following scale:

—Partial improvement in health or alleviation of disease
—Full restoration of health
—Disease prevention, nonfatal disease
—Life-saving, with disability
—Life-saving, with full recovery
—Disease prevention, fatal disease

Even this classification will be disputed. It is based on two assumptions: (a) to save a life is always better than to maintain or restore health, and (b) to prevent disease is always better than to cure it. It is easy to conceive of cases where these assumptions are inapplicable.

Summary

A given proposal for a health care investment can be crudely summarized by five measures, one of cost and four of benefit.

—The present value of annual expenditures
—The savings in expenditures of alternative means of care

—The number of persons who will benefit
—The age of persons benefitting
—The kind of benefit which will occur

Often it will be impossible to summarize a benefit in a single word, but a comment of a few sentences should indicate the expected benefits in terms of the dimensions given. The following illustration will serve to summarize the process of cost-benefit evaluation. The process of making the decisions, once these data are prepared, will be discussed in the following section.

Example

A hospital of 400 beds has had four major patient care projects proposed in the past several months. The hospital currently has an occupancy of 85 percent. Another large hospital in the same town has a much lower occupancy, and for that reason, proposals to invest in additional acute beds have been deferred. These projects, therefore, tend to ambulatory care programs.

Ambulatory Care Facility. It is proposed that an ambulatory care facility be constructed adjacent to the hospital to permit convenient office practice for full-time members of the medical staff and also to provide additional opportunities for postgraduate medical education. This facility will include 30,000 square feet in total, at a construction cost of $1,000,000. It will provide offices for up to fifteen physicians which will allow service to 60,000 visits per year. This volume of visits indicates about 12,000 to 15,000 patients each year. Consideration has been given to the possibility that the proposed facility will save inpatient beds, but it is concluded that there is insufficient evidence to justify assuming such a savings. The facility will serve a broad spectrum of the community, with a varying degree of success. Operating costs are estimated at $250,000 per year. A schedule of costs over the forty year life of the project is shown in table 9-1. The discounted present value of these costs is $5,749,800 at 4 percent.

Home Care Program. A program of organized home care is proposed which will require only moderate capital investment: $9,000 to renovate and equip a small office. This investment has an estimated life of ten years. Annual operating costs will be $46,000 per year once the program has been established. The program will benefit 250 persons per year directly, but it will result in freeing an average of eight hospital beds which will permit treatment of 300 new admissions each year. Since the average cost of treating these patients would be $500 each, the home care program will save $150,000 annually, less its operating cost.[e] Other

---

[e]This conclusion is based on the assumption that demand is present for beds at this hospital while not at the other hospital. Although the disparity in occupancy rates indicates that the assumption is correct, some interesting questions are raised about the savings from a total community viewpoint.

benefits will be limited. The patients tend to be elderly and the results of home care are supportive and palliative for most patients.

Dental Clinic. In the poorer areas of town, good dental care is almost totally lacking. A proposal has been made to establish a dental clinic through the hospital which will serve 1,200 families. About 6,000 persons will be served, most of them children or young adults. Stress will be upon prevention of loss of teeth through dental hygiene and prompt attention to caries. A small clinic space will be required, at a cost of $36,000. The major capital cost will be $104,000 for equipment. The life of this is expected to be ten years. Operating costs will be $160,000 per year.

Kidney Dialysis Unit. Patients with total renal failure are few in number, but they die unless transplants or mechanical substitutes for their kidneys are available. It is estimated that there are over thirty deaths per year in the city due to this cause at ages ranging from fifteen upward. Most of these patients can be kept alive by biweekly dialysis. The results are generally good; patients are able to work and live nearly normal lives. An inpatient facility can be designed to handle thirty patients at a cost of $63,000. Operating costs will be $156,000 per year. Most equipment will last ten years although some items must be replaced earlier at a cost of $4,000 in the fifth year.

The proposals, and their costs are summarized in table 9-3. Costs have been discounted at 4 percent. Because a debatable assumption regarding demand for beds has been made in calculating the savings from home care, both the net annual cost and the present value of cash expenditures have been shown. Table 9-3 does clarify the alternatives. Despite its low capital investment, kidney dialysis is clearly the worst opportunity on a cost per beneficiary basis. If the value of benefits per person in each facility is considered equal, then the cost per person per year, at present value, is:

Ambulatory facility	$ 12.00
Dental clinic	24.00
Home care (cost only)	152.00
Kidney dialysis	4,420.00

The ambulatory facility is clearly the preferred choice on this limited ground, with the dental clinic close behind. If the savings assumption for home care is accepted, the home care program becomes the first choice.

Sensitivity Analysis. Table 9-4 shows the impact of varying interest rate. Only the ambulatory facility is seriously affected. At interests of 4 or 6 percent it is markedly more attractive than the dental clinic. At 0 percent the present cost per beneficiary is $23 for the ambulatory facility and $29 for the dental clinic.

Table 9-3
Comparison of New Program Activities

(1)	(2)	(3)	(4)	(5)	(6)	(7)	(8)	(9)
Name	Life	Initial Capital	Annual Operating Cost	Present Value at $I = 4\%$ [a]	Average Annual Savings	Persons Benefitting Per Year	Cost per Beneficiary [b]	Comments
Ambulatory	40	$1,110,000	$250,000	$5,749,000	—	12,000	$12.00	Benefits are varied, both in age and kind. Facility will be helpful to teaching program
Home care	10	9,000	46,000	382,000	$150,000	250	152.00	Supportive care of the aged and convalescense of some middle-aged and young. Frees 8 beds/day, permitting 300 additional admissions per year. This saving yields return in excess of 50%
Dental care	10	140,000	160,000	1,438,000	—	6,000	24.00	Preventive dental care, heavy emphasis on young welfare recipients
Kidney dialysis	10	63,000	156,000	1,328,000	—	30	4,420.00	Life-saving benefit, with nearly (80%) total recovery of function

[a] Equals Capital Cost + Discounted Operating Costs
[b] Column 5 ÷ (Col. 2 × Col. 7)

Table 9-4
Net Present Cost per Beneficiary at Varying Interest

	0%	4%	6%
Ambulatory facility	$ 23.	$ 12.	$ 9.
Dental clinic	29.	24.	22.
Home care (costs)	187.	152.	139.
Kidney dialysis	5,410.	4,420.	4,040.

This reflects the weighting of near-term expenses for capital equally with heavy operating expenses. When the latter are discounted, the relative position of the ambulatory facility improves.

In view of the closeness of the cost of the dental and ambulatory proposals, it might be desirable to compare them on the same life, by extending the estimates of costs of the dental clinic to a forty year basis. The average operating cost for the remaining period will remain the same, but a regular influx of capital will be necessary to maintain the equipment. The same is true of the ambulatory facility, and the budgeted expenses have been tabulated and discounted in table 9-2. A similar procedure for the dental clinic yields total costs for forty years at present value of $3,450,000 at 4 percent, $2,648,000 at 6 percent. Under this assumption, the value at varying interest for the two projects remains nearly proportional. The sensitivity to interest rate has largely disappeared.

Net Present Cost Per Beneficiary
Dental Clinic Project Extended to Forty Year Life

Interest	Dental	Ambulatory
0%	$29.	$23.
4%	$14.	$12.
6%	$11.	$ 9.

This ambulatory clinic's advantage over the dental clinic holds up under sensitivity analysis regarding both interest and project life, although as the cost of capital increases, the advantage declines.

Although the analysis of cost and benefit is helpful, it does not fully answer the important question, "Which of these proposals should be accepted?" A method of reaching the decision, and thereby fixing the hospital's capital budget, is discussed in the following section.

Capital Budgeting Decisions

By developing careful budgets of proposed operating expenditures, potential savings, and capital requirements, and by describing the nature of health benefits, a hospital can prepare an orderly summary of the opportunities before it. By using the discounting formula

$$\sum_{t=1}^{T} \frac{c_t}{(1-I)^t}$$

the differences between capital and operating expenses can be reduced to a single value. Where the opportunity results in net cash inflow to the hospital, the value of this can be stated relative to the investment required. A serious management problem remains; to select which, if any, of these opportunities are "worth" the investment. The amounts of resources for capital and for operating expense are limited. Although all cost-saving projects which earn more than the return the hospital could get on securities, and all projects which save lives or improve health are presumably desirable, the hospital and the community in which it operates must select between competing projects of diverse kinds of benefits. Theoretically any monetary project which earns more than the interest rate at which the necessary capital could be borrowed should be undertaken; practically the solution is not so simple. Nonmonetary factors such as the load upon credit resources, the load upon management, the public or employee reaction to the project, and the availability of critical skilled manpower must be taken into account. In addition there is the possibility that some other unit in the community could provide the same benefit at lower cost. In short the calculations of present value and internal rate of return are aids to decision making, rather than decision makers.

Hospital Planning Committee

A systematic method of handling the decision would be one which prepares the quantifiable aspects of each opportunity (in the manner described in the preceding sections) and refers the final decision to a broadly constituted management group. This group should be a subcommittee of the board of trustees and should include strong trustee representation because the decisions it faces are directly concerned with the future of the institution. Medical and nursing advice will be necessary to reach many decisions. Both these professions should be represented. The development of detailed knowledge of the opportunities and of the coordination of many different kinds of activities and services is the job of administration (along with the assistance of various departments of the hospital). Administration should have a representative on the committee in addition to its role as committee staff. The functions of personnel and finance may also be represented. Trustee representation should include some overlap with the finance committee of the board.

Such a committee might function by receiving and encouraging proposals for new opportunities and by being acquainted with them both before and after their detailed investigation and evaluation. Periodically the committee must rank order the projects available to it and propose expenditures of capital funds for some or all of these. As a subcommittee of the board, its proposals should be in the form of recommendation for the full board. Its recommendation regarding each project must fall into one of three categories.

1. Immediate finance—those projects which should be implemented as soon as possible, in order of their desirability
2. Defer—projects which cannot be undertaken because of manpower shortages, because special situations inflate the capital requirements, or because the project requires preliminary action on some other proposal, although the project is believed to be of value
3. Reject—projects which are unsuitable for the hospital in the foreseeable future because their value is insufficient, because some other community agency can implement them with better results, or because their implementation is inconsistent with institutional goals

A second task of the committee would be to establish the interest rate to be used in evaluating nonmonetary proposals by considering the hospital's credit position and available capital. The committee should establish the rate because of the impact it has upon many of the decisions. Many projects will appear in a more favorable light at some rates than at others, and staff manipulation is possible unless the rate is a committee responsibility.

The final selection of projects should be the responsibility of the trustees, who will wish to take projects in the order recommended by the committee except in unusual instances. The number of projects which they accept, however, will depend upon their cost and the availability of funds. The recommendations of the committee, when approved by the trustees, become the capital expenditures budget of the hospital. The finance committee of the trustees and the controller are responsible for the operation of this budget. The capital budget and much other information regarding the new programs will have been specified in the proposal development.

Community Planning Committee

A growing number of communities require joint planning of hospital expansion among several hospitals in order to control the rate of growth of total hospital expenses and force an orderly pattern of growth. In such cases, a community-wide committee such as a planning council may approve capital expenditures of individual units. This committee might work directly with the reports of individual hospitals by approving individual capital proposals. In some instances, a planning council might wish to encourage competitive proposals on specific projects. Certainly one aspect of the committee's function will be to search for the most economical route to a given benefit.

Another aspect of the committee's work would be review of the interest rate. A combined hospital system might have substantially better credit possibilities and a lower interest rate. Some proposals for planning agencies include diverting the cash flow of hospitals over and above direct operating expenses to a pooled fund, which would give the central committee a revenue which it could commit directly to repayment of debt.[6] A committee which was representative of the community as a whole and which supervised capital planning of individual units by review of the unit's own capital proposals might retain control over a multiple hospital system while leaving substantial initiative to the individual institutions to design and implement both operational changes and expansions.

Additional Readings

Most recent texts on financial management for business contain extensive discussion of rates of return and investment decisions. For example:

Solomon, E.G., ed. *The Management of Corporate Capital,* The Free Press, New York, 1959, esp. pp. 13-55.

Anthony, R.N. *Management Accounting: Text and Cases*, 3d Ed. R.D. Irwin, Homewood, Ill., 1964.

Van Horne, J.C. *Financial Management and Policy*, 2nd Ed., Prentice-Hall, Englewood Cliffs, N.J., 1971.

Table 9-5
Present Value of $1 Received at the End of the "Year".

Years Hence	1%	2%	4%	6%	8%	10%	12%	14%	15%	16%	18%	20%	22%	24%	25%	26%	28%	30%	35%	40%	45%	50%
1	0.990	0.980	0.962	0.943	0.926	0.909	0.893	0.877	0.870	0.862	0.847	0.833	0.820	0.806	0.800	0.794	0.781	0.769	0.741	0.714	0.690	0.667
2	0.980	0.961	0.925	0.890	0.857	0.826	0.797	0.769	0.756	0.743	0.718	0.694	0.672	0.650	0.640	0.630	0.610	0.592	0.549	0.510	0.476	0.444
3	0.971	0.942	0.889	0.840	0.794	0.751	0.712	0.675	0.658	0.641	0.609	0.579	0.551	0.524	0.512	0.500	0.477	0.455	0.406	0.364	0.328	0.296
4	0.961	0.924	0.855	0.792	0.735	0.683	0.636	0.592	0.572	0.552	0.516	0.482	0.451	0.423	0.410	0.397	0.373	0.350	0.301	0.260	0.226	0.198
5	0.951	0.906	0.822	0.747	0.681	0.621	0.567	0.519	0.497	0.476	0.437	0.402	0.370	0.341	0.328	0.315	0.291	0.269	0.223	0.186	0.156	0.132
6	0.942	0.888	0.790	0.705	0.630	0.564	0.507	0.456	0.432	0.410	0.370	0.335	0.303	0.275	0.262	0.250	0.227	0.207	0.165	0.133	0.108	0.088
7	0.933	0.871	0.760	0.665	0.583	0.513	0.452	0.400	0.376	0.354	0.314	0.279	0.249	0.222	0.210	0.198	0.178	0.159	0.122	0.095	0.074	0.059
8	0.923	0.853	0.731	0.627	0.540	0.467	0.404	0.351	0.327	0.305	0.266	0.233	0.204	0.179	0.168	0.157	0.139	0.123	0.091	0.068	0.051	0.039
9	0.914	0.837	0.703	0.592	0.500	0.424	0.361	0.308	0.284	0.263	0.225	0.194	0.167	0.144	0.134	0.125	0.108	0.094	0.067	0.048	0.035	0.026
10	0.905	0.820	0.676	0.558	0.463	0.386	0.322	0.270	0.247	0.227	0.191	0.162	0.137	0.116	0.107	0.099	0.085	0.073	0.050	0.035	0.024	0.017
11	0.896	0.804	0.650	0.527	0.429	0.350	0.287	0.237	0.215	0.195	0.162	0.135	0.112	0.094	0.086	0.079	0.066	0.056	0.037	0.025	0.017	0.012
12	0.887	0.788	0.625	0.497	0.397	0.319	0.257	0.208	0.187	0.168	0.137	0.112	0.092	0.076	0.069	0.062	0.052	0.043	0.027	0.018	0.012	0.008
13	0.879	0.773	0.601	0.469	0.368	0.290	0.229	0.182	0.163	0.145	0.116	0.093	0.075	0.061	0.055	0.050	0.040	0.033	0.020	0.013	0.008	0.005
14	0.870	0.758	0.577	0.442	0.340	0.263	0.205	0.160	0.141	0.125	0.099	0.078	0.062	0.049	0.044	0.039	0.032	0.025	0.015	0.009	0.006	0.003
15	0.861	0.743	0.555	0.417	0.315	0.239	0.183	0.140	0.123	0.108	0.084	0.065	0.051	0.040	0.035	0.031	0.025	0.020	0.011	0.006	0.004	0.002
16	0.853	0.728	0.534	0.394	0.292	0.218	0.163	0.123	0.107	0.093	0.071	0.054	0.042	0.032	0.028	0.025	0.019	0.015	0.008	0.005	0.003	0.002
17	0.844	0.714	0.513	0.371	0.270	0.198	0.146	0.108	0.093	0.080	0.060	0.045	0.034	0.026	0.023	0.020	0.015	0.012	0.006	0.003	0.002	0.001
18	0.836	0.700	0.494	0.350	0.250	0.180	0.130	0.095	0.081	0.069	0.051	0.038	0.028	0.021	0.018	0.016	0.012	0.009	0.005	0.002	0.001	0.001
19	0.828	0.686	0.475	0.331	0.232	0.164	0.116	0.083	0.070	0.060	0.043	0.031	0.023	0.017	0.014	0.012	0.009	0.007	0.003	0.002	0.001	
20	0.820	0.673	0.456	0.312	0.215	0.149	0.104	0.073	0.061	0.051	0.037	0.026	0.019	0.014	0.012	0.010	0.007	0.005	0.002	0.001		
21	0.811	0.660	0.439	0.294	0.199	0.135	0.093	0.064	0.053	0.044	0.031	0.022	0.015	0.011	0.009	0.008	0.006	0.004	0.002	0.001	0.001	
22	0.803	0.647	0.422	0.278	0.184	0.123	0.083	0.056	0.046	0.038	0.026	0.018	0.013	0.009	0.007	0.006	0.004	0.003	0.001	0.001		
23	0.795	0.634	0.406	0.262	0.170	0.112	0.074	0.049	0.040	0.033	0.022	0.015	0.010	0.007	0.006	0.005	0.003	0.002	0.001			
24	0.788	0.622	0.390	0.247	0.158	0.102	0.066	0.043	0.035	0.028	0.019	0.013	0.008	0.006	0.005	0.004	0.003	0.002	0.001			
25	0.780	0.610	0.375	0.233	0.146	0.092	0.059	0.038	0.030	0.024	0.016	0.010	0.007	0.005	0.004	0.003	0.002	0.001	0.001			
26	0.772	0.598	0.361	0.220	0.135	0.084	0.053	0.033	0.026	0.021	0.014	0.009	0.006	0.004	0.003	0.002	0.002	0.001				
27	0.764	0.586	0.347	0.207	0.125	0.076	0.047	0.029	0.023	0.018	0.011	0.007	0.005	0.003	0.002	0.002	0.001	0.001				
28	0.757	0.574	0.333	0.196	0.116	0.069	0.042	0.026	0.020	0.016	0.010	0.006	0.004	0.002	0.002	0.002	0.001	0.001				
29	0.749	0.563	0.321	0.185	0.107	0.063	0.037	0.022	0.017	0.014	0.008	0.005	0.003	0.002	0.002	0.001	0.001	0.001				
30	0.742	0.552	0.308	0.174	0.099	0.057	0.033	0.020	0.015	0.012	0.007	0.004	0.003	0.002	0.001	0.001	0.001	0.001				
40	0.672	0.453	0.208	0.097	0.046	0.022	0.011	0.005	0.004	0.003	0.001	0.001										
50	0.608	0.372	0.141	0.054	0.021	0.009	0.003	0.001	0.001	0.001												

Source: Robert N. Anthony, *Management Accounting: Text and Cases* (3d Ed.: Homewood, Ill.: Richard D. Irwin, Inc., 1964), p. 743.

Table 9-6
Present Value of $1 Received Annually at the End of Each "Year" for N Years

Years (N)	1%	2%	4%	6%	8%	10%	12%	14%	15%	16%	18%	20%	22%	24%	25%	26%	28%	30%	35%	40%	45%	50%
1	0.990	0.980	0.962	0.943	0.926	0.909	0.893	0.877	0.870	0.862	0.847	0.833	0.820	0.806	0.800	0.794	0.781	0.769	0.741	0.714	0.690	0.667
2	1.970	1.942	1.886	1.833	1.783	1.736	1.690	1.647	1.626	1.605	1.566	1.528	1.492	1.457	1.440	1.424	1.392	1.361	1.289	1.224	1.165	1.111
3	2.941	2.884	2.775	2.673	2.577	2.487	2.402	2.322	2.283	2.246	2.174	2.106	2.042	1.981	1.952	1.923	1.868	1.816	1.696	1.589	1.493	1.407
4	3.902	3.808	3.630	3.465	3.312	3.170	3.037	2.914	2.855	2.798	2.690	2.589	2.494	2.404	2.362	2.320	2.241	2.166	1.997	1.849	1.720	1.605
5	4.853	4.713	4.452	4.212	3.993	3.791	3.605	3.433	3.352	3.274	3.127	2.991	2.864	2.745	2.689	2.635	2.532	2.436	2.220	2.035	1.876	1.737
6	5.795	5.601	5.242	4.917	4.623	4.355	4.111	3.889	3.784	3.685	3.498	3.326	3.167	3.020	2.951	2.885	2.759	2.643	2.385	2.168	1.983	1.824
7	6.728	6.472	6.002	5.582	5.206	4.868	4.564	4.288	4.160	4.039	3.812	3.605	3.416	3.242	3.161	3.083	2.937	2.802	2.508	2.263	2.057	1.883
8	7.652	7.325	6.733	6.210	5.747	5.335	4.968	4.639	4.487	4.344	4.078	3.837	3.619	3.421	3.329	3.241	3.076	2.925	2.598	2.331	2.108	1.922
9	8.566	8.162	7.435	6.802	6.247	5.759	5.328	4.946	4.772	4.607	4.303	4.031	3.786	3.566	3.463	3.366	3.184	3.019	2.665	2.379	2.144	1.948
10	9.471	8.983	8.111	7.360	6.710	6.145	5.650	5.216	5.019	4.833	4.494	4.192	3.923	3.682	3.571	3.465	3.269	3.092	2.715	2.414	2.168	1.965
11	10.368	9.787	8.760	7.887	7.139	6.495	5.988	5.453	5.234	5.029	4.656	4.327	4.035	3.776	3.656	3.544	3.335	3.147	2.752	2.438	2.185	1.977
12	11.255	10.575	9.385	8.384	7.536	6.814	6.194	5.660	5.421	5.197	4.793	4.439	4.127	3.851	3.725	3.606	3.387	3.190	2.779	2.456	2.196	1.985
13	12.134	11.343	9.986	8.853	7.904	7.103	6.424	5.842	5.583	5.342	4.910	4.533	4.203	3.912	3.780	3.656	3.427	3.223	2.799	2.468	2.204	1.990
14	13.004	12.106	10.563	9.295	8.244	7.367	6.628	6.002	5.724	5.468	5.008	4.611	4.265	3.962	3.824	3.695	3.459	3.249	2.814	2.477	2.210	1.993
15	13.865	12.849	11.118	9.712	8.559	7.606	6.811	6.142	5.847	5.575	5.092	4.675	4.315	4.001	3.859	3.726	3.483	3.268	2.825	2.484	2.214	1.995
16	14.718	13.578	11.652	10.106	8.851	7.824	6.974	6.265	5.954	5.669	5.162	4.730	4.357	4.033	3.887	3.751	3.503	3.283	2.834	2.489	2.216	1.997
17	15.562	14.292	12.166	10.477	9.122	8.022	7.120	6.373	6.047	5.749	5.222	4.775	4.391	4.059	3.910	3.771	3.518	3.295	2.840	2.492	2.218	1.998
18	16.398	14.992	12.659	10.828	9.372	8.201	7.250	6.467	6.128	5.818	5.273	4.812	4.419	4.080	3.928	3.786	3.529	3.304	2.844	2.494	2.219	1.999
19	17.226	15.678	13.134	11.158	9.604	8.365	7.366	6.550	6.198	5.877	5.316	4.844	4.442	4.097	3.942	3.799	3.539	3.311	2.848	2.496	2.220	1.999
20	18.046	16.351	13.590	11.470	9.818	8.514	7.469	6.623	6.259	5.929	5.353	4.870	4.460	4.110	3.954	3.808	3.546	3.316	2.850	2.497	2.221	1.999
21	18.857	17.011	14.029	11.764	10.017	8.649	7.562	6.687	6.312	5.973	5.384	4.891	4.476	4.121	3.963	3.816	3.551	3.320	2.852	2.498	2.221	2.000
22	19.660	17.658	14.451	12.042	10.201	8.772	7.645	6.743	6.359	6.011	5.410	4.909	4.488	4.130	3.970	3.822	3.556	3.323	2.853	2.498	2.222	2.000
23	20.456	18.292	14.857	12.303	10.371	8.883	7.718	6.792	6.399	6.044	5.432	4.925	4.499	4.137	3.976	3.827	3.559	3.325	2.854	2.499	2.222	2.000
24	21.243	18.914	15.247	12.550	10.529	8.985	7.784	6.835	6.434	6.073	5.451	4.937	4.507	4.143	3.981	3.831	3.562	3.327	2.855	2.499	2.222	2.000
25	22.023	19.523	15.622	12.783	10.675	9.077	7.843	6.873	6.464	6.097	5.467	4.948	4.514	4.147	3.985	3.834	3.564	3.329	2.856	2.499	2.222	2.000
26	22.795	20.121	15.983	13.003	10.810	9.161	7.896	6.906	6.491	6.118	5.480	4.956	4.520	4.151	3.988	3.837	3.566	3.330	2.856	2.500	2.222	2.000
27	23.560	20.707	16.330	13.211	10.935	9.237	7.943	6.935	6.514	6.136	5.492	4.964	4.524	4.154	3.990	3.839	3.567	3.331	2.856	2.500	2.222	2.000
28	24.316	21.281	16.663	13.406	11.051	9.307	7.984	6.961	6.534	6.152	5.502	4.970	4.528	4.157	3.992	3.840	3.568	3.331	2.857	2.500	2.222	2.000
29	25.066	21.844	16.984	13.591	11.158	9.370	8.022	6.983	6.551	6.166	5.510	4.975	4.531	4.159	3.994	3.841	3.569	3.332	2.857	2.500	2.222	2.000
30	25.808	22.396	17.292	13.765	11.258	9.427	8.055	7.003	6.566	6.177	5.517	4.979	4.534	4.160	3.995	3.842	3.569	3.332	2.857	2.500	2.222	2.000
40	32.835	27.355	19.793	15.046	11.925	9.779	8.244	7.105	6.642	6.234	5.548	4.997	4.544	4.166	3.999	3.846	3.571	3.333	2.857	2.500	2.222	2.000
50	39.196	31.424	21.482	15.762	12.234	9.915	8.304	7.133	6.661	6.246	5.554	4.999	4.545	4.167	4.000	3.846	3.571	3.333	2.857	2.500	2.222	2.000

Source: Robert N. Anthony, *Management Accounting: Text and Cases* (3d Ed., Homewood, Ill.: Richard D. Irwin, Inc., 1964).

Part III
Control Systems

10 Nature and Application of Control Systems in Hospitals

Concept of Control Systems

A control system is a set of activities or devices which maintains ongoing assessment of the achievement of a process in terms of previously established goals and attempts corrective action when achievement is different from expectation. Any process may have a control system if it is complex enough that the outcome is in doubt, and if it can be manipulated with a resulting change in outcome. Most human endeavors have control systems of some sort. Two sophisticated but dissimilar examples are the guidance systems of lunar rockets and the control functions embodied in government. A very simple example is the automatic sprinkler system used in fire control. Control systems are common in biological and mechanical systems as well. The general theory of control systems is called *cybernetics*, and the systems themselves are sometimes called *cybernetic systems*.[a] The principal purpose of all but the most rudimentary control systems is two-fold: (a) to provide control of the process, so that results are consistent with expectations, and (b) to generate a warning signal when control is not being achieved. By inference, when a warning signal is not generated by a working control system, there is assurance that goals are being achieved.

The second purpose of control systems permits a reduction in the quantity of information which is required to monitor a complex process. While the direct monitoring of the process, called the *primary control*, requires substantial information, the secondary monitoring, called the *super control*, requires only a warning signal when the primary control fails. This signal is called an *exception report*.

The nature of control systems was shown graphically in chapter 1 (see fig. 1-2). The monitor within the heavy lines is the primary control. The second monitor is a super control.

Components

In figure 1-2 (chap. 1), the primary control process summarized in the section labeled monitor can be expanded and described, as shown in figure 10-1. In this figure, the monitor activities have been divided into three components.

---

[a]*Cybernetics* is derived from a Greek word meaning steersman or helmsman. The helmsman provides the directional control system of a moving vessel.

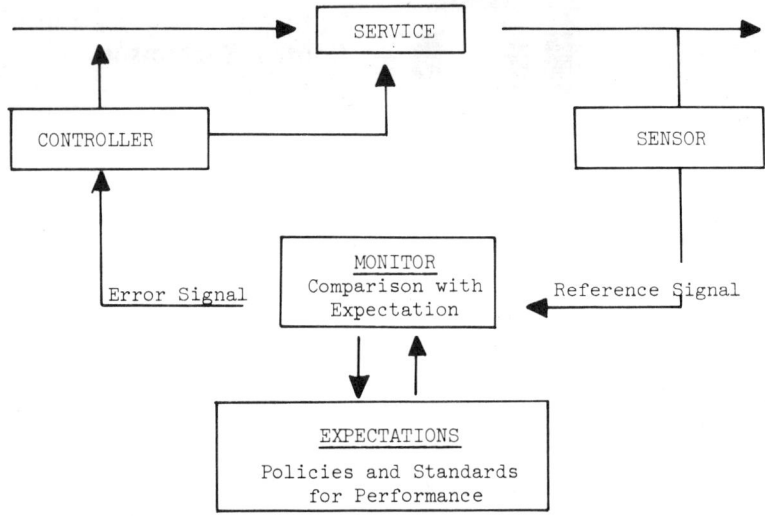

Figure 10-1. Components of Monitor Process.

1. *Sensor*, which identifies the state of the process under control. Its output is called the *reference signal*
2. *Monitor*, which compares the reference signal against the expectations for the process and generates an *error signal*, which is some measure of the difference between performance and expectation
3. *Controller*, which takes corrective action aimed at reduction of the error signal

All three of these components must be present and working for a control system to be effective. If any is missing, the system fails. Also, the total performance of the control system is limited by the weakest component. If the sensor generates an incorrect reference signal, the error signal will be wrong, and the action of the controller will be wrong. Similarly, if there are no statements of performance expectation, there can be no error signal and no control.

Response Time

There is an additional opportunity for control system failure which can occur when all three components work well. This condition occurs when delays in the control system cause the controller to act after the condition which caused the error signal has changed. This condition may occur in any kind of process and control, but it is easiest to illustrate in an electronic amplification network. This process takes an input signal which may vary in strength and produces an output signal which is supposed to be at a controlled constant strength. Suppose a sudden, large burst occurs in the input. The output strength increases rapidly, and the sensor passes this information back through the monitor to the controller which reduces the amount of amplification. By this time, however, the burst has passed. The output then drops suddenly well below the desired level. This is detected by the sensor and amplification is increased. The result is the creation of two (or more) fluctuations in the output as a result of a single change in input. Thus the time necessary to operate the feedback loop is an important characteristic in its success.

One way to attack this problem is to reduce the length of the *feedback cycle*, or *response time*—the time required from reference signal change to controller action. Another is to construct the monitor so that it does not generate an error signal until a change in the reference signal has reached a certain combination of magnitude and duration. In the example cited, the monitor could be constructed to ignore small variations entirely and to issue error signals on large variations only if they persisted for a certain length of time. The result would be imperfect control; the output signal would fluctuate slightly from time to time and would occasionally transmit a burst of much larger output. This result is superior, however, to the first case where the amplifier overreacted to transient bursts and increased the overall variation in output signal. This example has numerous analogues in human systems. Its impact can be summarized in a rule of thumb: "The longer the response time of a control system, the less precision can be achieved in control."[1]

Implicit or Intuitive Control Systems

Organizations, including hospitals, can be viewed as being partially control systems of complex processes. Supervisors, for example, are explicitly responsible for the control of the processes they supervise. Consider the operations of a laundry manager acting as a primary control system. He embodies all three operations of the system, although each operation can be identified as he performs it. His eyes and ears are the principal sensors, and if he does his job well, they cover all aspects of the laundry operation. He learns by observation how much soiled linen is available, how many personnel reported for work, and which machines are operating. He knows from experience if nothing else how much clean linen is expected from the laundry and what rate of production he must achieve in various sections of the laundry to meet this goal. He has some standard, or expectation, as to quality of production—how clean a sheet should be, how it should be folded, etc. This information, based on expectations, permits him to check actual production and detect errors or deviations. Finally, he has certain control mechanisms available to him so that he can take corrective action—have a machine repaired, change the order of production, change personnel assignment, etc. It is worth noting that none of this information must necessarily be quantitative or even explicit. He can perform these functions at a level which is completely intuitive, and in fact he may do so very well.

Explicit Systems and Super Controls

Certain problems inevitably arise, however, when the supervisor's primary control performance is entirely intuitive. Can the process be improved by reducing the ratio of input resources to output (efficiency)? Can the causes of failure to meet production goals be identified? Can the system be adapted to changes in the goals, such as an increase in the output required? Can someone else replace the laundry manager when he is absent and perform the control function? In general, can management be sure the primary control function is adequately performed? It is on questions of this kind that intuitive control systems founder. They have some important advantages, however. They can be fast in response time, inexpensive to operate, and in some situations astonishingly flexible and effective. It is safe to say that the primary controls in most hospital activities consist of nonexplicit human systems of this kind. While they may be inadequate for all the needs of the organization, they are often essential for some needs. Their strengths should be recognized and supported by more formal and explicit control systems.

One of the difficulties of nonexplicit control systems is their extreme dependence upon the performance of an individual. This performance varies, and when several individuals perform essentially the same job, super controls are usually desirable to see that some minimum level of performances is maintained. When primary control systems are entirely intuitive, super control systems become very difficult to maintain. As a second example, consider that head nurses perform primary control functions analagous to the laundry manager's. However, the output of their process is largely intangible, a set of services rendered to patients, many of which leave no trace after a few minutes or hours. In the typical nursing organization, head nurses report to supervisors who are responsible for controlling their performance. This is a super control system. The supervisor is in a position of disadvantage, compared to the head nurse or the laundry manager. She is not in constant visual contact with her processes, and she cannot inspect them periodically and fully determine what activity has occurred. She can and does continue to use an intuitive control process, but she must begin to augment it with substantial quantities of explicit information. The more precision she desires in her control, the more explicit information she will require. Thus in a typical nursing organization, all levels of personnel keep a variety of records and reports which can be used to assess the performance. The more tightly performance of different head nurses is controlled, the more explicit and elaborate the control systems become.

General Considerations in Control Systems

There are certain general considerations in the design of control systems which can provide a framework for understanding both details of system design and specific hospital applications. These include the differentiation of control systems from closely related organizational activities, the range of applicability, problems connected with each of the components—sensor, monitor, and controller—and the cost and sensitivity of systems.

Control systems should be distinguished from certain closely related activities such as structural controls and research. In designing organizations it is desirable to build in certain features which help achieve certain goals. For example, it is considered desirable to have separate persons receive checks by mail and post accounts receivable because it closes a way to embezzlement. Other examples are certain licensing and certification requirements, such as rules requiring registered nurses for certain tasks and policies recommended by the Joint Commission on Accreditation of Hospitals. These structural features are not control systems. Although they aid in goal achievement and may also facilitate design of control systems, they lack the component of ongoing monitoring of the process. Educational activities in an organization are not the same as control systems, either, for the same reasons. Research is a similar example. Processes may be studied in detail, on an *ad hoc* basis, and perhaps completely redesigned. Research activities eventually terminate, however. When this occurs, the ongoing assurance of performance is lost unless specific control systems have been designed. Budgeting and other planning activities might also be confused with control systems, but they too lack essential components. The budget or plan can be used as a standard or expectation in a control system, but the preparation of a budget or plan is not in itself sufficient. The element of corrective action is missing.

Applicability

Control systems of at least intuitive types are implicit in organizational structures for most important processes. Systems can be designed for subprocesses and components as well. There can be control systems on subprocesses for scheduling demand which detect excessive waiting time, bookings over capacity of the process, changes in random demand processes, and excessive idle time of the process. A critical element in these systems is often the ability to control. There can be no control system over random obstetrical demand, for example, when the supply of facilities is fixed and there is no way to divert demand to some other institution.

Resource supply processes can be subject to control systems. Lot testing of delivered goods against purchase specification is an example common to both hospitals and industry. Deliveries which fail to meet specifications are refused, thus controlling the quality of the procurement process output. Human resources can be subject to control systems as well. The selection process in hiring is a form of primary control. Surveys of personnel attitudes and job satisfaction can be used in control systems maintaining the quality of supervision. Records of maintenance cost of equipment can be used to monitor equipment performance, and control systems can eliminate troublesome pieces.

Processes of various kinds can be controlled through partial measures of goal achievement. Thus efficiency of performance and cost per unit of output can be subject to a control system. Quality of many processes can be subject to control using implicit or explicit systems. Quality control systems may be separate from efficiency or cost controls, or operated together with control systems on these elements of the process.

It is important to recognize the interlocking nature of these subprocess control systems. In a process where demand is stochastic, efficiency is affected by demand variation. Thus an efficiency control system in these processes must either control demand or adjust resources to demand variation. Quality frequently depends upon the availability of resources. The installation of more explicit control systems in one subprocess frequently requires attention to all aspects, lest the goals of the process as a whole become distorted toward meeting the needs of the control system. When careful controls are imposed upon the use of resources, it is often necessary to improve the control systems for quality. The quality control systems provide assurance that the achievement of goals in this area has not deteriorated as a result of the stress upon efficiency and economy.

Sensor Considerations

There are many data systems in the hospital which are currently used as explicit sensors for control systems. Some representative examples of these are:

1. Turnover, absenteeism, and injury statistics—used as monitors of the work force, its morale, and health. These are sometimes used to infer changes in the supervisory process generally or in specific departments. Injury statistics are used to monitor accident prevention and safety processes.
2. Manhours, manhours/output unit, and dollars/output unit. These are used to control quantity of inputs and to control efficiency.
3. Occupancy and idle capacity rates. These can be used to monitor scheduling processes. They are measures of efficiency of capital equipment and facilities use.
4. Error, accident, failure, and complaint rates. These can be used to assess some aspects of nursing quality and other patient services. Transfusion reactions are used as a control of laboratory cross match procedures. Equipment breakdown rates can be used in maintenance quality control.

Failure to follow policy, as in obtaining admission lab procedures or written consent to surgery, can be used in quality control procedures.
5. Professional activity measures. These include rates such as consultation rates and autopsy rates and have been used in medical quality measurement for several decades, although their unsophisticated use has been questioned.
6. Waiting lists and average waiting time—measures of unmet demand. They can be used to control systems for scheduling processes such as the admitting and outpatient scheduling systems. Unfilled positions and average time to fill positions are measures of personnel department performance.
7. Output measures. Output measures are most commonly used in conjunction with resource input measures, in ratios of output/man-hour, etc. The two measures, output and input, are used to calculate efficiency, the ratio of actual to potential output where potential output is a function of inputs. Certain departments have extensive control over their output, so that direct measures of volume of output become reference data for control systems. The number and amount of accounts processed by credit and collections is one possible example. In medical care processes, unfavorable or unexpected outcomes are quality sensors. Hence, infant mortality rates, normal surgical tissue rates, etc.

These measures all have the characteristic of being immediately calculable from empirical data. Other than relatively simple definitions, they require no criteria or judgment in data collection. Quantitative data are often available as a by-product of accounting, payroll, or medical records information systems.

Despite the number and variety of these measures, they fail to cover many important areas for control. In these cases, more elaborate and specialized systems must be constructed. One of the important areas not well covered is efficiency. Efficiency of human systems requires the construction of standards for performance which translate input to potential output. While it can be calculated in the monitor or comparator process, it cannot be measured directly except in purely mechanical conditions. A second control measure of widespread importance is quality. While some of the measures above can be used to control quality of various processes, more elaborate sensors are often necessary.

Specialized sensors collect additional data for control systems by processes such as inspection, abstracting, surveying, and specialized records. They often involve the use of additional forms and personnel. Data are frequently collected through various sampling procedures. Information processing and data reduction procedures are often necessary to translate raw data to useful reference signals. A widely used example is the PAS case abstract and processing routine for medical care quality control. Surveys of employee morale and attitude are another example. So are inspection surveys of elements of quality which have recently come into use in housekeeping, dietary, and nursing processes. Pathology laboratories use blind samples with known values to provide absolute checks on the quality of test results. In processes generating a tangible product, such as the pharmacy, product inspection systems can be used to generate quality scores which become reference signals. Examples of these specialized sensors and their use in quality control systems will be discussed in the following chapters. Despite the increased costs involved, these devices are steadily gaining acceptance.

Costs. In the design of complex sensors as well as in the selection of available information to be used for reference signals, several considerations are important. Cost is obviously one of these. Specialized forms and processing are costly in themselves, and the use of trained personnel to collect data by inspection or abstracting further increases the control system cost. The sophistication of control systems should parallel the value of control itself; an inexpensive process does not justify expensive controls. By the same token, a process with many elements which can be only poorly controlled does not justify expensive sensor systems. Only when the value of the realizable improvement is great should expensive systems be established. Many hospital processes have high realizable improvements, however. Improvements in the quality of medical care, for example, are generally considered to be worth substantial expense to obtain. The cost of unnecessary manpower is high enough to justify large control expenses. Similarly eliminating delays in patient care and reducing length of stay result in large savings, and justify elaborate controls.

The cost of control systems is often hard to estimate. Apparently expensive explicit systems may actually replace intuitive control systems which have absorbed large "hidden" costs in supervisory staff time and medical staff effort. A system like PAS-MAP, with the length of stay package (described in a later chapter), costs thousands of dollars a year, but it may be justified on three different grounds: it produces certain information which the hospital would have to compile anyway; it may reduce the ineffective time spent on control by the medical staff because it presents data in a better organized form, with some preselection of areas requiring attention; and finally, it may be more effective, resulting in better control of quality and length of stay.

Reliability and Validity. All measurement systems must be considered in terms of their reliability validity and bias. *Validity* is the extent to which a measure accurately reflects the true state of its subject. *Reliability* is the extent to which a measure gives consistent values when applied to a constant situation by different observers, or by the same observer at different times.

An example of a room thermometer and temperature measurement may serve to illustrate these definitions. If the thermometer has been assembled in such a way that it consistently reads a high or a low value, it may be said to be *invalid*.

Similarly, the measurement may be invalid (biased) if the thermometer is located near a radiator or in an isolated area of direct sunlight or in some other nonrepresentative portion of the room. If, in addition, the thermometer is so small or so difficult to read that a reasonable number of observers disagree as to the exact reading of the thermometer at the same time, then it may be said to be *unreliable*. The degree of the unreliability is represented by the distribution of readings obtained from varying observers at the same thermometer setting. The degree of invalidity can only be obtained by comparison against the actual temperature of the room as measured by a known standard. In general, the more sophisticated the measurement device is, the more troublesome these two errors become.

In estimating the quality of the medical care and nursing care processes, the problem of validity is particularly difficult. The lack of clear standards and the lack of demonstrated relationships between components of the process and the outcome leave many measures without proven validity. It is often the case that the validity of a measure is tested against an interim standard or criterion which is in turn judged to be valid by competent professional authority. An example is the determination of admission hematocrit or hemoglobin levels. It is assumed by most professional groups, including the Joint Commission, that good care will result if this test is performed on all patients when they are admitted. There is no formal proof, however, that better care results when the tests are done and recorded in the medical history.

Problems of validity of measures of quality of care can occasionally be solved by reference to outcome studies involving control groups. The proof of a number of procedural and structural standards lies in published research. Thus the desirability of Papanicolaou smears for women was established by analysis of survival rates of matched groups of women who received the examination and the indicated treatment, versus those whose treatment was not begun until clinical symptoms appeared. Similarly, the value of prenatal care was established by demonstrating increases in the percentages of favorable outcomes. For many common quality measures, however, such proof is lacking and probably unobtainable. Professional judgment is the sole justification of the use of the measure as well as of the standard of achievement.

Reliability of measurement is generally tested by special studies. These usually compare measures obtained from the same population as they are recorded by different observers or by differing measurement techniques. If an identical population is available, it is also possible to compare scores by the same observers at different times.

Sensitivity and Bias. Related to the problem of reliability are problems of sensitivity and bias. *Sensitivity* is the ability of a measure to detect a given change in the process under measurement. Obviously a measure can only be sensitive to the extent it is reliable. *Bias* is a loss of reliability or validity in a constant direction. Measurements taken under certain conditions which represent only a special fraction of the process under study may be biased. Certain observers may report biased results either accidentally or deliberately. Bias is reduced by careful attention to the measurement process, including sampling, method of observation, and the selection and training of observers.

Monitor Considerations

The task of the monitor can be separated into two steps, comparison against the standard, and generation of the error signal.

Standards. Standards, or expectations, represent the goals of the organization for the process and can be either implicit or explicit. When they are explicit they can be quantitative or nonquantitative. They derive from the policies of the institution, as reflected in budgets, planning documents, procedure manuals, research reports, and other statements reflecting organizational agreement on goals or desired achievement. Some examples of such standards are:

1. The x-ray department will provide 25 examinations per hour
2. The staffing standard for social service is 2 professional, 5 nonprofessional personnel
3. Patients having surgery shall have signed consent form A (with certain specified exceptions)
4. Cleaned floors shall be free of surface dirt, moisture, and litter
5. Expected laundry production is 100 pounds per manhour
6. Each patient shall have white blood cell, hematocrit, and urinalysis determination within 24 hours of admission

Standards can be constructed by authority, by agreement, by empirical study, or by reference to past performance. In general *any* quantitative reference signal generates one possible standard, its own expected value over time. This may not be entirely satisfactory however. For the laundry production standard, (5), the expected value of past performance in the absence of a standard may have been greater or less than 100 pounds per hour. Empirical study by industrial engineers may have been employed to establish the standard. Presumably the system will come "under control" after the standard has been in use for a while. Then the expected value of the reference signal will equal the standard. Budget standards are agreements if the budget is negotiated with the primary control supervisor and he accepts it. Standards such as the clean floor standard may be reached by consensus within the organization or by reference to authority. Many medical standards are set by authority because of a lack of basic knowledge about the validity of certain practices. Standard 6 is adopted from the Joint Commission requirements. Standard 3 is recommended by all legal authorities.

As a general rule, as much consensus should be gained on standards as possible. Participative management requires that all persons responsible for the application of a process not only understand the standard but have the opportunity to comment upon it. Despite the strong legal authority for standard 3, there are cases (emergencies, children, drunken and drugged patients, etc.) where its application is far from routine. Persons enforcing the standard should aid in identifying the appropriate exceptions and alternatives. The same process is desirable in setting standards by empirical study. The supervisor should participate in the study design and in the adoption of its conclusion.

The separation of sensors and standards is to some extent arbitrary. While some reference signals such as laundry production per man hour exist independent of the standard, others as a practical matter are generated by application of the standard to the process itself. There is no practical reference signal on clean floors in the absence of observer judgment. Many reference signals are defined by the standard. Standards 1, 2, 3, and 5 clearly indicate the nature of the reference signal required, although the signal is independent of the standard itself.

The fact that the standard is not quantitative does not prohibit a quantitative reference signal. Either "number of floors not clean" or "floors not clean divided by floors observed" is a quantitative error signal. This type of signal, where the output of the process is compared to a standard and either passes or fails, is called an *attributes measure*. Attributes measures can even be generated against intuitive standards ("number of floors the chief housekeeper did not judge to be clean"), although such a procedure would be of questionable reliability and might produce substantial bias. Quantitative standards, such as the x-ray and laundry output standards, generally are independent of the reference signal which obviously must be quantitative as well. Measures of this kind are called *variables measures*. These error signals, instead of being binary counts or ratios (number failed or fraction failed) are numerical scores. (Laundry output was 98, 97 and 101 pounds per manhour, etc.). This permits a different and more sensitive statistical analysis.

Error Signal. Given a sensor and a standard, comparison of the two generates a signal expressing some amount of difference. If attributes measures are used, the difference signal will be either an integer (the number of units which failed) or a ratio (the proportion of failures to all units). If a variables measure is used the signal can be either the numerical difference between the reference signal and the standard or the ratio of reference signal to standard. In all of these cases, the basic question is, "Should an error signal be generated?" When the difference is zero, or the ratio 0.0, the answer is no. This, however, will rarely occur. Most processes which require control are stochastic. That is, they are subject to random variation which is caused by fluctuations in demand, in inputs, or in imperfections in the process itself. At some level, these fluctuations are too small for the controller to adjust successfully. It is usually necessary to establish *control limits* which allow differences below a certain magnitude to occur without initiation of an error signal.

Control limits are set balancing two opposing tendencies:

1. Tendency to issue an error signal to the controller when the process variation is too small to be controlled—a *false positive* or Type I error
2. Tendency to issue *no* error signal when the process variation can be controlled—a *false negative* or Type II error.

The narrower the control limits, the greater the chance of false positive signals. The broader the control limits, the greater the chance of a false negative signal. The false positive creates unnecessary activity for the controller and can in some situations make the process unstable by continually adjusting when no adjustment is desirable. The false negative permits the process to fluctuate more than is necessary before control is actuated.

Control limits can be established arbitrarily and they frequently are. They also can be established arbitrarily and then adjusted by trial and error. There is also a third method, however, called *statistical quality control*. This technique assumes that the reference signal from a stochastic process is a random variable, and that the standard is the expected value of the random variable. This permits an unbiased test of the null hypothesis:

> The current value of the reference signal does not differ from the universe of historical values of the signal.

Stated less rigorously, it tests whether the process has deviated from past performance, or whether the value of the reference signal is within the variation expected from random or uncontrollable factors. The test constructs the probability distribution of the reference signal and permits calculation of the probability of both Type I and Type II errors for a given control limit. Its advantages lie in the ease with which calculations can be made automatically or by computer, and in the ability to predict the results of a given control limit in terms of false negative and false positive error signals. The elements of the statistical technique will be described in a following section.

Controller Considerations

In simple, mechanical systems, the function of the controller is almost automatic. When the compass indicates a deviation to starboard, the helm is adjusted to port. When the temperature-sensing device in the fire control sprinkler melts, water pours from the sprinkler. In more complex systems, the controller's functions are more difficult. The first step is to attempt to identify the cause of the deviation. This often requires special studies or analyses, perhaps in identifying certain elements of the process by instituting special studies of the reference signal or by establishing new, *ad hoc*, data collection systems. If a control system for patient accidents indicated an increased rate of accidents, studies might investigate which patients were involved, which nursing units, or which time of day. Inspection of sites of accidents might be undertaken, or interviews of witnesses or victims. If no cause could be identified, the error signal might be dismissed as a false positive signal.

Once the apparent cause of process change has been decided, the appropriate corrective action can be selected and implemented. In complex systems, it is impossible to state all the possible corrective actions. They include education and retraining, changes in personnel, incentives, discipline, and adjustments in procedures. While it is usually desirable to ascertain the cause of the failure, trial-and-error approaches are sometimes appropriate. In very complex process, such as nursing and medical care, control actions tend to be studied in advance, and carefully safeguarded against accepting a false positive signal. This implies that the controller actions will be slow and expensive, but that is consistent with the low reliability and validity of reference signals and standards.

Statistical Quality Control Techniques

Hospitals can generate a large number of individual statistics where each statistic is a measure of some limited aspect of quality or efficiency of the total process. An effective information-handling system must be able to process the incoming statistics. Since the number of statistics is large, the processing must be simple, nearly automatic, and require a minimum of skilled attention. Even at the primary control level, only those cases where there is a high probability of finding an unusual situation can be studied in depth, and the first job of the system is to identify these cases. Techniques have been developed to do this job based upon relatively simple statistical analyses. These are called quality control techniques, although they are applicable to any continuing process measure, whether it is concerned with quality or other aspects of the process.

Almost any complex process will have some variability in the degree to which it achieves its goals. Certainly this will be the case with all hospital processes and medical care processes. Uncontrollable variations in the environment, such as changes in the demand for services and differences in education and attitude of personnel, occur both with the passage of time in a single institution and between two or more institutions compared at the same time. Thus any measure that tries to represent the quality of process will naturally show some variability. The management problem is to isolate those instances of variation where there is a high probability of a change within the system that can be identified and corrected, without meanwhile investigating too many cases of "random" or uncontrollable variability. Statistical quality control can be used to evaluate the probability that a given change in a measurement statistic represents an exceptional situation worthy of further analysis. These methods are described below. Although they are all the same in principle and are applications of the tests of whether different samples are from the same population, they differ in calculation by the nature of the measurement statistics.

Analysis of Variables Measures

Variables measures generate a quantitative reference signal which is continuous[b] or which can be treated as continuous. These can be analyzed by a process of grouping small samples from the same process, usually those taken on a daily or other short-term periodic basis, and treating the resulting distribution of grouped data as a normally distributed population. The reference statistic is compared against its own expected value. Measures from hospital experience which fit this procedure include percentage scores from various kinds of audits, percentage scores from patient questionnaires, occupancy percentages, and total numerical values such as the number of outstanding open accounts or the dollar value of accounts receivable or the quantity or value of inventories. Some of these measures do not fit the strict mathematical definition of continuity, but they have the characteristic that the difference between any two possible values of reference signal (as for example between 356 and 357 open patient accounts or between a test score of 73 and one of 74), is trivial and may be ignored.

Variables measures are collected for a sample of individual cases of an identifiable ongoing process over a specified period of time. Thus for example, a nursing audit routine may be applied to five patients on a nursing floor on each day, the value of outstanding accounts may be reported from a trial balance each Friday of the month, etc. The result will be a set of values for each successive time period. There should be three or more observations each in each set. For each of these sets the mean and standard deviation can be estimated according to the usual formulae:

$$\bar{x} = \frac{\sum x}{n}$$

---

[b]A continuous variable is one which is not subject to interruption or discontinuity. Specifically, if the variable can be conceived of as a line, there is a single value for every point on the line, and if any two nearby points on the line are compared, their values become equal as the distance between them goes to zero. The most common form of discontinuous variable is the *discrete variable*, which can take on only certain values, as for example, integer values. Some common examples of continuous variables are temperature and time. Discrete variables are persons, telephone calls, and deaths. When the value of a discrete variable is large, e.g. 1000 persons, it is common to treat it as though it were continuous, since the distinction becomes unimportant.

$$s^2 = \frac{\sum (x_i - \bar{x})^2}{n - 1}$$

where x is the value of the variable to be measured and n is the number of measurements in the subgroup. According to the Central Limit Theorem, the distribution of means and standard deviations of the sets collectively will approximate the normal distribution even if the distribution of the original parameter is not normal. The closeness of the approximation will depend upon the shape of the underlying distributions and the size of the sample. For many situations, the approximations become quite reliable for n's as small as 3, although if the underlying distribution is highly skewed, larger n's are necessary. Grouping the data in this way has two advantages: first, it permits application of the Central Limit Theorem and the assumption that the subgroup values will be normally distributed *despite the distribution of values in the original population*, and second, study of the data on a daily basis can be made using both the standard deviation, s, and the mean, $\bar{x}$, so that changes in either of these two quantities can be evaluated as to their statistical significance.

The student should note that a statistic of this type can change in either its mean or its standard deviation, and that these two changes may be independent. A change in the mean, of course, reflects either higher or lower achievement on the quality scale. A change in the standard deviation reflects an increase or decrease in the uniformity with which the quality is obtained within the subgroup. For example, if five patients are selected for nursing audit from a nursing unit each day, the mean audit score may remain at 75 while the standard deviation of the audit scores may increase from five to ten. Such a finding would reflect larger numbers of scores with greater distances from mean value, or a decline in the uniformity of quality on the floor. Of course, the change can be due either to random occurrences or to some change in the process which is worthy of investigation.

Statistical limits for given levels of probability can be assigned to both $\bar{x}_i$ and s_i, where i designates the subgroup. If N subgroup values have been calculated,

$$\bar{\bar{x}} = \frac{\sum_{i=1}^{N} \bar{x}_i}{N}$$ and an unbiased estimate of the standard deviation of $\bar{x}$ is given by the formula:

$$s_{\bar{x}} = \frac{\sum_{i=1}^{N} s_i / N}{\sqrt{n}},$$

where N = number of subgroups, and s = standard deviation for the subgroup of size n. Values of $\bar{x}$ deviant from $\bar{\bar{x}}$ can be assumed to occur with the probability indicated by the normal distribution. That is, unless there has been a change in the underlying process, values of ($\bar{x} - \bar{\bar{x}}$) greater than $1s_{\bar{x}}$ will occur 32 percent of the time and values greater than $2s_{\bar{x}}$ will occur slightly less than 5 percent of the time. Confidence limits of $3s_x$ are commonly used in industry, and these will occur only twice per 1,000 trials.

It is a common procedure to plot quality control information on a graph. The graph usually shows a grand mean of $\bar{x}$, that is $\bar{\bar{x}}$, and confidence limits based on $s_{\bar{x}}$. Individual values of $\bar{x}$ which occur outside the confidence limits have only the indicated probability of occurrence by pure chance and are selected for individual analysis. Once the cause of unusual values of $\bar{x}$ is determined and corrected, it is acceptable to recalculate the values of the grand mean of $\bar{\bar{x}}$ and $s_{\bar{x}}$ excluding the unusual values.

A similar technique can be used to find significant variations in the standard deviation of the subgroups. The individual values of s_i will have a standard deviation, s_s:

$$s_s = \frac{\bar{s}}{\sqrt{2n}}.$$

where s = standard deviation of all values of x taken individually, and n remains the subgroup size

$$s = \frac{\sum_{i=1}^{N} s_i}{N}$$

This distribution can be approximated by the normal distribution, for many applications.[c]

Example. The following example will clarify the analysis of variables measures. This example comes from a hospital where the CASH nursing audit[d] is used. The audit results in a numerical total score for each patient to which it is applied, and the hospital has arranged for application to three randomly selected patients on a given floor on a daily basis. A trained supervisor visits the floor and applies the audit. Her scores, for 20 days, are as follows:

---

[c]Statistical quality control references contain more accurate approximations of the distribution of s_s.

[d]Described in a following chapter.

Audit scores

Day				Day			
1 –	71,	62,	86	11 –	94,	85,	81
2 –	85,	82,	77	12 –	48,	74,	67
3 –	76,	86,	95	13 –	61,	71,	76
4 –	89,	70,	62	14 –	78,	45,	90
5 –	91,	75,	80	15 –	61,	59,	71
6 –	74,	82,	78	16 –	67,	76,	78
7 –	79,	68,	64	17 –	74,	82,	76
8 –	65,	70,	75	18 –	85,	74,	86
9 –	95,	68,	83	19 –	91,	100,	86
10 –	82,	85,	70	20 –	74,	89,	70

The values of the mean, x_i, and standard deviation, s_i, are calculated from the usual formulae:

Day	Mean ($\bar{x}_i$)	Std. Dev. (s_i)
1	73.0	12.1
2	81.3	4.0
3	85.7	9.5
4	73.7	13.9
5	82.0	8.2
6	78.0	4.0
7	70.3	7.8
8	70.0	5.0
9	82.0	13.5
10	79.0	7.9
11	86.7	6.7
12	63.0	13.5
13	69.3	7.6
14	71.0	23.3
15	63.7	6.4
16	73.7	5.9
17	77.3	4.2
18	81.7	6.7
19	92.3	7.1
20	77.7	10.0

The grand mean, $\bar{\bar{x}} = 76.6$ and the overall standard deviation, $\sigma = 11.1$. The standard deviation of $\bar{x}$ is

$$s_{\bar{x}} = \frac{\sum_{i=1}^{N} s_i/N}{\sqrt{n}} = 5.1 \quad ,$$

where $N = 20$ and $n = 3$. The days where the chance of a random ocurrence of $\bar{x}$ is only 5 percent have values of $\bar{x}$ such that $\bar{x} \leq \bar{\bar{x}} - 1.96 s_{\bar{x}}$ or $\bar{x} \geq \bar{\bar{x}} + 1.96 s_{\bar{x}}$. Figure 10-2 shows the individual values of $\bar{x}$ and the grand mean and control limits. It can be seen that days 11, 12, 15, and 19 exceeded the 95 percent control limits.

The standard deviation of s is

$$s_s = \frac{\bar{s}}{\sqrt{2n}} = 3.6,$$

where $n = 3$, and the mean of s is

$$\bar{s} = \sum_{i=1}^{N} s_i/N = 8.8 \quad ,$$

where $N = 20$. Figure 10-3 shows the daily values of s, with $\bar{s}$ and the 95 percent control limits. The deviation of the sample values exceeded these limits on day 14.

The days 11, 12, 14, 15, and 19 are apparently "out of control" and are worthy of more detailed investigation. An error signal is generated on these days. Note that it cannot be inferred that anything unusual has occurred on the floor. The values can occur as a result of expected variation, and on the average, one day of each twenty would appear outside the control limits without identifiable cause. If the nursing supervisor is promptly provided with the information of an "unusual" day, she can investigate it and report her findings. Such an investigation might consist of the following steps:

1. Recheck score calculations of the input data. Revise and reprocess data if an error is found
2. Otherwise, discuss situation with head nurse. Staffing levels, assignment of personnel to sampled patients, general floor conditions, and areas of audit indicating low performance might be included in this discussion
3. Identify cause of unusual score

A report of causes of unusual scores might be prepared by the supervisor for monthly review and discussion. The causes assigned, the trends in the means and

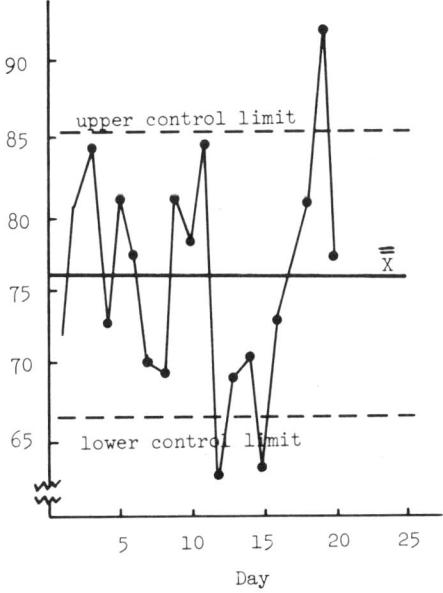

Figure 10-2. Nursing Audit Analysis: Daily Mean Values.

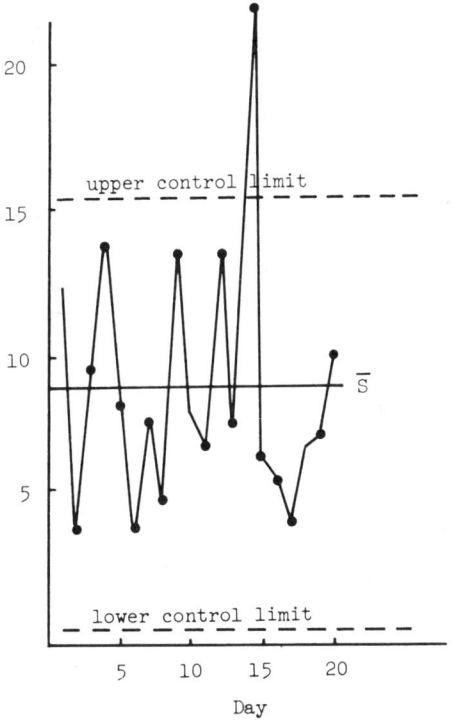

Figure 10-3. Nursing Audit Analysis: Daily Deviations.

control limits, and possible corrective actions could be reviewed. It should be remembered that 5 percent of the unusual cases will have no cause, and for an indeterminant number, the supervisor will have been unable to find the cause. One goal of the system would be to keep this number as low as possible. Another would be to keep $\bar{\bar{x}}$ and $\bar{s}$ stable at levels determined by nursing policy.

Super control statistics. The reports which are generated monthly contain several statistics:

$$\bar{\bar{x}} \text{ and } s_{\bar{x}}$$

$$\bar{s} \text{ and } s_{\bar{s}} \quad ,$$

and a percentage of unusual cases, p, for which no cause has been found. For a large hospital, a report can be prepared for administration which is based on a reapplication of the same quality control techniques. This report would treat the monthly reports of several supervisors as a subgroup with a mean quality score Q and a mean deviation, D, where

$$D = \sqrt{\frac{\sum \bar{s}^2}{N-1}}$$

where N = number of supervisors' monthly reports. (This formula makes several simplifying assumptions, primarily that the sampling routine is the same for each supervisor, that the samples are from different patient groups which do not overlap, and that the expectation of the same value of $\bar{s}$ from each supervisor is reasonable. In actual practice, a considerably more complicated estimate of D might be required and would have to be developed by a skilled statistician.) If $p=$ percent of unusual cases for which no cause is found, a mean of $\bar{p}$ can be calculated. This is an attributes measure and must be analyzed in the manner described below.

Control limits can be set for each of these statistics, Q, D, and $\bar{p}$, based on past monthly experience, and unusual cases can be investigated by the director of nurses and discussed with administration. $\bar{Q}$, $\bar{D}$, and their control limits might also be reported to the board of trustees.

In this example the analysis of a continuous variable quality measure, a nursing audit score, has been traced through the elementary statistical analysis, and a system has been outlined which routinely isolates the unusual cases, analyzes them, and prepares second and third level reports of the operation of the basic system. The amount of work necessary to implement the investigations can be controlled by adjusting the control limits to varying levels of the Z statistic from the normal table. (For $Z = 1.96$, one case in twenty will be investigated, plus cases caused by changes in the true level of care; for $Z = 2.58$, one in a hundred will be investigated plus a smaller number of cases caused by a larger change in the true level.) The larger the level of Z, the less investigation will be required, but there will be a corresponding reduction in sensitivity of the test. The control system is reviewed in figure 10-4. Substantial volumes of clerical work are involved, almost all of which can be programmed for the computer. Practical use of a quality control system of this type apparently must await the development of computer processing, for the combination of the volume of calculation and the prompt response required seems to preclude manual systems.

Attributes Measures

Attributes measures are those generated where the reference signal is nonquantitative. A quantitative difference signal can be created by making a *count* of items failing to possess the desired attributes, or calculating a *rate* of failures divided by total items examined. The application of the calculations for variables measures becomes impossible (There is no way to calculate a mean or a variance within a set.). In this case, quality control limits must be established on the assumption of independent Bernoulli trials. These were discussed in chapter 3. Under the assumption of an independent probability of failure, which is equally likely for any member of the set, distribution of actual failures in successive sets will follow the binomial distribution. When the probability of failure for any single unit is very small, the binomial is approximated by the Poisson distribution. Control limits are calculated by different procedures in each case, and these are described below.

Measures Following the Poisson Process. Certain attributes measures within the hospital, particularly those which relate to unexpected results of the medical care process, conform to criteria of the Poisson process. Briefly stated, these criteria are for independence of each occurrence from all other occurrences, a low probability of occurrence and an equal probability of an occurrence in any given small time period. Many kinds of accidental occurrences, such as accidents occurring to staff members, accidents occurring to guests and visitors to the hospital, patient falls, and medication errors may be expected to follow the Poisson process. In addition it is possible that certain employee turnover statistics follow a Poisson process, and that at least certain forms of patient death statistics, particularly those where the risk of death is usually small, are Poisson. A given statistic can be tested for the closeness of a Poisson approximation by calculating the χ^2 value as indicated in chapter 3. The process is discrete, that is, it results in a series of specific integer values (counts of occurrences) and the difference between two adjacent values is not trivial. It should be noted, however, that assumption of a stationary Poisson process

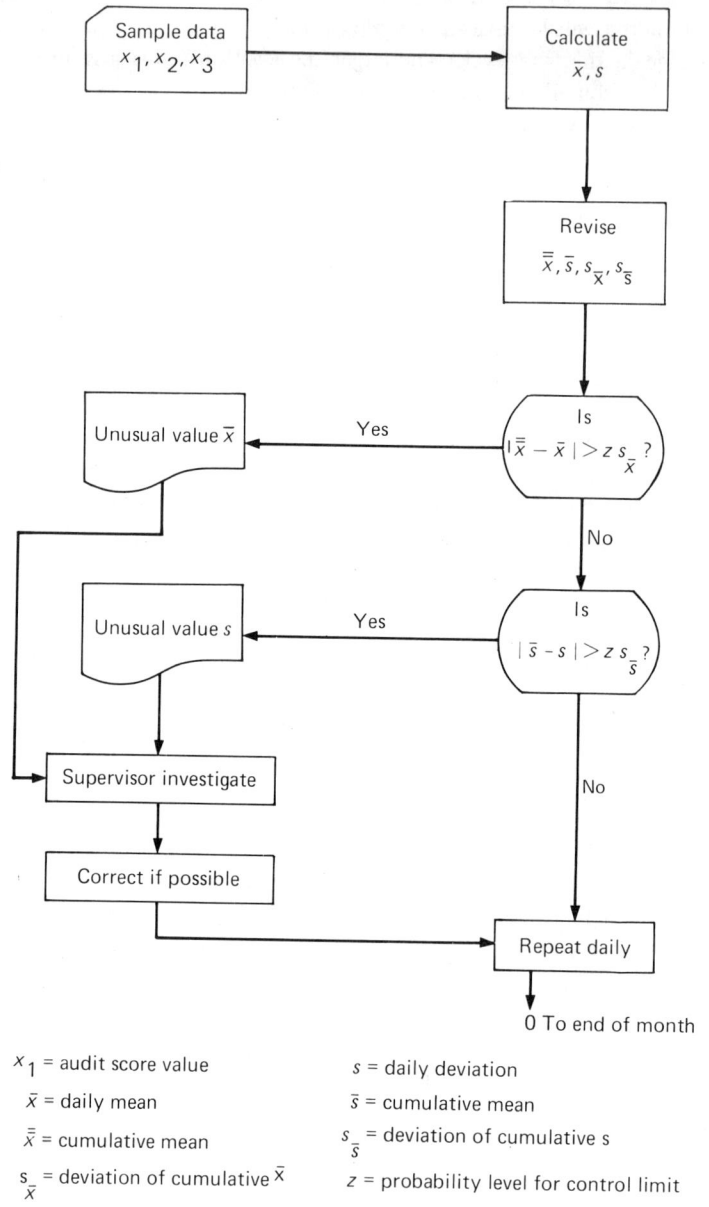

x_1 = audit score value
$\bar{x}$ = daily mean
$\bar{\bar{x}}$ = cumulative mean
$s_{\bar{x}}$ = deviation of cumulative $\bar{x}$
s = daily deviation
$\bar{s}$ = cumulative mean
$s_{\bar{s}}$ = deviation of cumulative s
z = probability level for control limit

Figure 10-4. Control System for Nursing Quality Part 1 — Daily, by Nursing Supervisor, for Each Floor.

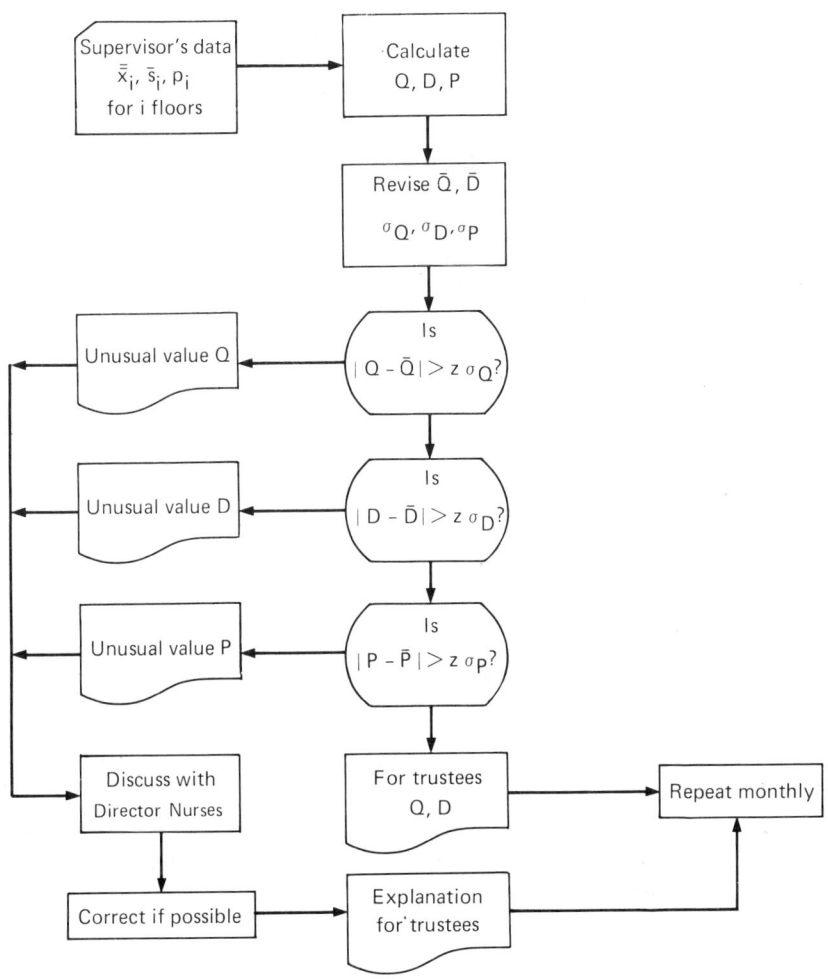

Q = hospital wide mean quality score

D = hospital wide mean deviation

σ_Q = deviation of Q about $\bar{Q}$

σ_D = deviation of D about $\bar{D}$

$\bar{Q}$ = historic mean of Q

$\bar{D}$ = historic mean of D

p_i = individual floor percent unexplained cases outside limits

P = mean of p_i for all floors for month.

Figure 10-4 cont. Control System for Nursing Quality. Part 2 — Monthly for Several Floors.

assumes stability in a population at risk. If for example a measure of turnover, the number of terminations per month, has been tested and found to follow a Poisson distribution but is then applied in a situation where the total work force is expanding, this statistic would reasonably be expected to drift upwards in value. This situation might still follow a Poisson process, but would be nonstationary.

If all conditions are met, a stationary Poisson process control statistic will be reported as an integer n_i over a series of equal time periods N. The mean or expected value of a Poisson distribution statistic will be:

$$m = \frac{\sum_{i=1}^{N} n_i}{N},$$

and the standard deviation

$$\sigma = \sqrt{m}.$$

The probability of occurrences different from the means by one, two, or three standard deviations does not follow the normal distribution, however, unless the mean is large. Control limits must be set by reference to tabulated values of the Poisson process. The only control limits are upon the individual n_i which have a known probability of occurrence given the assumption of a stationary Poisson process.

The following record of receipt of unusual incidents reports occurring to patients will illustrate. Each day r reports are received. The values are listed on chronological order by columns

2	3	2	1
3	0	1	2
0	2	1	1
0	2	1	1
0	2	2	2
1	0	4	0
0	2	0	1
0	0	3	0
1	1	1	0
0	0	1	1
1	0	1	3
0	1	0	1
1	0	1	1
1	4	4	1
4	4	1	1

$N = 60$. The total number of reports received

$$\left(\sum_{i=1}^{60} r_i \right)$$

is 74, and the distribution is as follows:

r	frequency
0	18
1	24
2	9
3	4
4	5
5	0

The estimate of the mean is

$$m = \sum_{i=1}^{N} r_i/N = 1.23 \quad ,$$

and the standard deviation

$$s = \sqrt{m} = 1.11 \quad .$$

The limits for quality control purposes can be set by reference to the Poisson distribution tables if this distribution actually represents a Poisson process. The usual χ^2 test can be performed against the Poisson distribution.

r	Frequency Actual	Expected ($\bar{x} = 1.2$)
0	18	18
1	24	22
2	9	13 $\chi^2 = 6.21$
3	4	5
4 or more	5	2

This value is within the $\chi^2_{0.05}$ value of 7.85 for 3 degrees of freedom. (An additional degree of freedom is lost by combining the values of r greater than 3.)

For a Poisson distribution with a mean of 1.2, the probabilities of each possible value are:

r	Probability	Cumulative Probability
0	0.301	1.000
1	0.361	0.699
2	0.217	0.337
3	0.087	0.121
4	0.026	0.034
5 or more	0.008	0.008

Values of r greater than 2 can be expected to occur 12 percent of the time, and those greater than 3 can be expected 4 percent of the time. An error signal might be established at this level. If values of 4 or more were investigated, there were five occurrences to investigate in this series. As was the case in the variables measure example, this frequency is higher than expected, indicating some possibility of deterioration in the control process.

As the populations at risk under a Poisson process become larger, the mean or expected value increases. Values of the Poisson formula are not tabulated for large means, but the distribution approximates the normal distribution. Use of the normal distribution to set control limits is usual for expected values greater than 25 and introduces no significant error in the control system.

Measures of Fraction Defective. A number of control measures do not meet the Poisson condition of low individual probability, but do meet the other assumptions of Bernoulli trials. The statistic of interest is presented as the fraction which meets (or the fraction which failed to meet) criteria for a given category. Some examples are the percentage of surgical tissue examined and found to be normal, the percentage of deaths undergoing autopsy, and possibly the percentage of personnel absent from work.

Where the Bernoulli process applies, a given sample of N items at risk will yield c items which fit the category of interest. A number of such samples will permit the calculation of an average fraction, $\bar{p}$:

$$\bar{p} = \frac{c}{N}.$$

p has a standard deviation:

$$\sigma_{\bar{p}} = \sqrt{\frac{\bar{p}(1-\bar{p})}{(N-1)}}.$$

where N is the size of the total population at risk in the particular sample or group of samples.

For a given shorter period of time, if n cases were at risk and c of these were in the category of interest, the fraction, p

$$p = \frac{c}{n} \quad \text{and} \quad \sigma_p = \sqrt{\frac{\bar{p}(1-\bar{p})}{n-1}} \ .$$

These values can be used to establish control limits and checked against $\bar{p}$. The values of p are distributed about $\bar{p}$ according to the binomial distribution. This distribution is tabulated for $n \leq 50$, and various $\bar{p}$ but except for very small values of $\bar{p}$ or n, the normal distribution is quite satisfactory as an approximation. The control limits for generating an error signal for p depend upon the sample size n. Charts for control limits of fraction defective are often established to show acceptable values of p at varying n. Alternatively, standardized control limits can be obtained by dividing the deviation in p by its own standard deviation. The resulting statistic has a mean value of 0 and a standard deviation of 1.

The formula which would be used is as follows:

$$\frac{p - \bar{p}}{\sigma_p} = \frac{p - \bar{p}}{\sqrt{\frac{\bar{p}(1-\bar{p})}{n-1}}} \ .$$

Example. A medium-sized hospital performed 140 appendectomies in the past year, or 11.7 per month. Pathology reports for the past year indicate that 20 percent, or 28 cases, were not justified on the basis of tissue examination. (Most authorities feel that this statistic should not be less than 15 percent because of the difficulties of diagnosis prior to surgery.)

$$\bar{p} = 0.20 \quad \sigma_{\bar{p}} = \sqrt{\frac{\bar{p}(1-\bar{p})}{N-1}} = \sqrt{\frac{0.20 \times 0.80}{139}} = 0.033 \ .$$

In the last month, 13 appendectomies were performed, with 4 not justified by the pathology.

$$p = \frac{4}{13} = 0.307 \quad \sigma_p = \sqrt{\frac{\bar{p}(1-\bar{p})}{n-1}} = \sqrt{\frac{0.2 \times 0.8}{12}} = 0.11 \ .$$

The 2 σ_p limits are $\bar{p}+.22$ (=0.42) and $\bar{p}-0.22$ (=0).
The value falls well within 2 σ limits of $\bar{p}$ for a sample of this size. For 13 cases, any value of normal tissue less than 6 would be within 95 percent control limits. Using the standardized formula,

$$\frac{p - \bar{p}}{\sigma_p} = \frac{0.31 - 0.20}{0.11} = 1.0,$$

indicating that this value falls one standard deviation from the mean p.

A variable control limit chart can be constructed for the control limits against which p is compared for varying sample sizes. If the control limit is to be 2σ, the acceptable values of p are as follows for various sample sizes:

n	σ_p	$\bar{p} + 2\sigma_p$	$\bar{p} - 2\sigma_p$	Acceptable c_{min}	c_{max}
10	0.13	0.46	0.00	0	4
15	0.10	0.40	0.00	0	6
20	0.09	0.38	0.02	1	7
25	0.08	0.36	0.04	1	9
30	0.07	0.35	0.05	2	10
35	0.07	0.35	0.07	3	11
40	0.05	0.30	0.10	4	12

These values can be plotted for easy reference, as shown in figure 10-5. Although the larger values of n are not likely to occur in a single month, it is possible and often desirable to combine the data for several consecutive months.

Testing the Difference between Two Quality Control Statistics

It is often desirable to compare performance as measured by quality control statistics between two different hospitals or two different nursing units or two different physicians. One possibility for this is to compare actual distributions of control score values on the two populations, and test the distributions themselves using chi-square. The conditions for the use of chi-square, namely that there be at least five entries for each cell in the matrix, must be met. An alternative test is to construct the t statistic for the difference between two means:

$$t = \frac{\bar{x}_1 - \bar{x}_2}{s \sqrt{\frac{1}{n_1} + \frac{1}{n_2}}},$$

and

$$s = \sqrt{\frac{(n_1 - 1)s_{x_1}^2 + (n_2 - 1)s_{x_2}^2}{n_1 + n_2 - 2}},$$

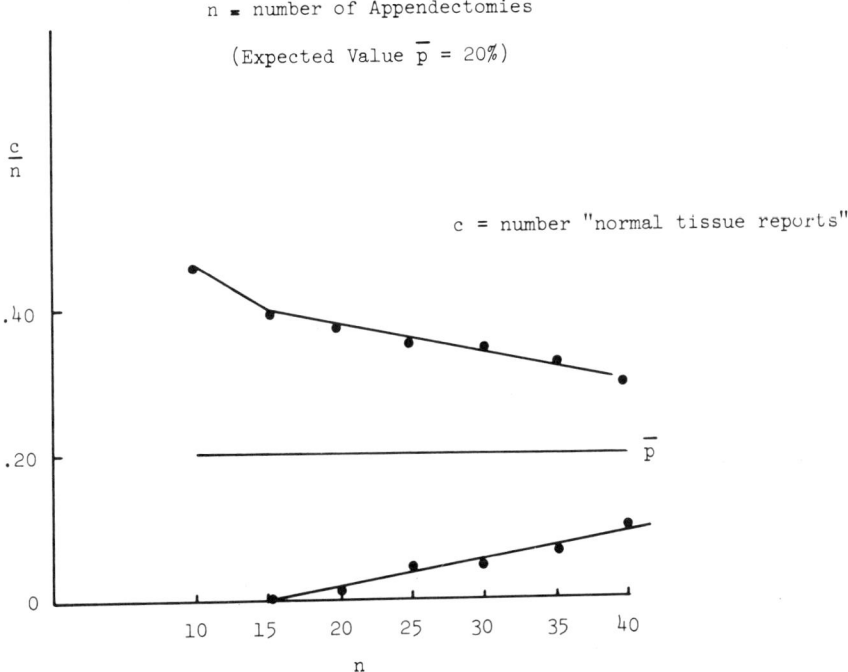

Figure 10-5. Control Limits on "Normal Tissue" Reports.

where the s_x values are estimated as indicated above. This statistic follows the student t distribution, for $(n_1 + n_2 - 2)$ degrees of freedom.

This formula can be solved for sample size if it is felt necessary to test the hypothesis that a statistically significant difference exists between the two means at a given level of confidence. The maximum sensitivity from the test is obtained when the two sample sizes n_1 and n_2 are equal. Solving the preceding equation under this assumption yields:

$$n = \frac{Z^2(\sigma_1^2 + \sigma_2^2)}{|\bar{x}_1 - \bar{x}_2|^2}.$$

An estimate of n can be made by postulating the amount of difference which will be acceptable and the level of confidence at which it must be tested (i.e., $Z = 1.96$ for a level of confidence of 0.05) and assuming values of σ_1 and σ_2 based on prior knowledge of the distribution of the statistic.

Meaning of Statistical Deviation

Great care must be taken in interpreting the results of a deviation which has been tested and found to be significantly different either from a series of past values of the same population or from the value of a similar population. The purpose of the statistical analysis is *to detect those cases where there is a high probability that further analysis will yield identifiable factors which differ in some manner from those in other cases.* No conclusion of "goodness" or "badness" can be inferred from any deviation no matter how significant it may be statistically. It is possible for statistically significant differences to be created by changes in the nature of demand for the service being tested as well as from changes in the way in which the service is delivered. It should also be noted that for any given level of significance there is a possibility of selecting a deviant case which, in fact, is caused by pure chance and situation. For example, if a level of significance of 10 percent is selected, then inevitably over the long run one out of every ten cases sampled will appear as deviant reports, but will not reveal any identifiable underlying factor when it has been analyzed. Similarly, if a significance level of 0.05 is selected, the chance will be one out of twenty. From a mathematical viewpoint, as well as from the viewpoint of sound organizational behavior, the only justifiable interpretation of a deviant value is that it is one that makes further study of the situation desirable. The correct interpretation of a deviant quality measure is always, "Were there identifiable causes of this situation which might be of value in improving the general level of quality in the future?"

It should also be noted that the statistical limits which are established by the nature of the process itself are entirely separate and distinct from any concept of a "minimal acceptable" level which may be set by some hospital policy. For example, assume that the process of obtaining autopsies on deceased patients is a Bernoulli process which has had a mean value over the past year of 0.33 in a hospital with 300 deaths per year. Over one year's time:

$$\bar{p} = 0.33$$

$$\sigma_{\bar{p}} = \sqrt{\frac{\bar{p}(1-\bar{p})}{N-1}} = \sqrt{\frac{0.33 \times 0.67}{299}} = 0.027$$

$$\bar{p} \pm 1.96\,\sigma_{\bar{p}} = 0.33 \pm 0.05 \text{ at } 95\% \text{ confidence.}$$

If the hospital accepts as a minimum acceptable level that no less than 25 percent of all deaths be autopsied in any one year, past performance is well above this level. For any given year the chance of a value of p of 0.25 or less is:

$$Z = \frac{|\bar{p} - 0.25|}{\sigma_p} = \frac{0.08}{0.027} = 2.962 \quad .$$

From the normal table, Z is less or equal to 2.96 with a probability of 0.9985. Thus a value of $\bar{p}$ less than 0.25 will occur 15 times in 10,000 years. However, for any average month:

$$\sigma_p = \sqrt{\frac{0.33 \times 0.67}{24}} = 0.094 \quad .$$

A value of $p = 0.25$ or less gives a Z statistic:

$$Z = \frac{|\bar{p} - 0.25|}{0.09} = \frac{0.08}{0.094} = 0.851 \quad .$$

From the normal table, such a value can occur 20 percent of the time. (The binomial distribution can be substituted for the normal for smaller n. The difference is not significant for the examples.)

The 0.05 confidence limit for values below the limit (remembering that the usual "0.05 confidence limits" is for values *above* and *below*) is at

$$Z = 1.645$$

$$1.645 = \frac{|\bar{p} - p_{LCL}|}{0.094}$$

$$1.645 \times 0.094 = |\bar{p} - p_{LCL}|, \text{ where } \bar{p} = 0.33$$

$$p_{LCL} = 0.33 - 0.15 = 0.18$$

Thus in any given month, if the medical care committee wishes to investigate reductions in the autopsy rate only when there is a 95 percent chance that some change could actually be detected in the process, they would not investigate monthly autopsy percentages unless less than 18 percent of the deaths which occurred were autopsied.

Considerably more is known about the interpretation of quality control statistics than has been presented in this brief review. For example, it is possible to refine the process of selecting likely situations for study by considering "runs" of quality control values. In the example above, although there is a 5 percent chance of getting an autopsy rate of only 18 percent without any change in the basic process in a single month given the assumption that it is a true Bernoulli process, the probability of getting 18 percent in two months successively is approximately 0.05 × 0.05 or 0.0025. Thus, if the committee is willing to accept an autopsy rate of 20 percent for one month, two successive values of 20 percent would be evidence of a situation well within their normal criteria for investigation, that is whenever there is a 0.05 chance of detecting some change in the process. Complete analysis of the probabilities of "runs" and of other refinements of quality control statistics is beyond the scope of this book, but the student is referred to established references on industrial quality control.[2]

Additional Readings

Bowman, E.H. and Fetter, R.B., *Analysis for Production and Operations Management*, 3rd Ed., R.D. Irwin, Inc., Homewood, Illinois, 1967, p. 164 ff.
The derivation of the formulae and industrial examples can be found in industrial quality control texts such as Duncan, A.J., *Quality Control in Industrial Statistics*, 3rd Ed., R.D. Irwin, Homewood, Ill., 1965.

11 Examples of Hospital Control Systems

Introduction

Given the basic concepts and techniques of control systems described in the preceding chapter, this chapter and the two which follow it will be devoted to examples of the development of explicit quantitative primary and super-control systems which are necessary to improve the effectiveness of hospital operations. Before beginning a review of the examples, it seems desirable to summarize the key points of the preceding chapter as these relate to the design of explicit control systems.

First, the purposes of control systems generally are to identify processes or conditions where organizational goals are not being achieved and also to provide assurance that the areas or processes not identified are working satisfactorily. Since these purposes are met in part by implicit and nonquantitative systems, the justification of explicit quantitative control systems lies in their ability to reduce the human resource effort necessary to achieve control and/or to improve the degree of control for a given effort at either the primary or super control level. Explicit quantitative control systems should be carefully designed to supplement and not to impede or replace effective human control systems.

Second, the benefits of explicit quantitative systems come principally in the sensor and monitor elements of control. At least in hospital systems, controller elements remain largely in the realm of human organizational behavior. The systems described below generally make their contribution by improving the reliability or sensitivity of the reference signal and by automating the monitor process which generates the error signal. Since these systems rarely, if ever, go beyond that point to controller activities, they are only partial control systems. Their output is an error signal which has a high probability of reflecting an actual change in the process under control. The measure of potential benefit is their ability to minimize the generation of a false-positive error signal for a given level of protection against the false negative signal. Their costs and time lags, both of which are often substantial, must be considered in the light of this benefit.

Third, the total systems, including sensor, monitor, and controller elements, must be measured by the value of the improved control which can be achieved. The decision to install or improve a given control system should ultimately judge the relation of the total additional cost to the value of the improved control.

The design of explicit control systems for hospitals has largely been an effort of recent years. Although the examples described are far less than a comprehensive list of all the efforts which have been made, quantitative control systems are almost all in experimental or early demonstration phases. Few, if any of the systems which will be described are working at a level approaching their apparent potential. Their development to this point has been facilitated by technological advances in computer science and medical science, and spurred by increasing social concern about the cost and quality of medical and hospital care. Since these factors are continuing and increasing, it seems likely that the development and application of quantitative control techniques will be accelerating over the next few years.

This chapter will review the development of systems for the control of resources (and costs) in hospitals and will describe the principal efforts towards controlling the quality of nonmedical processes including nursing. The two chapters which follow will review the development of quantitative systems for aiding in controlling the quality of the medical care process itself.

Resource Control Systems

Discussion

The resources or inputs to a process are the manpower, supplies, facilities, and equipment which are allocated to it. In most cases, they are monetary costs, and they are measured more or less accurately by the accounting process of the organization. Their use is controlled with a view to the outputs of the process. The notion is implied that for a given quantity of output there is an expected cost of inputs. This is a concept of efficiency, which can be defined as:

$$E = \frac{\text{actual output}}{\text{(expected output for a given quantity of resources)}}$$

The efficiency concept can be applied either to physical resources such as facilities and equipment or to human resources. The application to physical resources is easier. In many cases the expected output is immediately obvious. For example, if the hospital has 100 beds available, the expected output is 100 patient days per day. If the actual output on a given day is 80 patient days, the efficiency of utilization of the resources is 80 percent. Occupancy and statistics like it are measures of efficiency of utilization of physical facilities. In more complex cases, the expected output must be calculated by reference to a standard. If for example an x-ray machine is used for chest x-rays which take two minutes apiece, the expected output of the machine is thirty examinations per hour. As noted in the preceding chapter, the standard can be calculated by reference to the average of historic achievement or constructed by careful study of the procedure using industrial engineering techniques.

Problem of Stochastic Variation

Stochastic variation in demand or in the amount of resources required to service demand can interfere seriously with the achievement of high levels of efficiency. When demand varies in an unpredictable manner, resources are allocated to handle some level of peak load in demand. Over a period of time, the average efficiency will be the ratio of the average demand to the resources allocated for the peak load condition. Efficiency in these cases will be relatively low, as noted in chapter 7. In addition, the variation in efficiency will be high because it is directly related to the daily variation in demand. This difficulty occurs frequently in hospitals. When it does, the efficiency measure has a relatively low mean and high variance and is no longer useful for control purposes. The only solutions are systems which reduce the variance in demand by scheduling or deliberately varying resources. Efficiency controls for systems of this type usually measure both the performance of the original process and simultaneously the performance of the scheduling or staffing process.

Problem of Efficiency of Human Resources

The use of human resources in the processes under efficiency control introduces another problem area. One difficulty is the lack of direct measure of human resources. Standards established for human performance by industrial engineers are based on subjective comparisons of the amount of effort necessary to perform certain simple and well-described tasks as walking a given distance or moving a small object. In more complex processes such as are found in hospitals, the ability of the individual to influence the efficiency and quality of the result is quite great and depends importantly on his attitudes and motivation. Performances consistently 30 to 40 percent better than industrial engineering standards are often encountered in simple, easily measured tasks. It seems likely that contributions can be at least as great in more complex processes like most hospital activities.

Some effort has been devoted to the measurement of attitudinal states of the work force in hospitals and in industry.[1,2] There is evidence that the style of management has an important effect on motivation and performance.[3,4] Authoritative styles of management apparently reduce motivation and individual effort and may curtail performance, even though such styles tend to rely upon formal control systems and efficiency measures. More participative management styles may in the long run obtain greater performance. The way in which efficiency data are used seems to be important in this regard; it is likely that control systems which are viewed by primary controllers and employees as something for their assistance are most satisfactory. Careless use of error signals by the controller, or the establishment of insensitive or unreasonable standards, can create the danger of a negative result. These considerations should be taken into account in designing or evaluating an efficiency control system.

The examples discussed below represent four types of effort to control resource allocation or efficiency. The first, simplest and probably least applicable to the hospital situation is a straight forward measure of the efficiency of a department with a relatively deterministic demand. The second is a brief summary of the use of budgetary and accounting information as a control system on resource allocation. The third is an example of an effort to measure employee productivity by direct although essentially subjective measurement. The fourth is an example of a control system upon a staffing process which attempts to make variable adjustment of resources to varying demand.

Work Standards and Conventional Efficiency Measures

In situations where the demand upon a process can be made stable by scheduling in advance or by the creation of inventories of work awaiting processing, and where a standard of output per man hour or per hour of equipment availability can be established, measures of efficiency can be taken directly by comparing the actual output to the expected output. Historically, this form of control of resource allocation can be traced back to the nineteenth century. It has had reasonably widespread application in some industrial situations. For example, in job shop industries such as the printing industry, time estimates can be made with precision on each incoming job. The actual man hours and machine hours devoted to the job can be recorded as the work progresses and the efficiency comparison of actual to expected can be routinely made at the end of the process. Supervisors of a system of this kind generally manage several jobs over a time period such as a month. They can thus be given an average efficiency rating for the month. Since some stochastic elements remain, this score can be treated as a variables measure and analyzed by statistical techniques if desired. Alternatively, arbitrary standards can be set for the generation error signals. A supervisor might come under censure if his efficiency fell below 90 percent. The use of incentive is also common in situations of this kind. Employees may be expected to maintain efficiencies well over 100 percent and paid in some manner proportionate to their achievement.

Systems of this kind depend on both the stability of demand and a specific description of the work to be done which is unambiguous and understood by all levels of the organization. Even in relatively simple industrial situations, these conditions do not always occur. Ambiguities creep into the specifications, equipment breaks down, raw materials change in quality, and these factors interact with employee attitudes. The result is that the systems themselves require continuous supervision.[5] Few situations in the hospital meet the necessary conditions. Some production activities with relatively stable demand, such as routine maintenance and housekeeping, may be treated in this way. Some production departments which are well buffered by inventories, such as central supply and medical records, may also be considered for this form of control. Work standards exist for a number of departments—laundry, pharmacy, housekeeping, dietary and others—and these are used to estimate long-run manpower requirements.[6] Several factors limit the spread of this approach either to the full extent that it has been used in industry or to the full coverage of the hospital. One is the variation in daily demand, which as noted takes the control of the work output out of the hands of the work team. Another has been the recurring disfavor into which incentive pay schemes have fallen, even in industrial settings. This seems to be related to the attitudinal factors involved. The third and most important for hospitals is the impact of professionalism. Work standards developed from unit times for component tasks are of limited use when the employee has both the authority and the responsibility to vary the length of the task and the task itself to the needs of the patient. Such a situation exists in nursing, which accounts for about half the hospital work force, and in several other departments. Although unit times for individual activities have been carefully developed in some of these departments, including nursing, these are incomplete as control systems. Not only do unpredictable changes in demand reduce their utility. The professional nature of the work places the definition of the amount of the work to be done in the hands of the primary work group.

More flexible approaches are clearly necessary for large parts of the hospital. While conventional time standards are useful in many ways, they fall well short of the total need.

Use of Budgeting and Accounting Data

The typical hospital budget is a plan for resource allocation which can be used as a standard in control systems. Several closely related statistics such as a man hour budget, or a standard based on prior performance, or the performance of other hospitals, can also be used. The actual expenditures of resources, in dollars or units per output unit, revealed by the accounting department become the reference signal. It is common to report deviation from the budget or deviations from previous years as a rudimentary error signal. This raw form has several disadvantages. It is not adjusted to changes in volume which might be expected to cause changes in resource consumption per unit. The deviation is often reported in dollars without adjustment for changes in the prices of resources. The budget as a planning document requires many months to compile and is usually done on an annual basis. Deviations from budget prices, from expected volumes, and from procedural changes begin immediately and tend to cumulate so that the meaningfulness of the error signal deteriorates steadily. Other deviations are cyclical but are not included in budget standards. Correction of these difficulties may be theoretically possible but impractical. Even using computers, the preparation of accounting reports takes a great deal of time.

Reports often reach the primary controllers several weeks or months after the period being reported. Further sophistication can add to the total processing time, and the delay reduces their value.

A number of potential improvements are obvious and many of these have been tried in various situations with differing degrees of success. Reporting only certain elements of resources, such as man hours, permits a shortened response time and eliminates changes in price. These data can often be generated automatically as a by-product of computerized payroll systems. Expectations for manpower costs or usage can be adjusted to monthly variations by the use of cyclical indexes. In some situations it is possible to rebudget the use of certain critical resources so that changes introduced by process adaptations and similar activities are not ignored. When the time period over which the control is calculated is long enough to permit averaging of stochastic variation, accounting measures provide a highly useful control system. A reference signal of output per man hour, over a period of time long enough to smooth random demand variation, is probably the most important single control measure for hospital resources. It can be compared to an empirical standard based upon adjusted historic value or to a standard constructed as a budget item.

There has been continuing effort to refine the accounting document to make it a more sensitive indicator of departmental performance and also to permit comparisons between hospitals. To some extent, however, these activities must remain a secondary purpose of the accounting system. The primary purpose is to measure the expenditures of the hospital against the revenues and to provide data for pricing services both for individual sale and for sale under third party contracts.

Hospital Administrative Services. Hospital Administrative Services (HAS), a national service of the American Hospital Association, has attempted to develop central computer processing of accounting data to provide a set of control sensors.[a] Direct expenses, certain resource measures such as man hours, and certain output measures such as patient days, meals, and pounds of laundry are reported monthly to the central computer service. In return, the hospital receives automatic calculation of certain resource allocation measures for its own situation and comparison against the distribution of similar hospitals classified by size, geography, and function. Hospitals are grouped by function—general, special, or teaching—by size, under 50, 50 to 99, and by hundreds of beds—by region, and by states for comparative purposes. Special national and regional compilations are also prepared periodically. The routine output reports are shown in figures 11-1, 11-2, and 11-3. These are received by the subscriber hospital monthly.

Figures 11-1 and 11-2 report the same data for the member hospital. In figure

---

[a]Hospital Administrative Services, 840 North Lake Shore Drive, Chicago, Illinois, 60611. Descriptive material on the service is prepared periodically and is available on request.

11-1 comparison is against distributions of hospitals in the same district without regard to size, the same state and size category, and the nation for the size category. Figure 11-2, called the Internal Report, provides a comparison against the same month last year and the previous twelve months. Part A of each report provides thirteen basic statistics dealing with revenue and costs in the section entitled "Administrative Indicators." The balance of part A is devoted to percentages of revenue according to the various revenue centers of the hospital. Parts B and C of each report provide a variety of expense and resource measures organized according to major cost centers. For each cost center, the percentage of that center's expenses to the total expenses of the institution are given followed by specifically designed departmental indicators. These are usually either man hours per unit of output or dollars per unit of output or the arithmetic inverse of those statistics. Occasionally measures of utilization of physical capacity, such as the percentage of occupancy, are included, as are ratios of the relative demand for the specific service as compared to other services of the hospital (e.g., operating room visits per hundred medical and surgical admissions). The output measures themselves are shown in figure 11-3, part A and the direct man hours recorded by the cost centers are shown in figure 11-3, part B. The statistics in figure 11-3 are also compared against previous months.

The parts of figure 11-1 show additional statistics giving the quartile ranking of the hospital against the distribution of a comparison group. Thus for the first administrative indicator, inpatient revenue per patient day, the hospital shown in the figure was in the third quartile of the district, $6.58 above the median; but it was in the second quartile of hospitals in its size group in the state and $12.83 below that median. The two extreme quartiles, the first and fourth, are truncated by identifying the 96th and subsequent percentiles with the letter H and the first through fifth percentiles with the letter L. See, for example, anesthesiology and occupational therapy on figure 11-1, part A.

There are 114 lines of data given in figure 11-1 and these lines are repeated in figure 11-2 so that comparison can be made against nine different statistics—previous three months, previous twelve months, and this month last year; district, state, and national medians; and district, state, and national quartiles. There are seventy-six additional statistics in figure 11-3 compared against three standards—the last three months, the last twelve months, and this month last year. The report offers 190 separate control statistics and approximately 1200 standards against which these can be compared. To judge it as an information system for control purposes, one might first review the accuracy and scope of the control statistics and then turn to the standards. Finally, one might consider such items as timeliness and formatting of reports.

Statistics Selected. Turning to the statistics reported for "Your Institution," the accuracy of these columns is entirely within the control of the participating hospital. HAS makes every effort to identify gross errors at the time of processing and provides manuals, consultation, and instruction on definitions of statistics, ways in which the data may be gathered, and recurring problems with the statistics. Since many of the statistics are within the accounting data system of the hospital and are therefore subject to routine cross-checking and auditing, one might assume that they are not only accurate but also consistent. Some parts of the statistcs are more accurate than others, however. Payroll expenditures and accounts receivables tend to be carefully maintained, as do gross statistics, such as patient days of care, births, and discharges. Some other output measures are subject to problems of definition. Laboratory tests, for example, must be counted according to consistent definitions, and pounds of laundry processed must be measured at a standardized point in the laundry activities (wet laundry weighs more than dry). Often the auditing of these minor statistics is limited and the accuracy is subject to some question. One dietician at a HAS member hospital was asked how she calculated the number of meals served to patients. She replied that she always took the reported number of patient days and multiplied it by 2.8. No one could recall the source of the 2.8 figure and there were no data to show that a constant multiplier was an accurate measure of output.

Most of the specific statistics selected have a high degree of face validity. Any administrator would be interested in his revenue, his costs, his accounts receivable, his uncollectible accounts, and his payroll expenditures for non-productive hours. "Equivalent full-time employees per bed" is a standard comparative statistic among hospitals which has some years of use. The statistics which express resources per unit of output, which occur repeatedly in parts B and C of the first two figures, are common measures of efficiency and are probably important for any administrative control system. The various other ratios and statistics given on parts B and C are sometimes more questionable. One might speculate, for example, on what the number of operating room visits per 100 medical and surgical admissions means. Certainly one could not make any direct assumptions about this ratio or its impact upon operating room cost per visit.

About forty of the statistics are either expense or revenue percentages which show the fraction of total revenues or total expenses of the cost center versus the hospital total. The interrelated nature of these statistics makes interpretation of them anything but straightforward. As a general matter, it is of interest to know the relative sources of revenue and the relative uses of funds. It does not seem likely that these percentages are useful as a continuing control device, however. One of the first problems is the extreme disparity in the percentages. While medical-surgical units generate over 50 percent of the revenue in the hospital shown in the figure, other important activities, such as labor and delivery room, generate only fractions of a percent. A similar but less severe problem exists with the expense percentages. It should be noted that there are a

JANUARY 1972
PAGE 1

	YOUR INSTITUTION		COMPARATIVE MEDIANS FOR PREVIOUS THREE MONTHS			
	CURRENT MONTH	PREVIOUS 3 MONTHS	DISTRICT GROUP 50 GROUP 24 COMPARED	STATE GROUP 545 25 COMPARED	NATIONAL GROUP 935 326 COMPARED	
1 -----ADMINISTRATIVE INDICATORS-----						
2 INPATIENT-REVENUE PER PATIENT DAY	93.85	96.28	87.27 3	106.68 2	91.46 3	
3 -COST PER PATIENT DAY RCCAC	87.58	94.35	82.40 3	96.53 2	84.12 3	
4 ACCOUNTS+NOTES RECEIVABLE 1000'S	1,693.00	1,578.00	446.00 4	1,231.00 3	1,319.00 3	
5 -DAYS OF REVENUE IN ACCTS. REC.	72.41	70.02	67.76 3	59.59 4	65.60 3	
6 ALLOW FOR UNCOLLECTABLE REC 1000'S	87.00	121.00	72.00 3	121.00 2	182.00 2	
7 -PERCENT OF ACCTS. REC.	5.13	7.66	12.21 1	9.30 2	13.99 1	
8 ALL NURSING UNITS-EXPENSE PERCENT	25.62	24.51	25.62 2	25.18 2	25.26 2	
9 -PERCENT OF OCCUPANCY	80.37	75.46	75.00 3	76.22 2	78.43 2	
10 -LENGTH OF STAY	7.55	7.14	6.92 3	7.27 2	7.23 2	
11 -DIRECT COST PER PATIENT DAY	25.24	26.02	24.37 2	26.80 2	22.97 3	
12 -MANHOURS PER BED PER DAY	4.38	4.25	4.44 2	4.98 1	4.75 1	
13 HOL.+VAC. SICK PAY DOLLARS 1000'S	41.51	26.64	8.80 4	25.73 3	20.39 3	
14 -PERCENT OF SALARIES	9.61	6.16	6.16 2	6.18 2	6.44 2	
15 EQUIV. FULL TIME EMPLOYEE PER BED	2.52	2.52	1.98 4	2.33 3	2.29 3	
16 -----REVENUE PERCENTAGES-----						
17 OBSTETRICAL NURSING UNITS	2.3	2.8	3.5 1	4.2 1	3.4 2	
18 NURSERIES	1.3	1.7	1.8 2	2.2 1	1.6 3	
19 MEDICAL + SURGICAL NURSING UNITS	52.4	50.3	47.6 3	45.5 3	46.2 3	
20 DELIVERY AND LABOR ROOMS	.7	.9	1.1 2	1.4 1	1.0 2	
21 OPERATING ROOMS	5.3	5.5	3.8 4	5.6 2	5.5 2	
22 RECOVERY ROOMS	---	---	.6	.7	.8	
23 CENTRAL SERVICES + SUPPLY	2.5	2.4	2.7 2	2.6 2	2.8 2	
24 INTRAVENOUS THERAPY	.8	.8	.8 2	1.0 2	1.4 1	
25 EMERGENCY SERVICES	3.8	3.8	3.1 4	3.1 4	2.9 3	
26 LABORATORY-INPATIENT	8.7	8.7	7.8 4	8.1 3	5.1 2	
27 -OUTPATIENT	2.6	2.5	2.2 4	1.3 4	1.2 4	
28 BLOOD BANK	---	---	.2	.5	.5	
29 RADIOLOGY-INPATIENT	2.5	3.1	3.3 2	3.4 2	4.8 1	
30 -OUTPATIENT	3.8	4.0	3.5 3	3.5 3	2.8 3	
31 PHARMACY-INPATIENT	4.2	4.3	5.8 1	6.2 1	6.2 1	
32 -OUTPATIENT	.5	.5	.4 3	.3 3	.3 3	
33 ANESTHESIOLOGY	4.9	5.5	2.1 H	2.5 4	1.7 H	
34 INHALATION THERAPY	2.2	1.9	2.2 2	2.1 2	2.2 2	
35 PHYSICAL THERAPY	1.1	1.1	1.6 2	1.6 2	1.0 3	
36 OCCUPATIONAL + RECREATIONAL THERAPY	.1	---	.4 L	.4 L	.2 L	
37 CLINICS	---	---	---	.5	.7	
38 ALL OTHER PATIENT SERVICES	.1	.2	1.2 L	1.4 1	1.9 L	
39 GROSS INPATIENT REVENUE	88.7	88.7	88.6 3	90.1 2	90.9 2	
40 GROSS OUTPATIENT REVENUE	11.3	11.3	11.0 3	9.8 3	9.0 3	
41 TOTAL PATIENT REVENUE	100.0	100.0	---	---	---	
42 DEDUCTIONS FROM PATIENT REVENUE	-5.0	-4.5	-4.6 3	-6.4 3	-8.6 4	

Figure 11-1, Part A. Comparative Report, Statement of Revenues. Source: American Hospital Association, 840 North Lake Shore Drive, Chicago, Ill. 60611, Hospital Administration Services.

JANUARY 1972
PAGE 2

	YOUR INSTITUTION		COMPARATIVE MEDIANS FOR PREVIOUS THREE MONTHS			
	CURRENT MONTH	PREVIOUS 3 MONTHS	DISTRICT GROUP 50 24 COMPARED	STATE GROUP 545 25 COMPARED	NATIONAL GROUP 935 326 COMPARED	
1 ------NURSING DIVISION------						
2 NURSING ADM.-EXPENSE PERCENT	3.2	3.0	1.9| 4	1.6| 4	1.7|4	
3 -MANHOURS PER BED PER MONTH	26.23	25.15	8.87|4	7.13| 4	7.50|4	
4 ------OBSTETRICAL SERVICES------						
5 OBSTETRICAL UNIT-EXPENSE PERCENT	1.3	1.3	1.5| 2	1.6| 1	1.6| 2	
6 -PERCENT OCCUPANCY	38.97	46.50	50.00| 2	63.01| 1	57.53| 1	
7 -PERCENT OF TOTAL ADMISSIONS	7.25	9.70	11.84|4	15.06| 1	12.88| 1	
8 -AVERAGE LENGTH OF STAY	4.46	3.97	3.97| 2	4.23| 2	3.83| 3	
9 -OBSTETRICAL TURNOVER RATE	2.83	3.58	3.66| 2	4.28| 1	4.50| 2	
10 -NURSING MH PER PATIENT DAY	8.76	7.42	6.01| 4	5.53| 4	5.96| 3	
11 DEL.+ LABOR ROOMS-EXPENSE PERCENT	.7	.8	.7| 3	1.2| 1	1.1| 1	
12 -DIRECT COST PER DELIVERY	75.16	64.15	38.71| 4	75.00| 1	71.13| 2	
13 -DELIVERY+LABOR MH PER DELIVERY	14.47	12.62	6.78| 3	15.25| 1	15.15| 2	
14 NURSERY UNIT-EXPENSE PERCENT	1.1	1.4	1.0| 3	1.4| 2	1.3| 2	
15 -NURSERY MH PER BASSINET PER DAY	3.04	3.76	2.04| 4	2.49| 4	2.25| 4	
16 ------GENERAL NURSING UNITS------						
17 MED.+SURG. UNITS-EXPENSE PERCENT	20.0	18.8	22.3| 1	20.8| 1	20.5| 2	
18 -PERCENT OCCUPANCY	84.33	78.22	77.50| 3	80.83| 2	80.93| 2	
19 -AVERAGE LENGTH OF STAY	7.79	7.48	7.45| 3	7.81| 1	7.75| 2	
20 -MED.+SURG. TURNOVER RATE	3.46	3.18	3.04| 3	2.98| 3	2.99| 3	
21 -NURSING MH PER BED PER DAY	4.47	4.32	4.78| 2	5.01| 1	4.85| 1	
22 -NURSING MH PER PATIENT DAY	5.30	5.53	6.59|L		6.14| 2	
23 -PERCENT REGISTERED NURSES	---	---	29.00	33.64	37.00	
24 -PERCENT LICENSED PRACTICAL NURSES	---	---	18.78	20.43	19.09	
25 ------OTHER NURSING SERVICES------						
26 OPERATING ROOMS-EXPENSE PERCENT	3.7	3.8	2.9| 4	3.7| 3	4.1| 2	
27 -O.R. VISITS/100 M+S ADMISSIONS	48.10	51.75	37.27| 3	56.76| 1	56.08| 2	
28 -DIRECT COST PER O.R. VISIT	60.21	63.25	58.24| 3	61.26| 3	59.11| 3	
29 -MANHOURS PER O.R. VISIT	11.30	11.90	8.94| 3	9.52| 3	10.52| 3	
30 RECOVERY ROOMS-EXPENSE PERCENT	---	---	.4	.4	.4	
31 CENTRAL SERVICES-EXPENSE PERCENT	1.8	1.8	2.2| 2	1.9| 2	2.2| 2	
32 -DIRECT COST PER PATIENT DAY	1.74	1.93	2.08| 2	2.07| 2	2.08| 2	
33 -LINE ITEMS PER MANHOUR	---	---	3.16	4.01	3.75	
34 INTRAVENOUS THERAPY-EXPENSE PERCENT	.7	.7	.3| 4	.5| 3	.6| 3	
35 -DIRECT COST PER PATIENT DAY	.68	.71	.37| 3	.60| 3	.56| 3	
36 EMERGENCY SERVICE-EXPENSE PERCENT	2.4	2.3	1.9| 3	2.4| 2	2.2| 3	
37 -MANHOURS PER VISIT	1.85	1.84	1.21| 4	1.47| 4	1.51| 3	
38 NURSING EDUCATION-EXPENSE PERCENT	3.6	3.6	.6| 4	.5| 4	1.2| 4	
39 CLINIC-EXPENSE PERCENT	---	---	---	.3	.7	
40 -MANHOURS PER VISIT	---	---	---	---	1.63	
41 -VISITS PER BED PER MONTH	---	---	---	2.69	1.48	

Figure 11-1, Part B. Comparative Report, Statement of Expenses. Source: Same as Fig. 11-1, Part A.

JANUARY 1972
PAGE 7

	SAME MONTH PREVIOUS YEAR	AVERAGE OF PREVIOUS 12 MOS.	AVERAGE OF PREVIOUS 3 MOS.	AVERAGE OF PREVIOUS MOS.	CURRENT MONTH
1 ----OTHER PROFESSIONAL SERVICES-----					
2					
3 LABORATORY-EXPENSE PERCENT	10.1	9.7	9.6	9.6	9.5
4 -CLINICAL LAB-IP TESTS PER ADM.	62,823	63,117		65,796	63,960
5 -TESTS PER MH	35.55	37.47		37.42	37.34
6 -DC PER TEST EX-FEES	4.81	5.01		4.91	5.02
7 -PERCENT OP TESTS	1.43	1.43		1.61	1.47
8 BLOOD BANK-EXPENSE PERCENT	3.42	3.13		2.96	2.75
9 -MANHOURS PER UNIT DRAWN	---	---		---	---
10					
11 RADIOLOGY-EXPENSE PERCENT	5.3	4.8	4.9		4.4
12 -DIAGNOSTIC-PROCEDURES PER ADM.	33,112	30,913		33,499	30,002
13 -DC PER PROCEDURE	1.07	1.10		1.20	1.15
14 -MANHOURS PER PROCEDURE	7.78	7.58		8.93	7.59
15 -PERCENT OP PROCEDURES	1.37	1.73		1.91	1.69
16	64.14	64.11		61.68	61.33
17 PHARMACY-EXPENSE PERCENT	2.7	2.8	3.2		2.7
18 -LINE ITEMS PER MANHOUR	16,585	18,493		21,750	18,261
19 -DIRECT COST PER PATIENT DAY	11.65	9.96		10.31	9.55
20	2.33	2.89		3.38	2.66
21 ANESTHESIOLOGY-EXPENSE PERCENT	3.0	3.4	4.1		3.5
22 INHALATION THERAPY-EXPENSE PERCENT	18,754	22,157		28,180	26,231
23	1.0	.9	.8	5,373	6,204
24 PHYSICAL THERAPY-EXPENSE PERCENT	6,338	6,019			.9
25 -TREATMENTS PER MANHOUR	.6	.6	.7	4,602	4,135
26 SOCIAL SERVICE-EXPENSE PERCENT	3,952	4,193		1.50	1.59
27 -MANHOURS PER CASE ACCEPTED	1.32	1.34		5,519	4,281
28	.9	1.0	.8		.6
29 MEDICAL RECORDS-EXPENSE PERCENT	5,491	6,490			
30 -MANHOURS PER DISCHARGE UNIT					
31 -MANHOURS PER AVERAGE OCCUPIED BED	1.6	1.5	1.6	10,971	10,119
32 MEDICAL LIBRARY-EXPENSE PERCENT	9,663	9,774		2.85	2.76
33 OTHER PAT. SERVICES-EXPENSE PERCENT	2.60	2.51		12.55	11.34
34 LAB SURVEY-IP TEST PER ADMISSION	10.30	10.66		---	---
35 -PERCENT OP LAB TESTS	.3	.2	.2	1,638	1,701
36 -PERCENT QUALITY CONTROL	1,661	1,615		---	---
37 -PERCENT STANDARDS	---	---		---	---
38 -TOTAL TESTS PER MANHOUR	---	---		---	---
39 -TOTAL DIRECT COST PER TEST	---	---		---	---
40 WEIGHTED TEST UNITS-PER MANHOUR	---	---		---	---
41 -DIRECT COST PER UNIT	---	---		---	---
42 -RATIO UNITS/UNWEIGHTED TESTS	---	---		---	---

Figure 11-1, Part C. Comparative Report, Operational and Department Indicators. Source: Same as Fig. 11-1, Part A.

JANUARY 1972
PAGE 4

	YOUR INSTITUTION		COMPARATIVE MEDIANS FOR PREVIOUS THREE MONTHS			
	CURRENT MONTH	PREVIOUS 3 MONTHS	DISTRICT GROUP 90 / 24 COMPARED	STATE GROUP 545 / 25 COMPARED	NATIONAL GROUP 935 / 326 COMPARED	
1 ----GENERAL SERVICES----						
2 DIETARY-EXPENSE PERCENT	5.21	5.45	7.4 | 2	6.9 | 3	7.3 | 3	
3 TOTAL-MEALS PER PATIENT DAY	1.40	1.44	4.43 | 4	4.43 | 4	4.39 | 4	
4 -DIRECT COST PER MEAL	.71	.73	1.55 | 2	1.58 | 1	1.52 | 2	
5 -LABOR COST PER MEAL	3.65	3.57	.78 | 1	.85 | 1	.79 | 2	
6 -MEALS SERVED PER MANHOUR			2.93 | 4	3.30 | 4	3.14 | 4	
7 INPATIENT MEALS SERVED PPD	2.80	2.83	2.85 | 2	2.79 | 3	2.79 | 3	
8 CAFETERIA MEALS-PERCENT OF TOTAL	46.23	48.13	39.24 | 4	35.70 | 4	36.53 | 4	
9 -PER MANHOUR	12.48	13.70	---	8.84 | 4	6.84 | 4	
10						
11 PLANT ENGINEERING-EXPENSE PERCENT	4.9	4.3	5.0 | 1	4.7 | 2	4.7 | 2	
12 -DIRECT COST PER BED PER MONTH	120.25	107.89	99.56 | 3	121.55 | 2	103.32 | 3	
13 -DIRECT COST PER 1000 FEET	178.35	160.03	156.09 | 3	185.39 | 2	149.23 | 3	
14 -MANHOURS PER 1000 FEET PER MONTH	19.86	19.48	18.17 | 3	19.48 | 2	18.51 | 3	
15						
16 HOUSEKEEPING-EXPENSE PERCENT	3.0	3.1	3.5 | 2	3.5 | 1	3.4 | 2	
17 -DIRECT COST PER BED PER MONTH	73.64	76.63	73.80 | 3	92.90 | 3	74.35 | 3	
18 -DIRECT COST PER 1000 FEET	142.06	147.82	135.90 | 3	158.26 | 2	128.30 | 3	
19 -MANHOURS PER 1000 FEET PER MONTH	51.17	50.91	49.23 | 3	51.61 | 2	45.42 | 3	
20						
21 LAUNDRY + LINEN-EXPENSE PERCENT	1.6	1.5	1.7 | 1	1.5 | 2	1.8 | 1	
22 -LAUNDRY COST PER 100 POUNDS	8.44	8.29	10.17 | 2	10.06 | 1	8.74 | 2	
23 -LAUNDRY POUNDS PER MANHOUR	35.83	35.88	31.75 | 3	34.41 | 3	35.35 | 3	
24 -POUNDS PER PATIENT DAY	15.73	16.13	15.87 | 3	14.21 | 3	15.29 | 3	
25 -LINEN COST PER PATIENT DAY	.25	.28	.24 | 3	.25 | 2	.38 | 2	
26						
27 ADM. + FISCAL-EXPENSE PERCENT	5.8	10.9	11.7 | 2	11.2 | 2	11.0 | 2	
28 -DIRECT COST PER OCCUPIED BED	300.63	359.19	309.54 | 3	352.24 | 3	303.28 | 3	
29 -SALARIES PER AVERAGE OCCUPIED BED	185.07	213.88	186.48 | 4	203.32 | 3	175.88 | 3	
30 EMP. HEALTH + WELFARE-EXPENSE PERCENT	6.3	5.4	5.1 | 3	5.5 | 1	5.0 | 3	
31 -PERCENT OF SALARIES	9.78	8.56	9.15 | 2	9.70 | 1	8.49 | 3	
32 DEPRECIATION-EXPENSE PERCENT	3.1	3.1	3.6 | 2	3.0 | 3	4.1 | 1	
33 MISC. OPERATING-EXPENSE PERCENT	.8	.7	1.5 | 1	.7 | 2	1.5 | 2	
34						
35 -SALARIES A PERCENT OF TOTAL EXP.	63.81	63.19	57.56 | 4	59.98 | 4	58.33 | 4	
36 -PROF. FEES PERCENT OF TOTAL	2.26	2.36	4.05 | 1	4.64 | 1	4.81 | 1	
37 -OTHER DIRECT EXPENSE PERCENT	33.91	34.43	38.51 | 1	35.12 | 2	37.24 | 2	
38 ----ADDITIONAL PROGRAMS----						
39 HOME HEALTH CARE-EXPENSE PERCENT	---	---	---	---	---	
40 MEDICAL STAFF-EXPENSE PERCENT	---	---	---	---	.4	
41 RESEARCH EXPENSE PERCENT	---	---	---	2.4	1.4	
42 PERSONNEL QUARTERS-EXPENSE PERCENT	.2	.2	---	---	.3 | 2	

Figure 11-1, Part C. (Continued).

JANUARY 1972
PAGE 5

#		SAME MONTH PREVIOUS YEAR	AVERAGE OF PREVIOUS 12 MOS.	AVERAGE OF PREVIOUS 3 MOS.	CURRENT MONTH
1	------ADMINISTRATIVE INDICATORS------				
2	INPATIENT-REVENUE PER PATIENT DAY	84.13	91.25	96.28	93.85
3	-COST PER PATIENT DAY RCCAC	78.14	89.45	94.35	87.58
4	ACCOUNTS+NOTES RECEIVABLE 1000'S	1,816.00	1,756.00	1,578.00	1,669.00
5	-DAYS OF REVENUE IN ACCTS. REC.	83.95	79.39	70.02	72.41
6	ALLOW FOR UNCOLLECTABLE REC 1000'S	83.00	127.00	121.00	87.00
7	-PERCENT OF ACCTS. REC.	4.57	7.23	7.66	5.13
8	ALL NURSING UNITS-EXPENSE PERCENT	26.54	25.36	24.51	25.62
9	-PERCENT OF OCCUPANCY	82.98	77.39	75.46	80.37
10	-LENGTH OF STAY	7.84	7.08	7.14	7.55
11	-DIRECT COST PER PATIENT DAY	23.24	25.79	26.02	25.24
12	-MANHOURS PER BED PER DAY	4.46	4.43	4.25	4.36
13	HOL.,VAC., SICK PAY DOLLARS 1000'S	35.05	27.37	26.64	41.51
14	-PERCENT OF SALARIES	8.79	6.67	6.16	9.61
15	EQUIV. FULL TIME EMPLOYEE PER BED	2.50	2.49	2.52	2.52
16	-----REVENUE PERCENTAGES-----				
17	OBSTETRICAL NURSING UNITS	2.9 / 19,411	3.1 / 20,256	2.8 / 19,741	2.3 / 16,530
18	NURSERIES	2.4 / 15,949	2.0 / 13,255	1.7 / 11,788	1.3 / 9,671
19	MEDICAL + SURGICAL NURSING UNITS	51.9 / 348,278	49.7 / 329,749	50.3 / 351,654	52.4 / 379,461
20	DELIVERY AND LABOR ROOMS	.8 / 5,144	.9 / 5,938	.9 / 6,375	.7 / 4,950
21	OPERATING ROOMS	5.3 / 35,210	5.6 / 37,445	5.5 / 38,421	5.3 / 38,095
22	RECOVERY ROOMS	---	---	---	---
23	CENTRAL SERVICES + SUPPLY	2.1 / 14,286	2.4 / 16,125	2.4 / 16,787	2.5 / 17,836
24	INTRAVENOUS THERAPY	.8 / 5,411	.8 / 5,538	.8 / 5,461	.8 / 5,835
25	EMERGENCY SERVICES	2.8 / 18,899	4.0 / 26,508	3.8 / 26,301	3.8 / 27,715
26	LABORATORY-INPATIENT	8.9 / 59,449	9.0 / 59,630	8.7 / 60,732	8.7 / 62,929
27	-OUTPATIENT	3.1 / 21,109	2.7 / 18,137	2.5 / 17,354	2.6 / 18,590
28	BLOOD BANK	---	---	---	---
29	RADIOLOGY-INPATIENT	2.9 / 19,711	3.0 / 19,873	3.1 / 21,903	2.9 / 20,718
30	-OUTPATIENT	4.7 / 31,429	4.3 / 28,368	4.0 / 28,135	3.8 / 27,415
31	PHARMACY-INPATIENT	4.3 / 28,617	4.2 / 28,163	4.3 / 30,052	4.2 / 30,207
32	-OUTPATIENT	.3 / 2,002	.5 / 3,347	.5 / 3,223	.5 / 3,569
33	ANESTHESIOLOGY	3.9 / 26,449	5.0 / 33,250	5.5 / 38,254	4.9 / 35,836
34	INHALATION THERAPY	1.7 / 11,394	1.5 / 10,049	1.9 / 13,107	2.2 / 15,956
35	PHYSICAL THERAPY	.8 / 5,611	.9 / 5,896	1.1 / 7,438	1.1 / 7,782
36	OCCUPATIONAL + RECREATIONAL THERAPY	.1 / 707	.1 / 573	.1 / 546	.1 / 507
37	CLINICS	---	---	---	---
38	ALL OTHER PATIENT SERVICES	.2 / 1,449	.2 / 1,358	.2 / 1,200	.1 / 1,081
39	GROSS INPATIENT REVENUE	89.1 / 597,362	87.8 / 582,663	88.7 / 619,420	88.7 / 643,085
40	GROSS OUTPATIENT REVENUE	10.9 / 73,153	12.2 / 80,886	11.3 / 79,125	11.3 / 81,622
41	TOTAL PATIENT REVENUE	100.0 / 670,515	100.0 / 663,549	100.0 / 698,545	100.0 / 724,707
42	DEDUCTIONS FROM PATIENT REVENUE	-5.1 / -34,928	-4.9 / -33,004	-5.0 / -32,339	-5.0 / -37,110

Figure 11-2, Part A. Internal Report, State of Revenues. Source: Same as Fig. 11-1, Part A.

		SAME MONTH PREVIOUS YEAR %	AVERAGE OF PREVIOUS 12 MOS. %	AVERAGE OF PREVIOUS 3 MOS. %	CURRENT MONTH %
1	----------NURSING DIVISION----------				
2	NURSING ADM.-EXPENSE PERCENT	3.9	3.4	3.0	3.2
3	-MANHOURS PER BED PER MONTH	24,133 33.17	22,006 28.49	20,623 25.15	21,776 26.23
4	----------OBSTETRICAL SERVICES----------				
5	OBSTETRICAL UNIT-EXPENSE PERCENT	1.2	1.3	1.3	1.3
6	-PERCENT OCCUPANCY	7,586 50.94	8,437 52.50	8,605 46.50	8,655 38.97
7	-PERCENT OF TOTAL ADMISSIONS	9.20	9.58	9.70	7.25
8	-AVERAGE LENGTH OF STAY	4.30	4.19	3.97	4.46
9	-OBSTETRICAL TURNOVER RATE	3.62	3.75	3.58	2.83
10	-NURSING MH PER PATIENT DAY	6.10	6.71	7.42	8.76
11	DEL.+ LABOR ROOMS-EXPENSE PERCENT	.8	.9	.8	.7
12	-DIRECT COST PER DELIVERY	5,050 56.74	5,567 61.85	5,453 64.15	5,036 75.16
13	-DELIVERY+LABOR MH PER DELIVERY	11.14	12.03	12.62	14.47
14	NURSERY UNIT-EXPENSE PERCENT	1.2	1.3	1.4	1.1
15	-NURSERY MH PER BASSINET PER DAY	7,499 3.29	8,486 3.63	9,574 3.76	7,493 3.04
16	----------GENERAL NURSING UNITS----------				
17	MED.+SURG. UNITS-EXPENSE PERCENT	20.2	19.4	18.8	20.0
18	-PERCENT OCCUPANCY	125,796 86.03	125,745 79.77	128,644 78.22	135,057 84.33
19	-AVERAGE LENGTH OF STAY	8.22	7.40	7.48	7.79
20	-MED.+SURG. TURNOVER RATE	3.40	3.23	3.18	3.46
21	-NURSING MH PER BED PER DAY	4.59	4.52	4.32	4.47
22	-NURSING MH PER PATIENT DAY	5.34	5.67	5.53	5.30
23	-PERCENT REGISTERED NURSES	---	---	---	---
24	-PERCENT LICENSED PRACTICAL NURSES	---	---	---	---
25	----------OTHER NURSING SERVICES----------				
26	OPERATING ROOMS-EXPENSE PERCENT	3.2	3.7	3.8	3.7
27	-C.R. VISITS/100 M+S ADMISSIONS	19,997 47.90	23,804 53.02	26,187 51.75	25,168 48.10
28	-DIRECT COST PER O.R. VISIT	48.65	55.35	63.25	60.21
29	-MANHOURS PER O.R. VISIT	5.88	10.64	11.90	11.30
30	RECOVERY ROOMS-EXPENSE PERCENT	---	---	---	---
31	CENTRAL SERVICES-EXPENSE PERCENT	1.6	1.7	1.8	1.8
32	-DIRECT COST PER PATIENT DAY	5,942 1.40	11,292 1.76	12,436 1.93	11,968 1.74
33	-LINE ITEMS PER MANHOUR	---	---	---	---
34	INTRAVENOUS THERAPY-EXPENSE PERCENT	.3	.5	.7	.7
35	-DIRECT COST PER PATIENT DAY	1,598 .22	3,169 .49	4,602 .71	4,661 .68
36	EMERGENCY SERVICE-EXPENSE PERCENT	2.2	2.2	2.3	2.4
37	-MANHOURS PER VISIT	13,571 2.07	14,517 1.63	15,465 1.84	16,388 1.85
38	NURSING EDUCATION-EXPENSE PERCENT				
39	CLINIC-EXPENSE PERCENT	2.9	3.3	3.6	3.6
40	-MANHOURS PER VISIT	18,271	21,620	24,823	24,617
41	-VISITS PER BED PER MONTH	---	---	---	---
42		---	---	---	---

JANUARY 1972 PAGE 6

Figure 11-2, Part B. Internal Report, State of Expenses. Source: Same as Fig. 11-1, Part A.

JANUARY 1972
PAGE 3

	YOUR INSTITUTION		COMPARATIVE MEDIANS FOR PREVIOUS THREE MONTHS					
	CURRENT MONTH	PREVIOUS 3 MONTHS	DISTRICT GROUP 24 COMPARED		SO GROUP 25 COMPARED		STATE 545 GROUP 326 COMPARED		NATIONAL 935 COMPARED	
1 ---OTHER PROFESSIONAL SERVICES-----								
2								
3 LABORATORY-EXPENSE PERCENT	9.5	9.6	7.01	4	7.3	4	7.1	4
4 -CLINICAL LAB-IP TESTS PER ADM.	37.34	37.42	12.36	4	19.93	4	19.83	4
5 -TESTS PER MH	5.02	4.91	3.64	2	3.22	4	4.10	3
6 -DC PER TEST EX-FEES	1.47	1.61	1.97	1	1.82	1	1.46	3
7 -PERCENT OP TESTS	2.75	2.96	18.44	4	11.76	4	12.00	1
8 BLOOD BANK-EXPENSE PERCENT	---	---	.2		.4		.6	1
9 -MANHOURS PER UNIT DRAWN	---	---	---		1.67		2.71	
10								
11 RADIOLOGY-EXPENSE PERCENT	4.4	4.9	5.3	2	6.1	1	5.4	2
12 -DIAGNOSTIC-PROCEDURES PER ADM.	1.15	1.20	1.30	2	1.42	1	1.60	1
13 -DC PER PROCEDURE	7.95	8.93	6.36	4	7.80	3	7.93	3
14 -MANHOURS PER PROCEDURE	1.69	1.91	.99	H	1.16	4	1.23	4
15 -PERCENT OP PROCEDURES	61.33	61.68	57.52	3	52.94	3	43.03	4
16								
17 PHARMACY-EXPENSE PERCENT	2.7	3.2	3.3	2	3.1	3	3.3	2
18 -LINE ITEMS PER MANHOUR	9.55	10.33	10.33	2	9.71	3	11.42	2
19 -DIRECT COST PER PATIENT DAY	2.66	3.38	3.00	3	3.38	2	3.21	3
20								
21 ANESTHESIOLOGY-EXPENSE PERCENT	3.9	4.1	1.4	4	1.4	4	1.0	H
22 INHALATION THERAPY-EXPENSE PERCENT	.9	.8	1.0	2	1.0	2	1.0	2
23								
24 PHYSICAL THERAPY-EXPENSE PERCENT	.6	.7	.8	2	.9	2	.6	3
25 -TREATMENTS PER MANHOUR	1.59	1.50	1.59	2	1.58	2	1.45	3
26 SOCIAL SERVICE-EXPENSE PERCENT	.6	.8	.4	3	.3	4	.2	H
27 -MANHOURS PER CASE ACCEPTED	---	---	4.32		3.52		4.91	
28								
29 MEDICAL RECORDS-EXPENSE PERCENT	1.5	1.6	1.3	3	1.2	3	1.2	4
30 -MANHOURS PER DISCHARGE UNIT	2.76	2.89	2.12	4	2.49	3	2.26	4
31 -MANHOURS PER AVERAGE OCCUPIED BED	11.34	12.55	9.54	4	10.28	4	9.65	4
32 MEDICAL LIBRARY-EXPENSE PERCENT	---	---	---		.1		.1	
33 OTHER PAT. SERVICES-EXPENSE PERCENT	.3	.2	1.0	H	1.2	H	1.2	H
34 LAB SURVEY-IP TEST PER ADMISSION	---	---	---		30.11		21.40	
35 -PERCENT OP LAB TESTS	---	---	---		10.21		10.73	
36 -PERCENT QUALITY CONTROL	---	---	---		6.75		7.94	
37 -PERCENT STANDARDS	---	---	---		2.67		4.38	
38 -TOTAL TESTS PER MANHOUR	---	---	---		5.31		4.49	
39 -TOTAL DIRECT COST PER TEST	---	---	---		1.34		1.83	
40 WEIGHTED TEST UNITS-PER MANHOUR	---	---	---		41.58		37.43	
41 -DIRECT COST PER UNIT	---	---	---		.18		.22	
42 -RATIO UNITS/UNWEIGHTED TESTS	---	---	---		6.62		7.23	

Figure 11–2, Part C. Internal Report, Operational and Departmental Indicators. Source: Same as Fig. 11-1, Part A.

JANUARY 1972
PAGE 8

	SAME MONTH PREVIOUS YEAR	AVERAGE OF PREVIOUS 12 MOS.	AVERAGE OF PREVIOUS 3 MOS.	CURRENT MONTH
1 ------GENERAL SERVICES------				
2 DIETARY-EXPENSE PERCENT	7.6	7.5	7.4	7.4
3 TOTAL-MEALS PER PATIENT DAY	47,244	48,621	50,618	50,210
	5.23	5.32	5.45	5.21
4 -DIRECT COST PER MEAL	1.27	1.42	1.44	1.40
5 -LABOR COST PER MEAL	.70	.74	.73	.71
6 -MEALS SERVED PER MANHOUR	3.68	3.43	3.57	3.65
7 INPATIENT MEALS SERVED PPD	2.78	2.78	2.83	2.80
8 CAFETERIA MEALS-PERCENT OF TOTAL	46.74	47.71	48.13	46.23
9 -PER MANHOUR	4.99	11.77	13.70	12.48
10				
11 PLANT ENGINEERING-EXPENSE PERCENT	4.9	4.5	4.3	4.9
12 -DIRECT COST PER BED PER MONTH	30,444	29,079	29,672	33,069
	110.30	105.74	107.85	120.25
13 -DIRECT COST PER 1000 FEET	164.19	156.83	160.03	178.35
14 -MANHOURS PER 1000 FEET PER MONTH	19.35	19.14	19.48	19.86
15				
16 HOUSEKEEPING-EXPENSE PERCENT	3.0	3.0	3.1	3.0
17 -DIRECT COST PER BED PER MONTH	18,495	19,797	21,074	20,253
	67.01	71.98	76.63	73.64
18 -DIRECT COST PER 1000 FEET	133.62	140.91	147.82	142.06
19 -MANHOURS PER 1000 FEET PER MONTH	50.48	50.07	50.91	51.17
20				
21 LAUNDRY + LINEN-EXPENSE PERCENT	1.8	1.6	1.5	1.6
22 -LAUNDRY COST PER 100 POUNDS	11,215	10,448	10,470	10,881
	8.08	8.07	8.29	8.44
23 -LAUNDRY POUNDS PER MANHOUR	36.17	36.52	35.88	35.83
24 -POUNDS PER PATIENT DAY	14.62	16.18	16.13	15.73
25 -LINEN COST PER PATIENT DAY	.39	.33	.28	.25
26				
27 ADM. + FISCAL-EXPENSE PERCENT	9.7	10.1	10.9	9.8
28 -DIRECT COST PER OCCUPIED BED	60,552	65,505	74,536	66,449
	264.38	307.78	359.19	300.63
29 -SALARIES PER AVERAGE OCCUPIED BED	180.57	197.90	213.88	189.07
30 EMP. HEALTH + WELFARE-EXPENSE PERCENT	36,455	44,483	37,644	42,233
31 -PERCENT OF SALARIES	9.14	10.64	8.56	9.78
32 DEPRECIATION-EXPENSE PERCENT	3.4	3.1	3.1	3.1
	20,840	20,278	20,840	20,840
33 MISC. OPERATING-EXPENSE PERCENT	.7	.6	.7	.8
	4,509	3,566	5,000	5,336
34 -HOSPITAL 100 PERCENT BASE TOTAL	100	100	100	100
35 -SALARIES A PERCENT OF TOTAL EXP.	63.98	63.07	63.19	63.81
36 -PROF. FEES PERCENT OF TOTAL	3.32	2.92	2.36	2.26
37 -OTHER DIRECT EXPENSE PERCENT	32.69	34.00	34.43	33.91
38 ------ADDITIONAL PROGRAMS------				
39 HOME HEALTH CARE-EXPENSE PERCENT	---	---	---	---
40 MEDICAL STAFF-EXPENSE PERCENT	---	---	---	---
41 RESEARCH EXPENSE PERCENT	---	---	---	---
42 PERSONNEL QUARTERS-EXPENSE PERCENT	.2	.2	.2	.2
	1,168	1,237	1,458	1,319

Figure 11-2, Part C. (Continued).

295

JANUARY 1972
PAGE 5

#		SAME MONTH PREVIOUS YEAR	AVERAGE OF PREVIOUS 12 MOS.	AVERAGE OF PREVIOUS 3 MOS.	CURRENT MONTH
1	-----NURSING DIVISION STATISTICS--				
2	OBSTETRICS - ADMISSIONS	87	90	86	68
3	- DISCHARGES	88	90	87	65
4	- TOTAL Pt. DAYS OF CARE	379	378	346	250
5	- BEDS - OBSTETRICS	24	24	24	24
6	NEWBORN - NUMBER OF DELIVERIES	89	90	85	67
7	- TOTAL NEWBORN DAYS OF CARE	520	432	368	303
8	- BASSINETS - NEWBORN	24	24	24	24
9	MED + SURG - ADMISSIONS	858	811	800	869
10	ADULT - DISCHARGES	817	811	813	842
11	+ - TOTAL Pt. DAYS OF CARE	6,721	6,007	6,087	6,562
12	CHILD - BEDS - ADULT + CHILD	252	251	251	251
13	OPERATING ROOM VISITS	411	430	414	418
14	RECOVERY ROOM VISITS	384	405	396	391
15	CENTRAL SUPPLY LINE ITEMS SOLD/ISSUED	---	---	---	---
16	EMERGENCY DEPARTMENT VISITS	1,624	2,351	2,326	2,492
17					
18	-----OTHER PROFESSIONAL SERVICES----				
19					
20	LABORATORY - CLINICAL TESTS - INPT	33,597	33,761	33,157	34,992
21	- CLINICAL TESTS - OUTPT	1,190	1,094	1,014	993
22	- PATHOLOGY TESTS	478	477	431	470
23	- AUTOPSY	7	5	5	11
24	BLOOD BANK UNITS DRAWN	---	---	---	---
25					
26	X-RAY - DIAG. PROCEDURES - INPT	1,018	995	1,066	1,078
27	- DIAG. PROCEDURES - OUTPT	1,821	1,778	1,716	1,710
28	- THERAPEUTIC PROCEDURES	---	---	---	---
29	- NUCLEAR MEDICINE PROCEDURES	---	---	---	---
30					
31	PHARMACY LINE ITEMS SOLD/ISSUED	14,196	13,376	13,956	13,487
32	ANESTHESIOLOGY CHARGE SLIPS	446	440	426	432
33	PHYSICAL THERAPY TREATMENTS	1,628	1,588	1,762	1,719
34	HOME HEALTH CARE VISITS	---	---	---	---
35	SOCIAL SERVICE CASES ACCEPTED	---	---	---	---
36	CLINIC VISITS	---	---	---	---
37	-----GENERAL SERVICES----				
38	NUMBER OF MEALS SERVED - PATIENTS	19,800	17,788	18,213	19,214
39	- CAFETERIA	17,379	16,236	16,900	16,524
40	PLANT FOOTAGE	185,412	185,412	185,412	185,412
41	HOUSEKEEPING FOOTAGE	138,411	140,487	142,564	142,564
42	POUNDS OF LAUNDRY PROCESSED	103,829	103,328	103,801	107,792

Figure 11-3, Part A. Internal Statistical Report. Source: Same as Fig. 11-1, Part A.

JANUARY 1972
PAGE 1C

	SAME MONTH PREVIOUS YEAR	AVERAGE OF PREVIOUS 12 MOS.	AVERAGE OF PREVIOUS 3 MOS.	CURRENT MONTH
1 ---------MANHOURS PAID--------	---	---	---	---
2 NURSING SERVICE -ADMINISTRATIVE	9,157	7,836	6,919	7,215
3 -OBSTETRICAL UNITS	2,313	2,537	2,565	2,541
4 -NURSERY UNITS	2,451	2,620	2,803	2,269
5 -MED.+ SURG. UNITS	35,897	34,073	33,675	34,830
6 REGISTERED NURSES-M+S	---	---	---	---
7 LICENSED PRACTICAL NURSES-M+S	---	---	---	---
8 OTHER NURSING PERSONNEL-M+S	35,897	34,073	33,675	34,830
9 -DELIVERY AND LABOR ROOMS	992	1,083	1,073	970
10 -OPERATING ROOMS	4,063	4,577	4,928	4,727
11 -RECOVERY ROOM	---	---	---	---
12 -CENTRAL SERVICES AND SUPPLY	2,057	2,197	2,202	2,284
13 -INTRAVENOUS THERAPY	---	257	569	405
14 -EMERGENCY SERVICES	3,367	3,833	4,254	4,633
15 NURSING EDUCATION	3,343	3,808	4,180	4,162
16 -TOTAL NURSING MANHOURS	63,640	62,821	63,212	64,036
17 LABORATORY	8,156	7,755	7,837	8,081
18 BLOOD BANK	---	---	---	---
19 RADIOLOGY	3,902	4,810	5,321	4,729
20 PHARMACY	1,218	1,342	1,351	1,412
21 ANESTHESIOLOGY	1,270	1,085	961	900
22 INHALATION THERAPY	1,452	1,547	1,397	1,299
23 PHYSICAL THERAPY	1,231	1,180	1,172	1,077
24 OCCUPATIONAL + RECREATIONAL THERAPY	348	346	350	353
25 HOME HEALTH CARE	---	---	---	---
26 SOCIAL SERVICE	1,027	930	722	625
27 MEDICAL RECORDS	2,360	2,269	2,605	2,508
28 MEDICAL LIBRARY	---	---	---	---
29 RESEARCH	---	---	---	---
30 CLINICS	---	---	---	---
31 ALL OTHER PATIENT SERVICES	---	---	---	---
32 DIETARY-PATIENT SERVICES	6,609	8,523	8,584	8,467
33 -CAFETERIA	3,480	1,379	1,234	1,324
34 PLANT ENGINEERING	3,589	3,549	3,513	3,684
35 HOUSEKEEPING	6,987	7,035	7,258	7,295
36 LAUNDRY	2,870	2,829	2,892	3,008
37 LINEN	---	---	---	---
38 PERSONNEL QUARTERS	547	519	591	473
39 ADMINISTRATION + FISCAL	10,807	10,935	10,947	10,771
40 MISCELLANEOUS OPERATING	---	---	---	---
41 MISCELLANEOUS NONOPERATING	---	---	---	---
42 TOTAL MANHOURS REPORTED	119,493	118,865	120,056	120,042

Figure 11–3, Part B. Internal Report, Manhours Paid. Source: Same as Fig. 11–1, Part A.

number of blanks on the form representing services that the hospital does not have. If the hospital were to add one of these services, the entire array of percentages would be adjusted. Similarly, if some of the services, such as emergency and outpatient laboratory and x-ray, were growing much more rapidly than others, the percentage of revenue and expense for these lines would be trending steadily upwards. All the other departments would be trending steadily downwards as a result of the shift. But the actual revenues or expenses might have changed only for one department. The sensitivity of these indicators varies greatly. A change of two-tenths of 1 percent in the absolute value of medical and surgical nursing revenue will appear on the form. But any change of less than 50 percent will go unrecorded in occupational therapy. It would appear that these percentagized figures in revenue and expense have less value as control statistics than do the raw numbers themselves.

Interhospital Comparisons. Comparisons of the experience of one institution against the pooled values for several others present a number of difficulties. It is well known that many parameters of the health care system are subject to extreme variation across the United States. Supplies of key professional manpower, of acute hospital facilities, utilization rates of facilities, and wage rates of manpower differ quite substantially from east to west and north to south across the nation. The same factors tend to show almost the same variation within many of the larger industrial states. Hospitals in Buffalo, New York, for example, operate in an economic environment which probably compares more closely with Erie and Pittsburgh, Pennsylvania than it does with New York City. On the other hand, the district, such as western New York, will have so few hospitals in it that it will not be possible to adjust for size variation. It is also well known that hospitals tend to have substantial increases in costs as they grow in size and complexity. The HAS answer to this has been to present all three possibilities and to permit the user to choose the one which pleases him most.

Comparability depends in part upon the item being studied. It would seem likely, for example, that hospitals treating the same kind of illness should use approximately the same amount of nursing care per patient day. This is one of the comparative statistics reported in part B. However, this assumption may not be correct. Some hospitals may be coping with what they feel are severe shortages, lowering the median and quartile levels. The generally desired standard, as opposed to the actual performance, may be a value in the third or fourth quartile of the distribution. In some areas covered by the performance measures, such as laundry and housekeeping, the amount of capital investment will strongly affect the performance. Poor relative performance of an indicator like pounds per man hour is not in itself sufficient argument to justify the additional capital investment, although it is admittedly a good indicator of the need to investigate such opportunities. After investigation, the possibility of changing the system may be rejected. At this point there is no further use in the comparison to other hospitals. Whenever this occurs, the opposite occurs as well. The datum from that subscriber is meaningless to other subscribers. It is still carried in the distribution, however, and to a certain extent it distorts the output. A number of very inefficient subscribers creates false confidence for others, yet past the initial revelation of inefficiency, the data do nothing for the inefficient subscribers.

In some of the HAS statistics, comparability is reduced in other ways. The figures show percentage distributions of expenditures and revenues by categories and comparative standings for the current month. The interpretation of these data is unclear. The report depends heavily on the reliability of input data of the comparison hospitals which will be discussed below. Even granting accuracy of this, the meaning of an error signal (e.g., a high quartile standing on a specific expense) is ambiguous. Consider a hospital which has arranged extensive outpatient radiology services, for example. Its relative expenditure and revenue for radiology will be high, although no out-of-control situation exists. Correspondingly, since percentages are used, the standing of every other classification of its report will be lowered slightly. The chances of a better rating are improved for these departments. Thus the possibility has been created for both false positive (radiology) and false negative (other departments) error signals. Another example which can be considered is the absense of a department which most other hospitals have. This increases the percentage for all the remaining departments, enhancing the probability of false signals. Where some of the services of the missing department are performed by one existing department (as might occur if inhalation therapy services were performed by nursing), the chances of a high rating for that department are increased substantially.

The second group of assumptions, regarding the reliability of the reference distribution, is also subject to question. It actually depends upon a series of conditions which must be met: (a) unambiguous rules for the assignment of expense to categories; (b) accurate compliance with these rules; (c) stability over time of the reference population; and (d) reasonable homogeneity of the reference population.

Rules for classification of expenses and revenue are prescribed in the AHA Chart of Accounts,[7] which has wide acceptance. There are, however, easy opportunities for error. Housekeeping costs for the operating and delivery suites, linen repair costs, costs of preparation of intravenous fluids (which may be incurred either in "Medical and Surgical Service" or "Pharmacy" depending on the system used) and the cost of patient meal service (either nursing or dietary) represent some of the areas for ambiguity or error.

Stability of the reference population is, at least at present, open to question. The service has been growing steadily, so that new hospitals are added regularly. In addition, certain hospitals are excluded from the reports each month. Exclusions may occur because of late reporting or because of apparently erroneous reports. State distributions have particularly noticeable variation from month to month in the number of hospitals included in the reference distribution.

In summary, it is important to ask if the reference distribution is meaningful. Sanders, in an analysis of the comparative position of one hospital against state and national medians over a period of years, showed that for several performance indicators quartiles were not stable over time, with both seasonal cycles and secular trends.[8] The distributions were skewed in some cases, so that the relative sensitivity of the quartiles varied. Finally the ranges were often quite large. On national data for meals per man hour for 19 months, high values sampled from a five-year period ranged from 189 percent of low values (4.26 vs. 2.26) to 272 percent (5.01 vs. 1.84). Much higher relative ranges were reported for laboratory procedures per man hour, x-ray procedures per man hour, and laboratory tests per man hour.[9] With ranges this large and unstable, it is reasonable to question whether a common underlying process exists, and therefore whether control system notions are applicable. The data provide interesting comparisons for use by an upper level of management to indicate broad areas of difference between hospitals. This is a different function, however, than the detection of variation from prior performance or anticipated performance inherent in the usual concept of control.

Historic Comparisons. While the problem of using the historic comparisons within the hospital are not as great as those involved in the selection of reference groups, there is still room for substantial improvement. The use of the statistic "this month last year" is not a substitute for a seasonally adjusted value for the reference statistics. Because of data-processing limitations, it is not possible to adjust historic statistics for agreed upon changes in various activities. There is no possibility offered for comparison to a budget. In addition, it should be noted that these statistics are nothing other than the hospital's own statistics which have been processed by the HAS computer. A hospital with its own computer could undoubtedly devise a more meaningful format, shorter turn around time, and possibly less data-processing costs. It would also be possible to establish control limits and to flag automatically those departments apparently deserving special attention.

The final criticism of HAS data would be the formatting and time lag. The report shown in the figures is dated January 1972. It was processed by HAS on March 1st and reached the hospital a few days thereafter. Assuming that it could be distributed to the department heads almost immediately, they would still be dealing with information on cost control which is five weeks out of data. The delay, of course, is caused by the slowness of reporting which must await the accumulation of a reasonable comparison group and is thus geared to the slowest report. Finally, the format of the report does not target specific date for each department head and present him exclusively with that data, but instead shows each cost center on a page with several others.

Despite these weaknesses, it should be understood that HAS is a pioneering effort. It has established the major parameters of cost and revenue control, developed standard definitions and data-gathering systems for these, and shown the possibilities of use of the computer in both interhospital and historical comparisons. There has been steady improvement in the system since its inception and it is likely that this improvement will continue. It is likely that HAS will provide the most feasible and economical data service for small hospitals for some years to come.

Alternative Systems. What is needed for accounting-based resource control systems is speed of reporting and realistic standards. HAS is limited in both respects by its interhospital approach. (Certain delays are built in to give all members of the reference group time to report.) There is considerable interest in alternative systems.

One alternative is the variable or flexible budget. This approach assumes that unit cost is a function of output. Instead of using dollar totals as the standard of comparison from the budget, it uses dollars per unit of output. A variety of assumptions are possible: that some costs are fixed and some are variable, that variable costs are truly linear, or that they are linear only over certain ranges, and so forth. This approach does improve the realism of the standard and the possibilities for control. However, it can be slow and expensive. Many items of cost are entered only after a series of month-end accounting transactions. Delays of two weeks or more appear inevitable under this approach. Besides, hospital primary controllers generally do not deal with dollars. They deal with actual resources, of which the dominant one is almost always man hours (which fact HAS designers have long noted).

The dominance of man hours in hospital costs has led many managers to concentrate on it as a major control device. It is easily accounted, and priced if desired, in the payroll accounting system. Other constraints force both rapid and accurate data processing. It is usually among the earliest hospital information systems to be automated. Once automated, the data for a control system is usually an inexpensive by-product. Further, if output data are collected on a similar cycle, it is possible wherever desirable to express output per man hour.

One of the efforts to develop this type of information into an efficiency control system is the Management Monitoring Systems Project of the University of Michigan Bureau of Hospital Administration. Under this system:

1. Manhours and output measures are accumulated for each primary responsibility center in the hospital. In general, a primary responsibility center is a primary controller. The accounting system accumulates direct costs for each responsibility center
2. Output per manhour statistics are calculated historically and graphed. In uncontrolled situations, these show considerable fluctuation

3. Supervisors select from historical output per manhour statistics the level of manpower necessary to perform at acceptable quality levels. This selection is carefully reviewed by hospital administration, which may adjust it upwards or downwards. The final decision, called the Manpower Input Decision, or MID, becomes the basis of the annual budget. It is multiplied by seasonally adjusted forecasts of annual volume and expected wage rates to gain the monthly expenditures for the budget
4. Supervisors are aided in the control function by a two-period, short-term forecast of volume, which helps them foresee manpower requirements calculated from the MID and to use attrition, vacations, part-time, overtime, and transfer labor to adjust the work force
5. Responsibility centers where demand fluctuations are unpredictable (obstetrics, for example) or where the work force is unable to respond effectively to volume variations (one and two person centers, for example) are controlled by traditional budget approaches of either total man hours or total dollars. (These departments are not usually a budgetary control problem)
6. Supervisors are judged by their ability to meet the MID rather than their overall budget performance. Feedback on performance is rapid, lagging only one to five working days behind the period itself
7. The next annual budget reviews the process. Supervisors are encouraged to reduce MIDs where they can do so without impairing quality. Upward adjustments in the MID can only be justified in terms of quality or performance of unmeasured services

Experience with this approach is still being accumulated. Final reports are expected in 1973.[10] Preliminary findings from one demonstration hospital are promising. They reveal, however, considerable mechanical problems. Both basic accounting practices and payroll procedures required improvement. The number of primary cost centers had to be increased. Hours of individual personnel, particularly in nursing, had to be correctly reported to cost centers (each nursing unit is a cost center). The traditional twelve-month year meshed badly with the twenty-six pay periods and created unnecessary forecasting difficulties (the number of week days per month varies more than the number of days). A thirteen-period year is clearly cheaper, but it requires revision of a large number of statistical and accounting reports and activities. Short-range, two-period forecasts could be prepared for many departments, with substantial variance reduction. Seasonal (monthly) indices and exponential smoothing are usually necessary. The parameters appear to be a function not only of the individual hospital but also of the department. Thus, substantial data gathering and analysis are necessary to start.

The method appears most promising in the long run, however. It is easy to maintain, once computerized payroll systems are established, and flexible enough to accommodate both seasonal variation and changes in method. (The same calculations which yield internal rates of return on capital investments can easily be translated to reductions in the MID.) Finally, in initial trials it paid off. Reductions of over $150,000 per year were made by supervisors preparing the budget for the demonstration hospital.[11]

Work Sampling Efficiency Measures

Some effort has been made to assess efficiency by work sampling. This technique involves the random observation of employees in the work situation and recording the nature of their activities. Employees found idle or engaged in nonproductive activities are counted as such, and an efficiency measure is the number of "productive" work observations divided by the total number of observations. The work sampling technique has been frequently used in hospitals for special studies,[12] but application to routine work surveillance is rare. Williams and Donaldson cite industrial applications of the technique and propose application to dietary departments.[13] Their proposal for rating the department includes not only recording of idle and nonproductive time and the identification of its major causes, but also the application of pacing estimations. Pace is the relative degree of effort or speed being exerted by the worker under observation. It has been used for many years by trained industrial engineers. Under proper conditions (principally good training and continuous practice including practice under controlled conditions), a reasonable degree of reliability can be maintained. The routine use of work sampling techniques, with or without pacing appears unlikely. The cost of data collection is high. Repeated use of the technique may lead to distortion or bias of activities by the department under study. Pacing, while it may improve reliability, increases cost and requires specially trained observers. The technique will continue to be used as a basic manpower planning device, however. It is particularly useful in measuring current practice of nursing and other professional activities.

Efficiency Control of Scheduling and Staffing Processes

One critical element in the control of efficiency in stochastic processes is the appropriate adjustment of resources and demand, under conditions where both may be subject to stochastic fluctuation. The design of systems of staffing or scheduling which make this adjustment is discussed in part II of this text. Assuming that such a system has been designed and installed, a control system can easily be designed to measure its effectiveness. Using nurse staffing as an example, the scheduling system requires specification of desirable standards for the total staffing per patient day and the fraction of total staff time provided by registered nurses. Deviation from these standards is the reference signal. Since each nursing unit is staffed for three shifts, there are six reference signals per unit per day. For each shift, (Δ Hours) and (Δ % RN) will be generated, where Δ indicates the difference between actual and standard. A cheap and quick control system would specify a minimum value for each statistic. That is the standard for the shift may be 2.5 hours/patient times 30 patients or 75 hours. A minimum might be specified by Nursing Department of 2.25 hours/patient, or 67.5 hours. Any difference of 7.5 hours or less would be ignored, and the presence of larger variation treated as failure. It thereby becomes an attributes measure, subject to either Poisson or binomial control limits. A similar technique could be used on the RN percentage.

A more elaborate comparator process could be devised to adjust the standard to a reasonable number of positions to be staffed. Thus 76 hours might be the expected staff for 30 patients, to permit assignments of either 4 or 8 hours per person. Differences would be in 4-hour units, either positive or negative. Specialized statistical calculations would be required to handle probability limits for the difference distribution, since it is an integer distribution with a mean, presumably, of zero. However, these could be established by simulation if necessary. The "percent RN" statistic could be handled as continuous variable, although the central limit theorem could not be applied except by the grouping of several days into a sample (weekly, for example).

Regardless of the data reduction system selected, the function of the first super control will be to detect and correct failures in the primary control system which makes the actual assignment. The second super control will be interested in trends in the deviation scores, the overall personnel supply, the training of the person making transfers of personnel to balance demand, and in the standards themselves. Continued failure to meet standards may simply imply that they are unrealistic. As indicated in the preceding chapter, the reference signal of the second super control is the incidence of out-of-control shifts in the portion of the hospital covered by the first super control system.

Similar control systems can be devised for other staffing and scheduling processes. The principle followed is to use the degree of deviation from a previously established standard, or the number of occurrences of deviation as the reference signal. While the establishment of control limits may sometimes be troublesome, some solution to that problem always exists.

Quality Control Systems in Other than Medical Systems

The problem of quality measurement in hospitals is a difficult one, and relatively few sound measures have been developed. Much of the work which has been done has concentrated upon the medical care process. This unique application of quality control will be reviewed in the following chapter. Elsewhere in the hospital, ready measures are rare, and only recently has attention turned to development of sensor devices.

One of the few areas where sophisticated quality control systems exist is the laboratory. The practice of developing test values on "unknown" samples, whose value is actually carefully analyzed in advance, has gone on for many years. The difference between the test value and the true value is a variables measure. A sample of several unknowns can be treated according to the central limit theorem, and plotted in the manner shown in the preceding chapter. Such graphs are frequently prepared and displayed in the laboratory to encourage technicians to maintain high performance.

Other examples are hard to find. The so-called incident report which is commonly used in hospitals to identify an unusual and unfortunate occurrence, usually an accident, is discussed in chapter 10. The use of incidence of infection in a computerized control system has been reported.[14] These sometimes border upon epidemiologic detection and control systems which are more often community than hospital based. Some health departments take bacterial counts on silverware and establish statistical control limits. Similar procedures can be followed to test the cleanliness of linen. Lot samples (the test of the probability that the lot of goods purchased or manufactured is not different from specifications) are not uncommon in food purchasing, with elementary statistical limits calculations. Beyond this, little has been done. The mechanical problems of data reduction and the lack of clearly validated systems have probably discouraged most administrators.

Much of the recent attention to quality control in nonmedical systems can be traced to the Commission on Administrative Services in Hospitals (CASH). CASH was originally formed as a cost control program serving several hospitals in southern California. Its early concentration on control of nurse staffing soon indicated the need for corresponding attention to quality measurement. Significant reductions were made in nursing hours per patient day, and it was felt necessary to assure everyone concerned that these were not achieved at the expense of quality.

Three CASH quality scales have been reported, covering Housekeeping, Dietary, and Nursing services. The housekeeping and dietary measures will be reviewed here, with discussion of the technique of application. The nursing scale has been the subject of much interest and presumably improvement. A modified version of the CASH instrument, prepared for use in a research project, will be reviewed in detail. All three measures attempt to construct a numerical score based upon sampled situations. They are treated statistically as variables measures.

Housekeeping

The CASH housekeeping quality control checklist is an example of the use of subjective judgment—in this case without specified criteria—in attributes tests, applied to a reasonably large number of conditions, to construct an index score for each observation. Figures 11-4 and 11-5 show the observer's reporting form.[15] Three characteristics are reviewed: cleanliness, orderliness, and "condition," which is principally a check upon need for repair or replacement. Items which are fixed in place cannot be rated for order. Two different forms are used for patient rooms and general areas, reflecting the different housekeeping responsibilities. Provision is made for comment on the cause of unsatisfactory ratings, to permit correction or further analysis. Totals are taken by simple count.

Calculation of an index score could be made by adding all the items recorded "S" (for satisfactory) (83 in figure 11-4) and dividing it by the total number of entries (94 in the figure). This procedure would have resulted in equal weight for all negative checks. The misplaced dresser, item 35, would have the same effect upon the index as the dirty toilet bowl, item 44. CASH's committee of executive housekeepers elected instead to weight the three columns unequally, so that cleanliness contributed 70 percent to the final score, orderliness 10 percent, and condition 20 percent. Such a decision might reflect judgment of the importance of the responsibility or of the employee's ability to control achievement. "Order" can easily be changed by doctors, nurses, or visitors who may come into the room between the completion of the work and the inspection. Weighting of the data is accomplished by calculating each score separately and multiplying it by its fractional weight (that is, its relative weight divided by the total weight).

$$(\text{Component raw score}) \times (\text{Weight/sum of weights}) = \text{Component weighted score}$$

The sum of the component weighted scores is the total score. In the example shown, the weighted scores

Cleanliness	$(31/37) \times 0.7$	$= 0.59$
Orderliness	$(15/18) \times 0.1$	$= 0.08$
Condition	$(37/39) \times 0.2$	$= \underline{0.19}$
	Weighted total score $=$	0.86

The weighted total score forms a single data point for a subsample calculation under the central limit theorem. Observations can be grouped in various ways to generate the control statistic. Patient room data might be analyzed separately from other areas. Alternatively and preferably, scores might be calculated on the areas of responsibility of each housekeeping supervisor.

The frequency of observation of various areas need not be the same. Patient rooms may be sampled with several times the frequency of other areas. The data points are compiled to make the mean score and mean variance for the period.

FACTOR	Clean		Order		Cond.		FACTOR	Clean		Order		Cond.	
	S	U	S	U	S	U		S	U	S	U	S	U
1. Floor	✓				✓		31. Bed/Mattress	✓		✓		✓	
2. Baseboards		✓			✓		32. Overbed Table	✓		✓		✓	
3.				Do			33. Bedside Table		✓	✓		✓	
4.				Not			34. Dresser/Chest	✓			✓	✓	
5. Walls	✓			Rate	✓		35. Chairs	✓		✓		✓	
6. Doors	✓					✓	36. Linen	✓		✓		✓	
7. Sills	✓				✓		37. Waste Container	✓		✓		✓	
8. Wainscoting	✓				✓		38. Cubicle Curtains	✓		✓		✓	
9. Vents	✓				✓		39. Lamps/Shades	✓		✓			
10. Extinguishers			✓		✓		40.						
11. Pictures	✓		✓		✓		41.						
12.							42.						
13.							43.						
14.							44. Toilet		✓			✓	
15. Windows			✓	Do	✓		45. Tub	✓		Do		✓	
16. Sills	✓			Not	✓		46. Floors	✓				✓	
17. Screens	✓			Rate		✓	47. Walls		✓			✓	
18. Blinds	✓		✓		✓		48. Lights	✓		Not		✓	
19. Drapes		✓	✓		✓		49. Shower	✓				✓	
20. Drape Tracks							50. Holders/Bars	✓		Rate		✓	
21.							51. Plumbing	✓				✓	
22.							52. Towels	✓			✓	✓	
23.							53. Shower Curtain	✓		✓		✓	
24. Ceilings	✓				✓		54. Medicine Cabinet	✓		✓		✓	
25. Vents	✓		Do		✓		55. Tissue			✓		✓	
26. Air Conditioning	✓		Not		✓		56. Soap			✓			
27. Light Fixtures	✓		Rate		✓		57.						
28.							58.						
29.							59.						
30.							60.						

LOCATION: Floor 2   Nursing Unit 2N   Room No. 207   Date 10/15/65   Time 3:30 (am)(pm)

CULTURE: Yes ✓ No ☐   Satis· Yes ✓ No ☐   TOTAL RATINGS 31 | 6 | 15 | 3 | 37 | 2

Comments for Unsatisfactory Ratings	Comments for Unsatisfactory Ratings
Ref.	Ref.
2-C Dust in Corners	33-C Dust
15-C Streaked Inside	44-C Dirty Bowl
19-C Dirty	47-C Streak Around Med Cabinet
6-Co Paint Chipped	34-O Pushed Out Too Far Into Room
17-Co Torn Should Be Replaced	52-O Hung On Shower Bar
	56-O No Soap

Evaluated By: A. Smith   Approved: R. Brown

COMMISSION FOR ADMINISTRATIVE SERVICES IN HOSPITALS

Figure 11-4. Quality Control Check Sheet I Housekeeping Department (Patient Room/Bath).

LOCATION: ☑Corridor ☐Stairway ☐Lobby Other _____ Date 10/15/65
Building 1   Floor 2   Department _____ Time 11:00 (am)(pm)

	Clean S U	Order S U	Cond. S U			Clean S U	Order S U	Cond. S U
1. Floors	✓		✓	31. Tables				
2. Baseboards	✓		✓	32. Desks				
3.				33. Chairs				
4.		Do		34. Files				
5. Walls	✓	Not	✓	35. Bookcases				
6. Doors	✓			36. Lockers				
7. Sills		Rate	✓	37. Partitions	✓	✓	✓	
8. Wainscoting			✓	38. Linen				
9. Vents	✓		✓	39. Equipment	✓	✓	✓	
10. Extinguishers	✓	✓	✓	40.				
11. Pictures				41.				
12.				42.				
13.				43.				
14.				44. Elevator Floors		Do Not		
15.				45. Elevator Walls	✓	Rate	✓	
16. Windows		Do		46.				
17. Sills		Not		47.				
18. Screens		Rate		48. Toilet				
19. Blinds				49. Floors				
20. Drapes				50. Walls		Do		
21. Drape Tracks				51. Lights		Not		
22.				52. Plumbing		Rate		
23.				53. Towels				
24. Ceilings	✓	D	✓	54. Mirror				
25. Vents	✓	Not	✓	55. Tissue				
26. Air Conditioning	✓	Rate	✓	56. Soap				
27. Light Fixtures		✓	✓	57.				
28.				58.				
29.				59.				
30.				60.				

CULTURE: Yes☐ No☑   Satis: Yes☐ No☐   TOTAL RATINGS 10 3 2 1 19 1

Comments for Unsatisfactory Ratings
Ref.
1-C BADLY SCUFFED
24-C DUST ACCUMULATION
27-C GRILLES DUSTY
10-O 2 EXT. HANGING IMPROPERLY
5-C PAINT PEELING NEAR C.S.

Evaluated By: _____   Approved: R. Brown

COMMISSION FOR ADMINISTRATIVE SERVICES IN HOSPITALS

Figure 11-5. Quality Control Check Sheet II Housekeeping Department (General Areas).

In this process, the frequency of observation serves the same function as weighting. More frequently sampled areas will count more heavily in the total. The CASH executive housekeeper group which set up the quality control system suggested that frequency is best determined in the individual hospital. A list of the areas to be inspected should be studied, as should frequency of inspection according to their importance, frequency of cleaning, and other judgmental factors. Difficulty of cleaning should not be a criterion for setting frequency, unless it is recognized as such. Increased sampling of hard-to-clean areas will result in a mean score which is lower than a uniform sample would yield. Further discussion of sample size and techniques appears in the section, "Considerations in Inspection Samples."

Dietary

Figures 11-6 and 11-7 show a more elaborate form of quality control index which is based upon the same principle as the housekeeping forms. These again are composites of a number of attributes tests. Subsampling is required. Certain days and meals are selected at random, and trays are selected from the serving line. Specific foods or components of the tray preparation are selected for review. Some factors, such as taste, are left to the inspecting dietician's judgment, as was done with the housekeeping survey. Others, such as temperature and serving time have standards which were set in advance by the CASH dietary panel. These require the collection of numerical data to justify the attributes test.[16] The CASH inspection of trays, on the bottom of figure 11-6, permits the selection of separate trays or the same tray for the subsample. Separate trays are probably slightly preferable in order to gain better independence of the sample.

The sample size for each shift is variable in the CASH methodology. Higher percentage acceptables require samples of only five trays per category. Lower values are verified by increasing sample size, as indicated in table 11-1. This has the effect of reducing the probabilities of a false positive (Type I) error, while leaving a relatively high probability of false negative.

Figure 11-7 records a general inspection of the dietary department and its personnel. Except for the inclusions of personal inspection it is essentially the same as the housekeeping form.

In processing the statistic, percent acceptable scores are calculated for each of ten categories from the two forms. These are weighted in the total index. Food appearance, taste, temperature, and accuracy of tray preparation have weights of 15 percent. Food texture and equipment inspection are weighted at 10 percent each and all other elements at 5 percent. Although the triple check of housekeeping—cleanliness, orderliness and operational condition—has been carried through on the form (figure 11-7), the weights have been dropped. This is

						Date 10/15/65					
☑ Breakfast ☐ Lunch ☐ Dinner ☐ Special						Time (A, B, C) 7:15 (am)(pm)					
☐ Breakfast ☑ Lunch ☐ Dinner ☐ Special						Time (D) 11:00 (am)(pm)					

	CATEGORY	A		B		C			D						
R E F	FOOD (Select 5)	Appearance		Taste		Texture		R E F	(Select 5)	Food Temperature					
										Serving Line				Floor	
		S	U	S	U	S	U			Actual	Std	S	U	Actual Std	S U
1	Bacon	✓		✓		✓		1	Mixed Veg.	170	160	✓			
2	Sc. Egg	✓		✓		✓		2	Mashed Pot.	150	150	✓			
3	Milk	✓			✓			3	Coffee	185	170	✓			
4	Cream of Wheat	✓		✓		✓		4	Cream Puff	65	45		✓		
5	Orange Juice	✓		✓		✓		5	Stroganoff	165	160	✓			
6	Toast		✓		✓		✓								
Total Ratings		5	1	4	2	4	1	Total Ratings				4	1		

Comments for Negative Ratings	Comments for Negative Ratings
A-6 Slightly Burned	D-4 Not Sufficiently Chilled
B-3 Sour
B-6 Burned
C-6 Burned

Eval. By C. Brown   Approv. A.J.   Date 10/17

Food Service

							Date 10/17/65		
☐ Breakfast ☐ Lunch ☑ Dinner ☐ Special							Time (A, B) 5:15 (am)(pm)		
☐ Breakfast ☑ Lunch ☐ Dinner ☐ Special							Time (C) 11:30 (am)(pm)		

R E F	Category Diet Description (Select 5 Trays)	Trays				Tray Delivery				
		A		B		C				
		Appearance		Accuracy		Kitchen	Floor	Bedside	Rating	
		S	U	S	U	Time leave:	Time to:	Time to:	S	U
1	Bland Diet	✓		✓		11:30	11:45		✓	
2	Weighed Diet-Diab.	✓			✓	11:32	11:45		✓	
3	Salt Free Diet	✓		✓			11:45	11:50	✓	
4	House Diet		✓		✓		11:45	12:05		✓
5	Weighed Diet	✓		✓			11:45	11:52	✓	
Total Ratings		4	1	3	2				4	1

Comments for Negative Ratings	Comments for Negative Ratings
A-4 Silver Askew	C-4 Identification Missing - Checked Out
B-2 Fork Missing
B-4 Napkin Missing

Eval. By Ozman   Approv. A.J.   Date 10/17

Figure 11-6. Quality Control Check Sheet I Dietary Department (Food Preparation).

Location: KITCHEN
Evaluated By: ___
Time: 2:30 (pm)
Date: 10/15/65

Equipment (Select 5)	Clean S	Clean U	Order S	Order U	Operational S	Operational U	Clean Inside	Clean Out	Order Part	Order Place	Order Neat	Operational State Condition
Carts	✓		✓		✓					✓		
Cooking Units	✓		—		✓							
Dishes	✓		✓		✓							
Machines & Parts												
Pots/Pans												
Refrigerators	✓		—		✓		✓					
Serving Station	✓		✓		✓							
Sinks												
Storage-Equip. Supplies												
Clng. Supply												
Tables												
Trash Containers												
Utensils												
Lowerators	✓		—		✓		✓					
Total Ratings	4	2	2	1	6	0						

Area Maintenance (Select 5)	Clean S	Clean U	Reason for Negative Rating or Condition to be Reported for Further Attention
Baseboards	✓		
Doors	✓		
Floors	✓		
Floor Sinks			
Hoods			
Lavatory		✓	DIRTY TOILET BOWL
Lights			
Walls		✓	NEED CLEANING / PAINT
Ventilators			
Total Ratings	3	2	

Personnel (Select 2) Name	Uniform S	Uniform U	Cap S	Cap U	Hairnet S	Hairnet U	Apron S	Apron U	Hands S	Hands U	Nails S	Nails U	Skin S	Skin U	Hygiene S	Hygiene U	Reason for Neg. Rat.
1 H. JONES	✓		✓		✓		✓			✓	✓		✓				DIRTY
2 R. WHITE	✓		✓		✓			✓	✓		✓		✓				
3																	
Total Ratings	✓	0	2	0	2	0	2	0	1	1	1	1	2	0	2	0	

Approved: A.J.   Date: 10/17

Figure 11-7. Quality Control Check Sheet II Dietary Department (Housekeeping and Sanitation).

Table 11-1
Supplementary Sampling for Varying Percentages Acceptable

If Category Percentage Acceptable Is:	Additional Samples Required
100	0
95	0
90	0
85	1
80	2
75	3
70	5
65	8
60	11
55	15
50	20

Source: CASH, "A Quality Control Plan for the Dietary Department," p. 12.

apparently in recognition of the small contribution which these subordinate weights would make to the total, and in an effort to reduce calculating requirements. It may also reflect the greater importance of condition in food processing machinery. Figure 11-8 shows a chart for accumulating data on a weekly basis. The weighting calculation has been done in advance and tabulated on the lower section of the form.

Measurement of Nursing Quality

Nursing care resembles medical care in that the quality of the service depends heavily on professional judgment in the individual situation. To the extent that this is so, it should be possible to approach the problem of measuring nursing quality in the same way as the problem of medical quality. That is, the outcomes, the rates of performance of desirable procedures, or the scores of individual cases subjected to audits could be measured, and the results used to guide a continuing program of self study by the department. The statistical and managerial procedures described in chapter 10 could be routinely followed. As noted in the earlier discussion, some practical headway has been made toward this goal. There are at least prototype audit schemes which provide reasonably reliable results when they are carefully applied. However, these schemes have a number of limitations. The difficulties which have been encountered seem to have their roots in two problems. First, the process of nursing care is not as

Calculated By _Alice White_ Approv **A.J.** Week Ending _10/10/65_

Food Preparation	Total Ratings			Percent Acceptable	Index Conversion
	Satis.	Unsatis.	Total		
Appearance	16	4	20	80	12
Taste	17	3	20	85	13
Texture	17	3	20	85	8
Temperature	14	6	20	70	11
Food Service					
Tray Appearance	15	5	20	75	4
Tray Accuracy	16	4	20	80	12
Delivery	14	6	20	70	3
Housekeeping and Sanitation					
Equipment	37	8	45	82	8
Area	13	7	20	65	3
Personnel	52	8	60	87	4
			Overall Quality Index	▷	78

Index Conversion Chart

% Accept	Food Preparation				Food Service			Housekeeping & Sanitation		
	Appearance	Taste	Texture	Temp	Tray App	Tray Acc	Delivery	Equipment	Area	Personnel
100	15	15	10	15	5	15	5	10	5	5
95	14	14	9	14	5	15	5	9	5	5
90	14	13	9	14	5	14	5	8	4	4
85	13	13	8	13	4	14	4	8	4	4
80	12	12	8	12	4	12	4	8	4	4
75	11	11	7	11	4	11	4	8	4	4
70	11	10	7	11	3	10	3	7	4	4
65	10	10	7	10	3	10	3	6	3	3
60	9	9	6	9	3	9	3	6	3	3
55	8	8	6	8	3	8	3	5	3	3
50	8	8	5	8	2	8	2	5	2	2

Figure 11-8. Quality Control Plan: Dietary Department (Index Calculation Sheet).

clearly defined and modeled as the process of medical care. Secondly, nursing service traditionally includes responsibility for a number of activities which do not include an important component of professional judgment and which, in some cases, are not even related to the care of individual patients. There has been greater success with the housekeeping and nonprofessional components of nursing department activities than with the important professional ones.

Efforts to define the process of nursing care have generally resulted in only global statements. For example: "The nursing process may be simply defined as that which goes on between the patient and the nurse in a given setting."[17] Others tend to be not only lacking in any specifics, but are also circular: "The general duty nurse is aware of the total nursing needs of the patient and is responsible for seeing that they are fulfilled."[18] Although both of the quotations are parts of rather long lists of nursing functions and responsibilities, the two problems of lack of specificity and circularity occur repeatedly. Medicine suffered from similar problems. However, as scientific medicine evolved, it became possible to specify independently smaller elements of the process which could be identified and judged. It also became possible to reach consensus on the desirability of specific elements in relation to specified groups of patients. Progress is being made in this direction in nursing, particularly with the development of written care plans for individual patients, but the results are many years behind the achievements in medicine.

From one point of view, it is easy to say that the activities of the nursing department in a typical hospital include both the care of the individual patients and also the maintenance of the unit generally, the communication of orders between the doctors and other departments in the hospital, and the maintenance of the medical record for use of the physician and others. Most nursing departments are, in fact, charged with all these activities. From the point of view of quality measurement, however, quite different skills are involved, and it would not be reasonable to expect a perfect correlation between achievements in each of these areas. It is relatively an easier task to specify measurement devices in the areas other than patient care. Many approaches to the general problem of quality measurement, in fact, are heavily loaded with measurements of nonclinical aspects of nursing.

Efforts to measure the quality of nursing care can generally be classified into three groups. The most basic are measures of patient welfare or the outcome of nursing care. The second class are the application of various indirect statistics which are believed to relate to quality of nursing care. Thirdly, several efforts have been made to develop procedural measures of nursing quality which can be applied by auditing techniques. At the present time, it is the third group which has the most promise for routine management monitoring of nursing care.

Patient Welfare and Outcome Measures. One of the early efforts to measure the effect of nursing care on the patient and his welfare was undertaken at the State

University of Iowa in the late 1950s.[19] This study attempted to measure the impact of both larger nursing staffs and better in-service training preparation upon the quantity and quality of nursing care. Quantity was measured by work sampling techniques, and quality was measured by a patient welfare instrument. Such measures as the length of stay in the hospital, the number of days that the patient had an elevation of body temperature, the amount of narcotics and sedatives, the patient's mental attitude, physical independence and mobility, the patient's skin condition and his own opinion of the nursing care he received were included in the Iowa welfare measures.[20] Most of these measures were judged by nurses. There were criteria and quantitative measures for some of these items, while a few were simply subjective estimates. The opinion of the patient's physician about the quality of nursing care was also included. Data collection also included reports from the ward staff and the charge nurse, interviews with the patients, and observation by members of the study staff. Thus the cost of collecting the data was not insignificant. The sensitivity of the measure which was developed remains essentially untested. The measure was not sensitive enough to detect changes in quality as a result of the adjustment in the staffing levels and training made in the experiment, even though these changes were fairly large. One can infer either (a) the changes which were made in training and staffing did not change care, or (b) the patient's welfare is insensitive to nursing care, or (c) this measurement instrument was insensitive to the patient's welfare. One point which must be noted is that almost all of the measures used were largely under the control of other members of the medical care team than the nurse. The patient's doctor and the nature of his disease are important in each of the measures which were selected. Thus the measurement score is subject to a great deal of variation which is essentially random from the point of view of the nursing care system.

One measure of the outcome of nursing care, patient's skin condition, has received a substantial amount of attention. Patients who are bedridden for a fairly long period of time can easily develop deterioration of areas of their skin. It is generally believed that the quality of nursing care is an important factor in the extent of the deterioration that occurs. Elaborate criteria have been developed for the measurement of the single phenomenon.[21] Although this measure is in itself of substantial value, it tends to be useful only among long stay patients. Thus it does not appear promising as a general monitor of quality.

It should be noted that the absence of a sensitive, reliable and valid measure of the outcome of patient care seriously hampers the development of inferential measures of the procedural or structural forms. If outcome measures such as recovery rate, pain, condition on recovery, and the avoidance of complications, could be obtained, even though their measurement was a lengthy and expensive process, other simpler measures could be proposed and tested against these. Those which proved to be highly correlated with outcomes would be used to provide inexpensive continuing monitors of care. Since there are no such measures of outcomes, indirect and procedural measures have been developed "in the dark" related at best to what is subjectively believed to be "good nursing care."

Indirect Measures of Nursing Quality. Most hospitals have systems of reporting various unfortunate incidents which occur on the nursing floor. These vary from patient falls and visitor accidents to errors in medication. As noted in chapter 10, counts of these reports develop statistics which can be treated either as Poisson processes or as Bernoulli processes. The principal difficulty with these statistics is that the number of reports received reflects two processes: the process of giving nursing care and the process of preparing incident reports. It is generally recognized that the number of reports received is itself a function of the reporting system and the emphasis which is placed on the reports. Exactly what the relationship is, is uncertain. It is known that if great stress is put upon finding medication errors, large numbers can be uncovered. If no stress is put on this factor, only those errors which have obvious clinical importance tend to be reported. At the same time, floors which tend to be giving low quality of care may also tend to be poorly organized in regard to writing and completing of reports and may thus issue fewer reports for a given number of accidents than better managed nursing units. Lastly, it seems possible that increased tension and particularly criticism based upon the reports may adversely affect the tendency to prepare a report. Although these difficulties are not sufficient to rule out the use of reports of this type to identify problem areas in the quality of care, they do indicate the need for very cautious analysis of the results.

There is some indication that the opinions of nurses themselves, when carefully measured, provides an indicator of the actual quality of care. Turnover, absenteeism, and employee accident rates provide indicators of personnel satisfaction which can be used on an ongoing basis. Revans has shown that these factors are apparently related to the average length of stay in the hospital.[22] These measures should certainly be calculated for each nursing unit and in fact, for all other work force groups in the hospital as indicators of the general effectiveness of the team. Georgopoulos and Mann have shown, and attempted to validate, the use of a questionnaire on employee satisfaction as a measure of nursing care.[23] Abdellah and Levine have developed a similar instrument which probes the attitudes of both patients and nurses and includes a weighting scale for quantitative analysis of responses.[24] The cost, complexity, and nature of these instruments seems to limit their use to occasional applications.

Procedural Measures of Nursing Care. A number of efforts have been made to develop comprehensive or representative lists of procedures which should be performed on a nursing floor to use in deriving either a quantitative score of nursing quality or at least a subjective estimate of areas of relative strength and weakness. Some of these are attempts to describe the desirable level of performance in all areas of nursing service and to provide checklists for the subjective comparison of achievement to the criteria.[25] Because of their broad scope and subjective nature, these do not seem to lend themselves to ongoing monitoring systems. Other approaches have been more specific and have attempted to isolate specific procedures in nursing care and measure their performance on a sampling basis by observation of individual patients and nursing units. One of the first of these to be routinely used as a quality monitor was developed by the Commission on Administrative Services in Hospitals.[26] The CASH scale was later expanded by the Veterans' Administration and revised again in connection with a study of the impact of unit managers on nursing quality and efficiency undertaken at the University of Michigan, Bureau of Hospital Administration. Specimens of two sections of this instrument are attached as appendix to this chapter, with the explanatory information for the nurse administering the instrument.[27]

This instrument is designed to be applied to individual patients who are sampled from the floor census. The subparts of the questionnaire can be weighted to construct a single score for each patient sampled and the data can be treated exactly as demonstrated in chapter 10. The reliability of this type of survey instrument appears to be satisfactory when application is by trained observers, and when observers do not report on units for which they have managerial responsibility.[28] It should be noted, however, that instruments of this type have still received only limited use and study.

Weights are assigned to the five areas of the questionnaire shown in the appendix as follows:

Areas	Weights
1. General	15
2. Patient welfare and safety	15
3. Patient comfort	15
4. Patient room	05
5. Patient's chart	15
6. Nursing care plan	15
7. Nursing unit	05
8. Ward medical administration	10
9. Ward building management	05

A hospital applying the audit could, of course, modify the weights as it saw fit.

Although this procedural audit instrument appears to have sufficient sensitivity and reliability to be useful, and although its validity is apparently acceptable, there are a number of drawbacks to it. It can be viewed only as an interim step toward the development of a better measure. There appear to be four types of problems with the present form of the instrument. It is costly to apply; it has certain difficulties in the weighting of the items; the items themselves vary in importance and are sometimes ambiguous; and the instrument as a whole places too much importance on nonclinical aspects of nursing. There are 105 items in the University of Michigan version shown in the appendix. It is estimated that it takes a trained observer forty-five minutes to apply the questionnaire to a single patient. On the basis of a three-patient sample per floor per day, the instrument would require two and one quarter man hours per nursing unit. This may be an unrealistic requirement. Scoring the questionnaire and reduction of the statistics would be in addition to that time.

An immediate simplification is suggested by study of the nine areas of the instrument and the weighting factors which are given them. It should be noted that only five of the nine areas, or seventy-three questions, relate to the care of a single patient. The other four areas (1, 7, 8, and 9) are of activities which are constant for a single nursing unit on a given day. Section one, in fact, is apparently composed of items which would vary only slightly over time. The inclusion of these items in a routine quality audit has the effect of reducing the sensitivity of the scores because the average percentage score is reduced or inflated by a constant or nearly constant value over a substantial period of time. It should be noted that although parts 7, 8, and 9 are weighted only 20 percent, they will have the same value for each patient sampled on the floor. Thus they will be counted three times in calculating the overall floor score. Revised procedures can easily be developed where these sections are completed once for each floor and arithmetic adjustments of the weights are made in calculating the floor mean score.

The individual items differ substantially in their nature. This difference can be in several different dimensions. For example, in section 2, item 2, "Is the bedside table and other self-care equipment positioned for the convenience and safety of the patient?" is primarily an item of convenience, whereas item 6, "Are restraints and/or protective devices applied when indicated and in a safe, comfortable manner?" is an item which directly affects the patient's well-being. The first question of section 4, "Is the room appearance satisfactory?" is an example of an essentially subjective judgment. In this case, the backup information contains specific criteria to guide the observer. However, a very similar question, 3.01, "Does patient appear comfortable?" is indicated on the backup sheet as self-evident. It is not at all clear that each nurse inspector would tend to judge the same patient as "appearing comfortable" in view of the fact that they would almost inevitably tend to make differing allowances for the patient's disease and condition. In other words, a patient in his first postoperative day is expected to be uncomfortable. It seems likely that many, but not all, nurses would interpret the question as being "Does the patient appear as comfortable as his condition permits?" Certain questions are actually impossible for the observer to answer. For example, question 5.03, "Is intake and output correctly recorded?" can sometimes be answered no, based upon available information, but more often the observer will have no evidence as to whether it is correct or incorrect. Certain questions such as 6.12, "Does plan indicate need and time of smoking supervision?" are either ambiguous or place rather extensive demand on the technical knowledge of the nurse. Either the nurse must assume that this question is not applicable unless the doctor has made specific comment in the medical record, or she must be equipped to draw fine lines regarding the dangers of smoking with certain diseases. These problems with the individual items are inevitable in any attempt of this kind, particularly in the developmental stages. However, it is from these kinds of difficulty that losses in reliability of the score occur.

It should be noted that questions of a nonclinical nature occur throughout the questionnaire, although parts 1, 7, 8, and 9 are almost entirely nonclinical. In total, it appears that the items and their weights place far too much stress upon these characteristics. Despite their management importance, they do not relate directly to the quality of nursing patient care. This difficulty can be partially corrected by changing the weights or by eliminating certain questions. In part, however, it stems from the difficulty of writing specific unambiguous questions about the still undefined process of "nursing care."

Future Developments in the Measurement of Nursing Quality. Smith and others conducted an extensive application of the CASH instrument in connection with an evaluation of unit management systems.[29] Using these data, Smith performed an analysis of individual items in the questionnaire in terms of their sensitivity and discrimination. Much of the more clinical portion of the CASH questionnaire was found lacking in discrimination. Whole blocks of questions, especially section 6 on nursing care plans, drew uniform answers. Hospitals which have no nursing care plan can never receive credit for many items in this section. Other questions were found to be answered yes nearly 100 percent (or nearly zero percent) of the time. As a result of this analysis, Smith has concluded that the questionnaire is useful only for housekeeping and unit related (as opposed to patient related) activities. It is, however, sensitive and reliable for those purposes.[30]

The next step appears to be the development of better clinical or professional nursing evaluations. Possibilities appear to revolve around the patient care plan, where desired outcomes and necessary procedures can be specified for individual patients or groups of patients. It is possible, for example, to specify that any patient should receive normal bodily care and delivery of all prescribed tests and treatments, as well as being provided with a clean, orderly, and safe environment. Specific patients have other needs. Diabetics, for example, need instruction in diet, insulin administration, urine testing, and the relation of diet, activity and insulin. They also need more careful skin care; particularly of the feet. A diabetic with hypertension also requires daily blood pressure administration and other specific items of care or instruction.

Questions covering achievements in these clinical areas can be added to the

CASH instrument. It appears from early work by Smith and Horn that such an approach is feasible, but that there may be several thousand specific questions. Many of these will be related to the patient's disease. Other items will be more important for some diseases than for others. Elaborate sampling routines will be necessary to reduce the population of relevant questions to representative samples of both patients and floors which can be obtained at reasonable expense. Such a program, while promising, is several years from reality.[31] Until it has been developed, hospitals can use CASH-type approaches, but only with recognition of their serious limitations.

Considerations in Inspection Samples

There are several aspects of the CASH-type inspection samples (for both nursing and other departments) which should be considered independent of the specific application. These include calculating aids, sample size selection, setting control limits, and sampling and inspection techniques.

Data Processing. The workload involved in inspection samples of this type grows rapidly with the complexity of the service under study. While the housekeeping survey requires only counting and weighting of relatively few numbers, the modified nursing form has a large number of elements, and the dietary form involves recording quantitative data as well as preliminary calculations covering the sample size. Computer processing advantages and possibilities are obvious. It would appear that computer assistance is necessary to make widespread use of these techniques. The proposed nursing approach will not be feasible under manual systems except at long intervals (annually or quarterly, for example). Data processing will necessarily involve both sampling and analysis.

Sample Size Determination. In industrial production applications of quality control, sample sizes can be set relative to the cost or value of the failure rate improvement. The cost of conducting the necessary additional inspection can be calculated, as can the savings resulting from the corresponding improvement in control. (Unsatisfactory products are returned and must be replaced. The unit cost of doing this is often very high. Thus there is substantial value in reducing the number of unsatisfactory products passed.) Such an approach is conceptually of value in hospitals, even though the cost of unsatisfactory items is probably immeasurable.

The general approach is as follows. Consider that the population under the control system has a mean value of the reference signal, μ. It is being controlled by a sampling process, which over a length of N periods ($N > 1$) will result in a sample size nN if there are n samples per period. This sample will yield a grand mean $\bar{\bar{x}}$ and an overall standard deviation of $\sigma_x/\sqrt{nN}$. The relationship between μ, $\bar{\bar{x}}$, and σ_x,

$$t = \frac{\mu - \bar{\bar{x}}}{\sigma_x/\sqrt{nN}}$$

will follow the student's t distribution. If the difference, $\mu - \bar{\bar{x}}$, and the level of confidence desired, are specified, the value

$$nN = \left(\frac{\sigma_x t}{(\mu - \bar{\bar{x}})}\right)^2.$$

Early experience with the control system can use an arbitrary value for n and data can be collected for several periods to estimate $\bar{\bar{x}}$ and σ.

The specification of $\mu - \bar{\bar{x}}$ and the level of confidence are judgmental in the absence of cost data. The statement is "The control system will detect a given level of deviation $(\mu - \bar{\bar{x}})$ at a given level of confidence." The sample size is inversely related to the square of the deviation. Thus detection of small deviations requires very large samples. At some point the gain in control will not be judged worthy of the increase. The calculation should be made at several levels of $\mu - \bar{\bar{x}}$.

Control Limits. A similar procedure could be followed with the confidence level, but it seems desirable to select an appropriate level, probably either $\alpha = 0.10$ or 0.05, for initial operation. Industrial operation usually specifies a much higher confidence level. The factor of 3 is used to set control limits. For large samples, this gives an $\alpha = 0.002$. (Control limits are normally stated for a two-tailed test.) As control systems continue to operate, standard deviations generally decline. That, after all, is one of the goals of the systems. Thus a given sample size yields increasingly high levels of confidence for detection of a given change in the population value μ. At some point, recalculation and reduction of the sample size may be desirable.

Selection of Sample and Inspection. Considerable care should be taken to avoid bias in data collection. The samples (patients, rooms, trays, etc.) to be inspected should be selected independently in advance of the inspection. The use of a random number table or similar unbiased sampling device is required. The identity of samples should be concealed until the time of inspection. Inspectors should not inspect areas for which they have direct supervisory responsibility. Inspectors should meet periodically to review criteria, if any, and to test reliability by independent review of the same sample at the same time. As a final check on reliability, inspectors can be assigned to duplicate review of the same area. The two samples representing different inspections of the same population can be tested by the t test for the difference between two means:

$$t = \frac{\bar{x}_1 - \bar{x}_2}{\sigma},$$

where σ is the pooled deviation

$$\sigma = \sqrt{\frac{\sigma_1^2}{n_1} + \frac{\sigma_2^2}{n_2}}.$$

Area scores can be compared for differences between areas as well. If inspectors are randomly assigned to areas and data collected over a period of time, the mean scores and variances can be calculated in a two-way analysis.

The hypothesis to be tested is that the variance introduced by the observer is not significant. In an ongoing quality control system, routine checks of this kind are highly desirable to prevent the development of bias.

Chapter 11
Appendix

Specimen Figures and Supporting Explanations for a CASH-type Nursing Quality Instrument

The following information is from the University of Michigan Bureau of Hospital Administration version of the CASH-type nursing care quality survey instrument. Two sections have been selected from the total of nine for illustration. In each case the questionnaire itself is shown as an appendix figures 11-9 and 11-10. The text below gives the explanatory and definitional material which is available to the inspecting nurse.

Backup Information for Work Sheet Number 2—Patient Welfare and Safety

2. Patient Welfare and Safety
    1. Patient requires no immediate attention?
        1.1 Does the patient have a request?
        1.2 Are there signs or symptoms of a threat to patient's life (dyspnea, bleeding, diaphoresis, suicidal ideas, etc.)?
        1.3 Is the patient having pain, nausea, or vomiting?
        1.4 Is the patient tense and/or restless, angry, or disoriented?
        1.5 Is the patient depressed?
    2. Are the bedside table and other self-care equipment positioned for the safety of the patient?
        2.1 Is the patient able to reach his water?
        2.2 Are all the items needed by the patient available in or on the bedside stand?
        2.3 Can the bedside table be raised or lowered easily?
    3. Is the call light or other mechanical communication device within easy reach, working and in good condition?
        3.1 Can the patient reach his light without strain?
        3.2 Is the cord secured?
        3.3 Does the call light work?
        3.4 Is the type of call system appropriate for the patient?
        3.5 Is the cord clean and free of frayed areas?
    4. Is the bed in proper position?
        4.1 Is the bed in a therapeutic position if indicated? e.g.,
            a. Semi-Fowlers after a carotid angiogram
            b. Flat or trendelenberg after a pneumoencephalogram
            c. Fowlers with pulmonary edema

Hospital Unit_____ Bed No._____
Patient Social Security No._____ Date_____
Patient Number_____   Time_____

2. PATIENT WELFARE AND SAFETY

Factor No.

		YES	NO	NA
.01	Does the patient appear comfortable?			
.02	Is the bedside table and other self-care equipment positioned for the convenience and safety of the patient?			
.03	Is the call light or other mechanical communication device within easy reach, and in proper working condition?			
.04	Is the bed in proper position? (semi-Fowler, trendelenberg, etc.)			
.05	Are side-rails up, if indicated?			
.06	Are restraints and/or protective devices applied when indicated, and in a safe and comfortable manner?			
.07	Are dressing and/or supports applied in a safe and comfortable manner?			
.08	Does the patient have all the preventive or protective devices he needs? (Bedboards, footboard, trapeze, etc.)			
.09	Is the patient in optimal body alignment?			
.10	Are measures being taken to minimize the development of contractures, decubitus ulcers, footdrop, etc.?			
.11	Is the identification tag current, complete, legible, and applied to the wrist?			
.12	Are oxygen precautions being taken?			
.13	Are isolation precautions being taken?			
	TOTAL			

Observer comments (reference backup information if available):

Factor No.

Figure 11-9. Nursing Quality Instrument: Work Sheet Number 2.

Hospital Unit _____ Bed No. _____
Patient Social Security No. _____ Date _____
Patient No. _____ Time _____

5. PATIENT'S CHART | YES | NO | NA |

Factor No.

.01 Have medications and treatments been given as ordered
     and charted correctly? _ _ _ _ _ _ _ _ _ _ _ _ _ _ _ _
.02 Have vital signs been taken as ordered and recorded
     correctly? _
.03 Is intake and output correctly recorded? _ _ _ _ _ _ _
.04 If orders are not carried out, have pertinent
     comments been recorded? _ _ _ _ _ _ _ _ _ _ _ _ _ _ _
.05 Have all orders been dated and signed by physician? _ _
.06 Was notification and response of physician charted? _ _
.07 Are pertinent recurring activities charted? _ _ _ _ _ _
.08 Do the nursing notes reflect existing patient or
     family teaching? _ _ _ _ _ _ _ _ _ _ _ _ _ _ _ _ _ _
.09 Are reasons for and effect of PRN, STAT and one-
     time medications charted on nurses' notes? _ _ _ _ _ _ _
.10 Are nurses' notes legible? _ _ _ _ _ _ _ _ _ _ _ _ _ _
.11 Are approved abbreviations being used? _ _ _ _ _ _ _ _
.12 Are recorder's signature and initials noted? _ _ _ _ _ _
.13 Is the patient's full name recorded on the
     medication card? _ _ _ _ _ _ _ _ _ _ _ _ _ _ _ _ _ _

                                TOTAL   ____ ___ ___

Observer comments (reference backup information if available):

Factor No.

Figure 11-10. Nursing Quality Instrument: Work Sheet Number 5.

4.2 Is the bed positioned to facilitate respirations and circulation?
4.3 Is the bed at the proper height to facilitate patient activity?
4.4 Is the bed at the proper height for administering patient care?
5. Are side rails up if indicated?
    5.1 Are they up:
        a. following the administration of sedatives?
        b. following the administration of analgesics such as Demerol and morphine sulfate?
        c. following recent administration of anesthesia?
        d. when a patient is disoriented?
        e. when a patient has a history of Grand Mal seizures?
        f. when a patient has a history of vertigo, loss of consciousness, etc.?
6. Are restraints and/or protective devices applied when indicated and in a safe and comfortable manner?
    6.1 Are the siderails padded for restless, disoriented and/or seizure patients?
    6.2 Are hard restraints (e.g., leather) padded with soft, absorbent material?
    6.3 Have measures been taken to protect the skin from direct contact with jacket, kerlix, posey, etc., restraints?
    6.4 Are the skin areas in direct contact with restraining devices erythematous and/or broken (e.g., the axilla with a jacket restraint)?
    6.5 Have measures been taken to limit skin apposition which is secondary to restraint devices (e.g., are the fingers wrapped when mitten restraints are necessary)?
    6.6 Restraints should not be fastened to siderails.
7. Are dressings and/or supports applied in a safe and comfortable manner?
    7.1 Is the dressing adequate, clean, secure and as comfortable as possible?
8. Does the patient have all the preventive or protective appliances he needs? (Bedboards, footboards, trapeze, etc.) Self-evident.
    8.1 Are the equipment and appliances described in the medical and nursing care plans provided and used correctly?
9. Is the patient in optimal body alignment?
    9.1 Is the patient positioned to insure a clear airway and to facilitate respirations?
10. Are measures being taken to minimize the development and/or progression of contractures, decubitus ulcers, foot drop, etc.?
    10.1 Are range of motion exercises being given?
    10.2 Are pressure areas protected (e.g., bridged) if indicated?

10.3 Are affected limbs in proper position to prevent contractures and foot drop (e.g., are the feet placed firmly against a footboard when indicated)?

10.4 Are the necessary devices used to maintain optimal positioning (e.g., are sandbags or some other such measure being utilized to prevent external lateral rotation of the legs)?

11. Self-evident
12. Are oxygen precautions being taken?
    12.1 Are oxygen precaution signs obvious?
    12.2 Is the "no smoking" restriction enforced?
    12.3 When an oxygen tent is used, is the mattress covered with plastic with the sides of the tent properly secured?
    12.4 Are electrical devices grounded or disconnected?
13. Are isolation precautions being taken?
    13.1 Are isolation units clearly demarcated?
    13.2 Is the physical setting appropriate (e.g., is a patient with a respiratory infection in a private room)?
    13.3 Are gowns, masks, gloves, etc. readily available and in a clean area?
    13.4 Are adequate measures provided for disposing of contaminated linen, equipment and waste?
14. Self-evident

Backup Information for Work Sheet Number 5–Patient Charts

5. *Patient's Chart*
   1. Self-evident
   2. Have medications been charted correctly?
      2.1 Are the nurses initials in the proper space on the medication record indicating that medicine was given?
      2.2 Are the PRN, STAT, or one-time orders charted on nurses' notes?
      2.3 Are the route and site of administration of injections indicated on nurses' notes?
      2.4 Is the legal signature used?
      2.5 If unable to give medication, has the space on the medication record been circled and the reason indicated on nurses' notes?
   3. Are reasons for and effect of PRN, STAT and one-time medication charted on nurses' notes?
      3.1 Has the reason for patient's request for medication been elicited?
      3.2 Have the type, location, and severity of pain been identified and noted?
      3.3 Have the type, location, and severity of urticaria been indicated?

      3.4 Have location, type, and severity of rash been noted?
      3.5 Has time patient obtained relief of condition been noted?
      3.6 Are any untoward symptoms or reaction to drug noted?
      3.7 Has the medication's effectiveness been indicated?
      3.8 Are the time and type of treatment indicated?
      3.9 Are the type and amount of solution indicated?
      3.10 Have the effects and results of treatment been charted?
      3.11 Has the signature been used?
4. Self-evident
5. Self-evident
6. Have vital signs been taken as ordered?
      6.1 Have the vital signs been taken as frequently as ordered by the doctors and nurses?
      6.2 Have the vital signs been taken as frequently as indicated by the patient's condition?
7. Have vital signs been recorded correctly?
      7.1 Has the TPR been recorded on proper graph? (TRP graph, B/P graph, B/P record or nurses' notes?)
      7.2 Has the B/P been recorded on proper form? (TPR graph, B/P graph, B/P record, or nurses' notes?)
      7.3 Is the legal signature used?
8. Is intake and output record current?
      8.1 Has intake and output been recorded on proper forms?
      8.2 Have the time, amount, type and route of administration been indicated?
      8.3 Have totals for each shift been kept?
      8.4 Has 24 hour total been maintained?
      8.5 Is there a total for both intake and output?
9. If orders are not carried out, have pertinent comments been recorded?
      9.1 Has the reason been indicated on nurses' notes why treatment or medication was not given?
10. Have all orders been dated and signed by physician?
      10.1 Has the date been indicated in proper column on doctor's order sheet?
      10.2 Does a signature appear?
11. Was notification and response of physician charted?
      11.1 Has physician been notified of patient's condition as indicated?
      11.2 On admission?
      11.3 Any significant change in patient's condition?
      11.4 Any complaints of unusual pain?
      11.5 Any reactions or untoward symptoms to drugs, blood, etc.?
      11.6 Any questions or problems regarding medical care?
      11.7 Request by patient?

11.8 Has response of physician been indicated, including time, date, and reply, on nurses' notes?
12. Are pertinent, recurring activities charted?
    12.1 Has there been any charting within past 48 hours?
    12.2 Have signs and symptoms; observations of the patient been recorded?
    12.3 Have the type and time of special oral hygiene been indicated on nurses' notes?
    12.4 Has ROM been charted with indication of time given and part or parts exercised?
    12.5 Has incontinent, scrotal, or catheter care been charted indicating time, amount, type of solution, amount and color of drainage and effects?
    12.6 Have any of the patient's feelings and reactions to his illness, care and/or progress been noted on nurses' notes?
    12.7 Has any teaching done for patient and/or family been charted on nurses' notes?
    12.8 Any changes in patient's condition been noted?
    12.9 Has ambulation and exercise of patient been indicated if pertinent?
    12.10 Has turning of patient with or without skin care been noted?
    12.11 Has the kind and amount of fluid forced been charted?
    12.12 Does the chart indicate the frequency and type of stools?

    12.13 Do the notes indicate the type, frequency, time, appearance of wound and patient tolerance of each dressing change?
    12.14 Is the frequency of tracheostomy care indicated?
    12.15 Is the frequency of tracheal suctioning, along with the tolerance of the patient, and the amount, color, and consistency of the secretions noted?
    12.16 Does the chart contain information on the type of solution, amount, frequency, times, character of the returns and patient tolerance of irrigations?
13. Do the nurses' notes reflect existing patient or family teaching?
    13.1 Is there any notation of explaining care to patient and/or family?
    13.2 Is there any notation of instruction of patient and/or family regarding procedures (administration of insulin, care of colostomy, how to get in wheelchair, etc.)?
    13.3 Is there any notation of patient's acceptance and understanding of the nurse's teaching?
    13.4 Have any needs of the patient been identified thru interaction with the patient and nursing intervention been charted?
    13.5 Is there any evidence of how the patient is accepting his illness and how he feels about his prognosis?

13.6 Is there any evidence of how the patient feels regarding his progress and possible discharge?
14. Self-evident
15. Self-evident
16. Self-evident
17. Self-evident

Additional Readings

Various commissions and services have descriptive material available for interested persons free or at low cost.

Hospital Administrative Services, American Hospital Association, 840 N. Lake Shore Drive, Chicago 60611.

Commission on Administrative Services in Hospitals, 3345 Wilshire Blvd., Los Angeles, California.

Community Systems Foundation, 2200 Fuller Road, Ann Arbor, Michigan 48105.

Ludwig, P.E. *Dollars and Sense: An Approach toward Hospital Cost Containment and Quality Improvement through Management Engineering Programs.* W.K. Kellogg Foundation, Battle Creek, Michigan, 1971. Includes discussion of cost control systems established by state hospital associations.

12 Measuring the Quality of the Medical Care Process

Introduction

Efforts to measure the quality of the medical care process—that is, the diagnosis and treatment of individual patients—go back at least fifty years.[1] A variety of techniques have been used, ranging from direct observation of care to statistical abstracts from medical histories. These have universally revealed substantial variation in the quality of performance, even within large, apparently well-controlled hospitals. So frequent is the finding of poor quality that no reasonable person is justified in making or accepting statements about the quality of care (other than its likely variability) in a given institution without systematic evidence to support the claim.

Similarly, no board of trustees or medical staff can afford complacency in regard to the achievements of their institution unless formal systems for the routine measurement of quality of care are installed and working effectively. As Klicka says:

Whether we like it or not, someone must exercise control in our hospitals to assure that the quality of care is at the highest possible level. By statute this control is given to the trustees who are responsible to the public served by the hospital. Trustees exercise this control by delegation of responsibility to the medical staff which is organized so that each physician is supervised by a physician senior to him. The typical medical staff organization thus provides stability and assurances that the watchful eye of one physician upon another is always present. The extent to which this eye is alert definitely determines the manner in which medicine is practiced in that hospital.[2] (Emphasis in the original.)

At the same time, it is apparent that techniques exist which can be used to make explicit judgments on quality of care. Donabedian, who has made extensive study of the possibilities, has concluded:

At least the better methods have been adequate for administrative and social policy purposes that have brought them into being. The search for perfection should not blind one to the fact that present techniques of evaluating quality, crude as they are, have revealed a range of quality from outstanding to deplorable. Tools are now available for making broad judgments of this kind with considerable assurance.[3]

There are two goals in the review of quality of medical care in a hospital: to aid the medical staff in continuing study and improvement of the quality of medical care, and to guarantee that minimal standards are met. The great practical problem to be overcome is cost. Physician time is highly valuable, and physicians generally do not enjoy case review. On the other hand, explicit measures by themselves are frequently of low validity, and large numbers of attributes and variables must be taken into account. An appropriate system for continuing improvement includes the following components:

1. A fact finding system which identifies quality problem areas
2. A system of impersonal analysis of facts conducted by skilled physicians
3. An educational system which spreads the conclusions from the analysis to individual physicians and the staff as a whole
4. A continuing fact-finding system which monitors achievement of the system as a whole for the staff and for the trustees, to assure that it continues to function effectively in meeting both goals

The first and fourth components are those of the sensor and monitor in conventional control systems. They constitute an information gathering subsystem which does not require direct professional action. It is clear that at present levels of ability to measure medical quality, review of summarized information by physicians forms the central mechanisms of control and improvement. The information-gathering system plays a subsidiary role where automation can be used to gain economy.

Placing the information-gathering subsystem in this supplementary role reduces the danger of overzealous reliance on incomplete statistical interpretations of the quality of medical care, but frees the physician from the chores of routine review and data compilation. In doing so, it permits the practical design of the information system. Stated another way, only the combination of all necessary information plus reliable professional analysis can be used to judge the quality of medical care. The information system alone merely detects and assembles the necessary information for judgment in a convenient and expeditious form. In this context, the goal of the information handling system is sufficient speed, reliability, flexibility, and sensitivity to support and encourage the activities of reviewing physicians. Validity of the information, that is its proven relation to improved end results of care, is of less immediate importance because reliance is placed on physician judgment to establish this element.

The information subsystem supplies data to the clinical meetings of the staff and to the appropriate committees, such as the tissue, records, and utilization committees. When the total system is designed in this way, it is consistent with the statistical limitations inherent in the concept of identification of "unusual cases" and also with the limitations in understanding of the process of restoring health. It also is consistent with the philosophy of the Joint Commission on Hospital Accreditation and its member organizations.

The two aspects of the system cannot be entirely divided. Although data gathering and data reduction are largely chores which can be done by clerks and computers, the medical staff members who rely on a report should be familiar with the way in which the data are prepared. Good system design requires medical advice. There are a number of problems in the selection and definition of individual statistics which the medical staff should decide. Many of these require an arbitrary judgment which is best made by those who will use the statistics. The selection of standards and control limits is more a medical than a statistical process. In short, the system will work best when there is plenty of communication between the judgmental and the information-gathering components.

Sheps classified measures of medical care quality into three groups: *outcomes*, the results of care in terms of changes in health; *procedural*, the presence or absence, or the quality of performance of certain procedures deemed to be of benefit in a given situation; and *structural*, measures of organizational characteristics and policies believed to be conducive to high quality.[4] Structural mechanisms include the traditional patterns of medical staff organization and are clearly stated in documents like the *Principles of Accreditation* of the Joint Commission.[5] They provide organizational support for continuous review and control, but rarely provide useful reference measures. Quantitative structural measures exist (attendance records at meetings, documentation of prior experience, etc.), but their limited validity and static qualities make them unsuitable.

Outcomes measures, on the other hand, are relatively difficult to relate to specifics within the control process. Death rates, disease incidence rates, age at death, causes of death, unexpected results including complications and infections, and preventable disabilities are all outcomes measures of various aspects of health practices. Often, however, they reflect patient and community attitudes, dietary and environmental factors, and other elements well beyond the control of the hospital and the medical staff. In order to use outcomes measures as reference signals in the quality of medical care, reasonable relationship must be established between the outcome and the process. Some important measures have been established, primarily in death, infection, and diagnostic accuracy rates of specific procedures. Maternal and neonatal deaths in particular have been carefully studied.

The bulk of measures for medical quality control are procedural. Many elements of care have been established as desirable in general or in special cases. The selection is sometimes supported by authority and sometimes by studies of validity. While validity can be questioned in specific procedural measures or certain applications of a usually valid measure, the set of procedural measures appears to represent a fair consensus of current medical thought. There are a large number of procedural measures, but they do not represent all aspects of care equally well. The more definitive the treatment the more numerous the procedural measures. There are many in surgical care. Areas such as psychiatric care are correspondingly without good procedural measures. Thus the measurement problems—limitations on the availability of relevant measures—result in an incomplete and potentially distorted quality control system. The weakness, however, is almost as much in the extent of medical knowledge generally as it is in measurement systems per se.

Manual Information-Gathering Systems

A System of Structural and Outcome Measures

Limited opportunities exist to apply statistical information handling to manual data collection methods. The number of readily available measures is small, and the opportunities for counting or measurement are few. The items included in the "Professional Activities Report" or "Professional Performance Report" devised by MacEachern and others in the 1930s have not been amplified extensively in manual methods since that time.[6] One of the most elaborate examples of such systems was that proposed by Johnson and Vivaldo in 1960.[7] A large number of statistics relevant to the problem of hospital quality generally were included. Only a few additions were made to the Professional Activity Report—those statistics relative directly to physician performance. However, the system devised by Johnson and Vivaldo included description of the output of hospital systems, including admissions, discharges, and treatments of various kinds. In addition to these data, which form the base of various rate calculations, the system calls for the monthly assembly of the following information:

1. *Demand*

    - Waiting lists for admission, by medical specialty
    - Admissions by urgency (emergency, urgent, elective)
    - Admissions of disease categories of special interest:
        tuberculosis, contagious, obstetrics, spontaneous and therapeutic abortions, Cesarian section, sterilization, premature infants, erythroblastosis, infants delivered before admission.
    - Maximum and minimum census
    - Degree of patient illness (average by nursing unit—subjective 11-point scale)

2. *Input*

    - Sources of whole blood (commercial donor, volunteer, etc.)
    - Number of employees (full-time, part-time, temporary)
    - Terminations of employees (analysis by cause and length of employment)

3. *Structural Quality Measures*

    - Blood Bank (inventory, expirations, outdated blood, contaminations)
    - Medical Records (incomplete charts by cause and service)

- Physicians' orders counted by route of delivery (telephone, card, or in person)
- Operating room floor conductivity
- Pharmacy (orders from outside hospital, prescriptions filled by RN, unbalanced narcotic records)
- Radiology (spills of radioactive material, radiation exposure records of staff)
- Medical staff (consultations by service, publications and national annual meeting attendance, annual committee participation, annual staff meeting attendance, annual evaluation by service chief)
- Educational programs other than medical staff (hours or number of lectures for formal professional programs and for inservice education)

4. *Outcome Statistics*

- Deaths and autopsies
- Laboratory known samples (both number tested and number correctly interpreted)
- Surgical tissue analysis (including tissue interpreted by outside pathologist)
- Infections (by service and type)
- Accidents and errors
- Transfusion reactions

In addition to these statistics, reports of both a structural and procedural nature are offered for quality control of nonmedical processes such as engineering and housekeeping. In total, approximately 600 separate statistics would be calculated and reported monthly, with only moderate specificity and little opportunity for causal analysis. No standards or limits are offered, although two year-to-date totals and this-month-last-year values are reported on each statistic. The inclusion of items apparently reflecting unmet demand and need—waiting lists, admissions by urgency—is worth noting. Maximum and minimum census data reflect the interaction of resources with quality.

This proposal, which is probably the most comprehensive manual system ever reported, clearly illustrates the advantages of the quantitative approach:

1. Each of the statistics, with minor exceptions, can be accepted as a worthwhile indicator of some aspect of the medical care process
2. The manual compilation of the nonphysician-related information is spread among the department heads, who can detect unusual values subjectively
3. Much of the compilation of the physician-related statistics is the responsibility of the medical record librarian, who also is in a position to detect unusual values subjectively and report these for staff discussion
4. The administrator's office can follow all or some of the statistics and note unusual values for analysis and/or reporting to the trustees or the medical

staff. (With 600 statistics, it would seem that a practical upper limit has been reached, however)
5. The record of past performance is available for comparison with present performance. It provides a basis for planning future system changes, as well

On the other hand:

1. It is clear that many of the statistics are gross in terms of pinpointing problem areas. For example, normal tissue rates are reported in total, whereas the rates for a few specific procedures are of considerable interest. Death and autopsies are reported as numbers rather than rates. Statistics for subject areas of interest, such as perinatal care, are scattered on several pages because the report is organized for other purposes
2. Relatively few statistics are included which can be related directly to the medical care process
3. The use of statistical control limits, or in fact any consideration of the variance of the statistics, is excluded, and is probably unfeasible in view of the work involved

Despite its weaknesses, many of which could be overcome by elementary computer programs, the technique illustrates an objective form of quality control. A number of intelligent questions about quality can be answered, either routinely or by special studies which are made practical by having the data routinely and consistently available.

Other Limitations of Manual Systems

The limitations of manual systems have been repeatedly pointed out. Lembcke noted the major problems:

It was apparent as early as 1948 that the "Reports of Professional Activities," as these indexes were called, did not provide satisfactory answers. The various death rates were virtually meaningless because of variations in the proportion of different types of diseases and operations. There was no definite or constant relationship between death rates and the proportion of patients having reasonably complete records of history, physical examination, laboratory diagnosis, and consultation, the reason being that points important in some diseases were being obscured by lumping them with diseases in which such points were insignificant. Further, hospital care is undertaken only occasionally with the aim of preventing immediate death—hospital death rates rarely exceed 4 percent, regardless of the quality of care—whereas a majority of patients are being treated with such other aims as restoring function, preventing disability, or relieving pain.[8]

Myers noted that gross aggregates were unrevealing in 1954.[9] Parker evaluated a number of conventional statistics as compared to results of medical audits and as compared to each other. Significant correlations were rare, and only the size of the hospital correlated with audit scores.[10]

The Professional Activity Study: A Partially Computerized Procedural-Outcome Measurement System

Given the limitations in manual processing of statistics, and the resulting problem of aggregation and omission, there appear to be two fruitful lines of approach. One is to seek automated data-processing mechanisms in order to derive more precise statistics. The other is to pursue techniques of case-by-case analysis using professional judgment and evaluation. The two approaches are not in conflict; in fact they are highly complementary. The latter subject is not quantitative in nature, and thus lies beyond the scope of this work. The former approach historically was taken by the Professional Activity Study. The achievements of this project and of some of its recent imitators are worthy of careful review.

The work of MacEachern and others to develop statistics for routinely measuring the quality of medical care in an individual hospital was first applied to a group of hospitals by Lembcke in the Rochester Regional Hospital Council in 1946. In 1949, despite Lembcke's growing dissatisfaction with the approach, the Southwestern Michigan Hospital Council adopted the format with the financial support and encouragement of the W.K. Kellogg Foundation. Dr. Vergil N. Slee began in 1952 to experiment with punch card data collection and analysis routines. An early paper showed the improved utility of statistics if they could be kept by diagnosis and other parameters for individual physicians and hospitals. The accuracy of presurgical diagnosis of acute appendicitis was explored by age and sex, for example. This paper also introduced notions of statistical significance of deviation, which had been rare in prior literature. It was pointed out that "business machines" and nonprofessional help freed the physician from the labor of analysis.[11] The work attracted the attention of the American College of Surgeons and the American College of Physicians, as well as that of the American Hospital Association, and these organizations, together with the Southwestern Michigan Hospital Council, formed the Commission on Professional and Hospital Activities in 1955 with the continuing support of the Kellogg Foundation.

The commission has continued to work under Dr. Slee's direction using an abstract of the medical record of each hospital discharge as the basis for its data. The abstract form created by the commission, coupled with increasingly sophisticated electronic data processing routines, has demonstrated a method of overcoming the limitations of grossly aggregated indexes such as those of

MacEachern and Lembcke. Despite this achievement, the statistical properties of the system have never been fully developed. The commission holds steadfastly to the view that it does not in itself measure quality.

The mission and contributions of CPHA are not the actual appraisal of quality of care or the evaluation of the utilization of hospitals or services. The CPHA information system, PAS and MAP, is designed to assist in the improvement of quality of care rather than to measure and report on its quality. . . . PAS and MAP do provide a tool with which anyone could make some evaluation or measurement of quality. But this is a secondary use, the primary use being as information sources for the individual participating hospital. And the framework in which they best fit is the internal medical audit, which is a continuing education activity of the hospital medical staff. It is CPHA's official policy to avoid passing judgment on quality. The hospital itself may, but we don't. However, evaluation of quality is certainly legitimate, and we have designed the systems so that it will serve this as well as other purposes.[1,2]

To summarize the CPHA position, it can be said that they attempt to condense medical record information into a form which facilitates medical audit. In the process they have selected and generated a large number of individual statistics which measure aspects of the quality of medical care, but in both the statistical and the auditing presentations the judgment of quality has been left entirely to the local medical staff. Thus there are no inferences, either statistical or judgmental supplied with the reports.

The PAS Case Abstract Input Form

Figure 12-1 shows the coded case abstract which is the basic input document for all PAS and MAP analysis. The abstract is prepared by the participating hospital for each patient discharged. Abstracts are prepared by the medical record department of the hospital from information contained entirely within the medical record. The form is divided by the heavy lines into five basic categories. The top portion, containing the name of the patient and his doctor, is completed by the hospital and removed. This stub serves as a record of the preparation of the abstract. The balance is forwarded to the commission for processing.

Identifying Data. The first section of the abstract provides basic identification of the patient, including age, sex, race, dates of admission and discharge, and the coded identification of the hospital and attending physician. The patient's discharge status, including an indication of whether or not the patient was transferred to another hospital or an extended care facility, is reported. In the same question are categories of deaths, including the presence of autopsy. Provision is made for recording the number of consultations, the medical specialty or hospital service, the presence of infection and other complication,

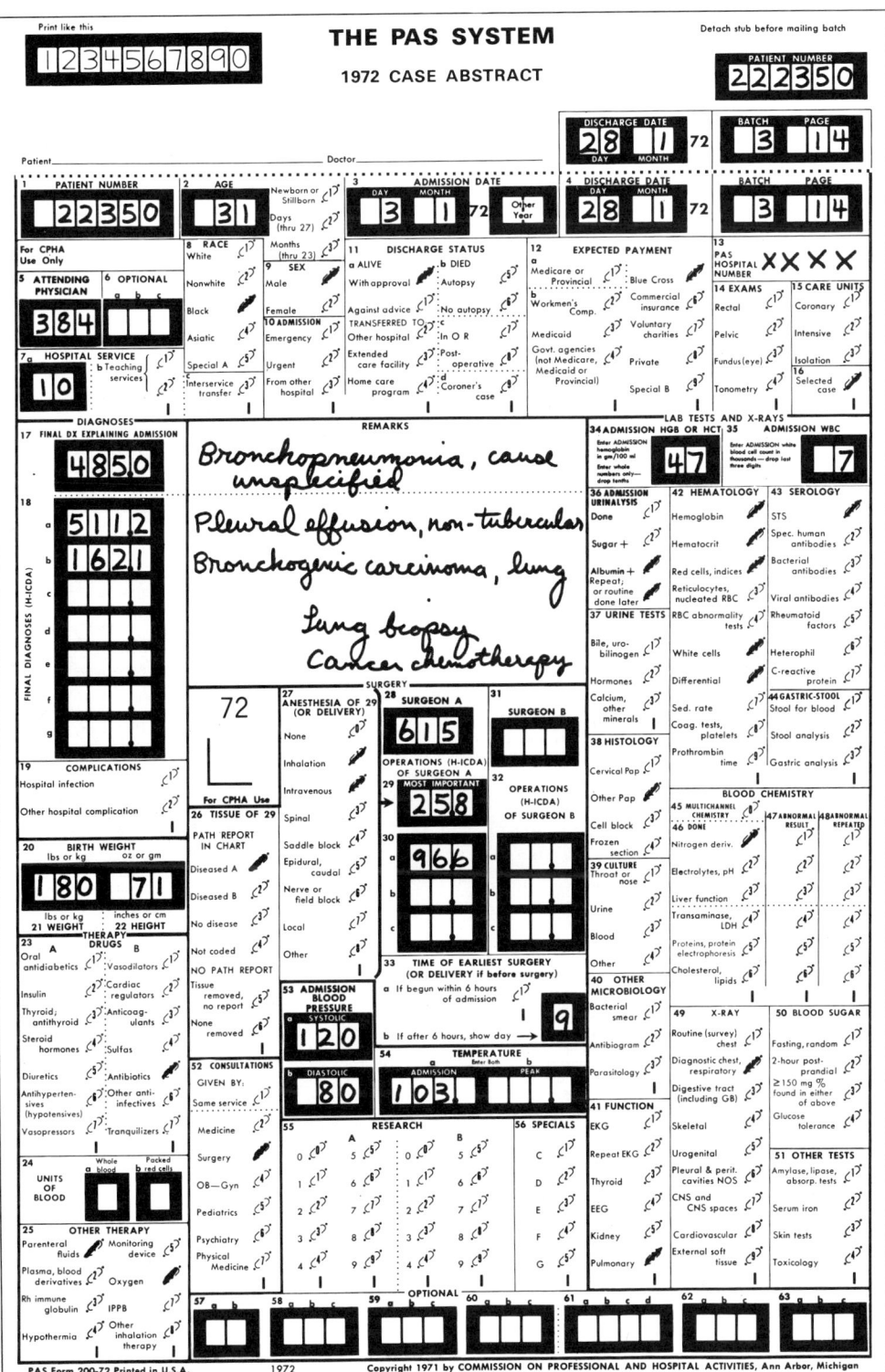

Figure 12-1. PAS 1971-72 MAP Case Abstract.

INFORMATION, INVESTIGATION, AND MANAGEMENT
RECORDED ON THE CASE ABSTRACT
FOR EACH PATIENT

PAS 1971–72 MAP
CASE ABSTRACT

The following information is recorded for every patient:

BASIC INFORMATION

Hospital
Patient } identity known only
Doctor* } to hospital
Clinical service*
Age
Sex
Race
Date of admission
Date of discharge
  (computer calculates length
  of stay, including not
  overnight)

Diagnoses (all)
  Cause of injury for
    trauma cases
  Tumor histology

Operations (all) including diagnostic
and therapeutic procedures such
as radiation therapy and psycho-
therapy
  Surgeon* (identity known
    only to hospital)
  Tissue pathology }
  Anesthesia   } for most
                      important
                      operation
  Time of earliest surgery or
  Time of delivery

Admission
  Emergency
  Urgent
  From another hospital

Complications
  Hospital infection
  Other hospital complications

Consultations from:
  Medicine
  Surgery
  OB-Gyn
  Pediatrics
  Psychiatry
  Physical Medicine

Discharged
  Alive
    With approval
    Against advice
    Transferred
      Other hospital
      Extended care facility
      Home care program

Died
  In operating room
  Postoperative
  Autopsy
  Coroner's case

Interservice Transfer

Source of payment (expected)
  Workmen's Compensation
  Medicaid
  Government agencies
  Blue Cross
  Commercial insurance
  Charities
  Private
  Special
  Medicare
  Provincial

INVESTIGATION DETAIL

Findings
  Admission (day of admission
    or the following day: pre-
    operative or pre-delivery
    for surgery or OB cases)
    Hemoglobin or hematocrit
    White blood count
    Urinalysis: positive findings
      Sugar
      Albumin
    Blood pressure
    Temperature
  Peak temperature
  Weight and height
  Birth weight for newborn

The following examinations are recorded:

Hematology
  Hemoglobin
  White cells
  Differential
  Red cells, indices
  Hematocrit
  Sedimentation rate
  Coagulation tests, platelets
  Prothrombin time
  Reticulocytes, nucleated RBC's
  Red cell abnormality
Urinalysis
  Admission only
  Repeated after second day
  Bile, urobilinogen
  Hormones
  Calcium, other minerals
Blood chemistry
  Nitrogen derivatives
  Electrolytes, pH

Liver function
  Transaminase, LDH
  Proteins, protein electro-
    phoresis
  Cholesterol, lipids
  Amylase, lipase, absorption
    tests
  Serum iron
  Sugar
    Fasting, random
    2 hour postprandial
    150 mg % found in either
      of the above
    Glucose tolerance
Screening
  Serological test for
    syphilis
  Multichannel chemistry
Serology
  Special human antibodies
  Bacterial antibodies
  Viral antibodies
  C-reactive protein
  Heterophile
  Rheumatoid factors
Microbiology
  Bacterial smear
  Culture (blood, throat,
    urine, other)
  Antibiogram
  Parasitology
Histology
  Cervical Papanicolaou
  Other Papanicolaou
  Frozen section
  Cell block
Gastric-Stool
  Gastric analysis
  Stool for blood
  Stool analysis
Radiology
  Chest, respiratory
  Skeletal
  Digestive tract (includ-
    ing GB)
  Urogenital
  Pleural and peritoneal
    cavities
  CNS and CNS spaces
  Cardiovascular
  External soft tissue

Function tests
  EKG (initial and repeat)
  EEG
  Kidney
  Pulmonary
  Thyroid
Other tests
  Skin tests
  Toxicology
Physical examination including
  Rectal
  Pelvic
  Funduscopic
  Tonometry

MANAGEMENT DETAIL

Drugs
  Oral antidiabetics
  Insulin
  Thyroid, antithyroid
  Steroid hormones
  Diuretics
  Antihypertensives
  Vasopressors
  Vasodilators
  Cardiac regulators
  Anticoagulants
  Sulfas
  Antibiotics
  Other anti-infectives
  Tranquilizers
Other therapy
  Parenteral fluids
  Blood
    Whole blood
    Packed red cells
    Plasma, blood derivatives
  Oxygen
  IPPB
  Other inhalation therapy
  Isolation
  Monitoring device
  Rh immune globulin
  Hypothermia
Care in special units
  Intensive care
  Cardiac care

Space is provided on the case abstract to allow incorporation of many items of special information. Residence of the patient, accommodation within the hospital, special therapy, selected laboratory findings, specific drugs, are just a few of the possible ways these optional items may be used. The hospital may initiate, change, or discontinue use of an optional item, upon arrangement with the Commission. As an extra-charge option, the abstract provides room for entering referring and consulting physicians, who will receive indexes of their cases every six months.

* A hospital may structure the codes for attending physician, surgeon, and hospital service to meet its particular requirements. This includes designation of teaching cases.

Figure 12-1. PAS 1971-72 MAP Case Abstract, (Continued).

and whether or not the patient was on an urgent or emergency basis. The major source of payment for the patient, as expected at the time of admission can be indicated. (This is frequently different from the actual source or sources, and thus of limited use in demand analysis. PAS feels that the anticipated source influences medical judgment more than the actual.)[13] There is also provision for various other identifications which may be assigned by the hospital.

Diagnosis and Surgical or Obstetrical Treatment. Provision is made for recording up to eight individual final diagnoses, coded according to the International Classification of Diseases. Space is provided for writing the name of the disease, and CPHA will provide coding assistance if necessary. Additional codes are available for classification of tumors or of analysis of external cause of injury. Identifying data are provided for up to seven surgical procedures with identification of the most important surgery. If subsequent surgery is done by a second surgeon, he may be identified. A supplementary data form permits additional diagnoses, surgical procedures, and surgeons without limit. The time of the first surgery can be indicated as well as the type of anesthesia and the tissue report of the most important surgery. (These need not be the same.) In the case of obstetrical patients the surgical section can be related to delivery, and provision is made for the birth weight of the infant on the newborn's case abstract. A separate abstract is prepared for the newborn.

Investigation. This section provides for the recording of selected pieces of information covering the patient's condition and the diagnostic workup. Generally speaking, the abstract includes a record of the presence of a test at some point during the patient's stay but does not include either the test result or the number of times it was performed. Exceptions to this are in the admission data which record quantitative scores for hemoglobin or hematocrit, white blood count, the presence of sugar and albumen in the urine, the systolic and diastolic blood pressure and the temperature in whole degrees. It is also possible to indicate a finding of 150 milligrams percent blood sugar at anytime during the stay, and it is possible to show the maximum temperature recorded for the patient.

Nonsurgical Management. The administration of blood, the use of a number of specific drug therapy routines, and the use of a number of other therapeutic devices or services can be shown, including showing the use of various specialized care units in the progressive patient care format. With the exception of blood, only the presence of a given therapeutic activity can be shown and not the frequency or quantity.

Additional Information. Several fields are left for inputting additional coded information for research or special studies designed by the hospital. These permit the addition of any data which can be coded. Zip codes, charges, consulting doctors, and other items are entered here by participating hospitals.

Commentary. An abstract must, by definition, select from the total available information. The PAS format presents one possibility of this kind which has been proven to be both practical and rewarding. The constraints under which it has been designed are that: (a) it is applicable to any discharge from an acute hospital in the United States or Canada regardless of geographic location or the nature of the patient's illness and treatment; (b) it can be prepared from information available in the medical record by clerical personnel who have had limited specialized training for this purpose; and (c) a relatively short amount of time (estimated by CPHA as two to five minutes) is necessary to prepare an individual abstract.

A number of possible expansions or revisions of the abstract form have been suggested. It would clearly be desirable to obtain quantitative information on diagnostic and treatment services, but collecting such information from the medical record would vastly increase the amount of time necessary to prepare the abstract and is probably beyond the capabilities of an abstracting process. It has been suggested that the abstract form be specialized by service.[14] Large sections of the form are irrelevant to the care of certain kinds of patients. For example, approximately half of the patients admitted to the hospital do not undergo surgery. The space devoted to surgery on the abstract form is lost on these patients. It could be devoted to specific information such as the Apgar score of newborn infants or data on prenatal care which would be of interest to obstetrical and pediatric services. Information on the findings of history and physical examination and laboratory workup which is important to assessing the quality of care in internal medicine is lacking, while at the same time a review of diagnostic tests used is probably more extensive than would be appropriate for common uncomplicated surgical diagnoses such as appendectomy and tonsilectomy. A number of additional items would be of value in studying the continuity of patient care including information on readmission rates, whether or not the admission was from another institution or agency, and identification of the referring agency or the agency to which the patient was referred.[15] Many of these problems can be handled by careful use of the optional fields.

PAS has responded to this problem in part, creating a supplementary (not a substitute) input device for the study of perinatal care. This is shown in figure 12-2. Its use and analysis are available to the Medical Audit Program users, but not to the basic PAS plan. Dr. Slee cites two problems with varying the basic input device: (a) it increases cost of training, programming, and other activities, (b) there are many ambiguous cases, such as the diabetic patient with a surgical problem.[16]

The PAS form is subject to regular review, usually every three years. The cost of inputting information, both from the record to the form and from form to

USE DARK PENCIL ONLY **1972 BIRTH ABSTRACT**

PAS PERINATAL STUDY

COMPLETE FOR ALL NEWBORN AND STILLBORN

(H-ICDA code for final diagnosis explaining admission in range Y20.0–Y32.3)
Also complete as much as possible for newborn admitted after birth

Doctor B. Smith

Detach stub before mailing batch

BABY'S PATIENT NUMBER: 1859

Patient Jones, Robert

BABY'S DISCHARGE DATE — Day 20 Month 9 — 1972

Batch 1 Page 1

1972

Batch 1 Page 1

1 BABY'S PATIENT NUMBER: 1859

2 BIRTH ABSTRACT: B

3 BABY'S ADMISSION DATE — Day 10 Month 9 Year 2

4 BABY'S DISCHARGE DATE — Day 20 Month 9 Year 2

5 PAS HOSPITAL NUMBER: XXXX

6 RESUSCITATION
0 ✓ None
1 ○ Under 5 min.
2 ○ 5-14 min.
3 ○ 15 min. or more

7 INCUBATOR
a Time:
4 ○ Under 8 hrs.
5 ○ 8 – 23 hrs.
6 ○ 24 – 47 hrs.
7 ○ 2 – 6 days
8 ○ 7 days or more
b If O_2 given, highest concentration:
9 ○ was over 40%

8 TOTAL APGAR SCORE
a At 1 minute: 10
b At 5 minutes: 10

9 MAXIMUM BILIRUBIN
Enter whole numbers only–drop tenths

10 ADMISSION TEMPERATURE
0 ○ Not recorded
1 ○ 95.9 F or less (under 35.5 C)
2 ○ 96 (35.5 - .9)
3 ✓ 97 (36.0 - .4)
4 ○ 98 + (36.5 +)

11 PKU TESTING
5 ○ Not done
6 ○ Phenistix (urine)
7 ✓ Blood test
8 ○ Positive result on 6 or 7

12 CHROMOSOMES
9 ○ Karyotype done

13 BABY'S BLOOD TYPE
0 ○ O +
1 ○ A +
2 ○ B +
3 ○ AB +
4 ○ O –
5 ○ A –
6 ○ B –
7 ○ AB –
Not grouped 8 ○ Rh +
9 ○ Rh –

14 EYE CARE
0 ✓ AgNO3
1 ○ Penicillin
2 ○ Other

15 MISCELLANEOUS
3 ○ Fetus died BEFORE admission of mother
4 ○ 1st
5 ○ 2nd } Birth sequence for multiple births
6 ○ 3rd
7 ✓ Vitamin K given baby
8 ○ Baby rooming in with mother
9 ○ Baby kept beyond normal discharge date for nonmedical reasons

16 TIME OF PERINATAL DEATH (for liveborn)
1 ○ Under 1 hr.
2 ○ 1-6 hrs.
3 ○ 7-12 hrs.
4 ○ 13-24 hrs.
5 ○ Over 24 hrs.

S

MOTHER

17 MOTHER'S PATIENT NUMBER
○ Infant born elsewhere, mother NOT admitted
1796

18 MOTHER'S DISCHARGE DATE — Day 16 Month 9 Year 2

19 GRAVIDITY (total pregnancies including this one): 3

20 PARITY (number of liveborn and stillborn including this pregnancy): 3

21 NUMBER OF PREGNANCIES WITH MULTIPLE BIRTHS (including this pregnancy)

22 NUMBER OF FETAL AND NEONATAL DEATHS (including this pregnancy)
a Abortion
b Stillborn
c Neonatal death

23 NUMBER OF CESAREAN SECTIONS (including this pregnancy)

24 MOTHER'S BLOOD TYPE
0 ○ O +
1 ○ A +
2 ○ B +
3 ○ AB +
4 ○ O –
5 ○ A –
6 ○ B –
7 ○ AB –
Not grouped 8 ○ Rh +
9 ○ Rh –

25a WEIGHT GAIN DURING THIS PREGNANCY lbs or kg: 17
– – – OR – – –
25b WEIGHT LOSS DURING THIS PREGNANCY lbs or kg: —

26 DATE OF LAST MENSTRUAL PERIOD
Day Month Year
– – – OR – – –
WEEKS OF GESTATION: 36

MATERNAL HISTORY

27
a PRIOR to this pregnancy:
0 ○ Venereal disease
1 ○ Venous thrombosis
2 ○ Urinary tract disease
3 ○ Toxemia
b INCLUDING this pregnancy:
4 ○ Convulsions
5 ○ Hypertension
6 ○ Heart disease
7 ○ Iso-immunization
8 ○ Diabetes
9 ○ Birth weight ≥ 10 pounds

28
DURING this pregnancy:
0 ○ Venereal disease
1 ○ Venous thrombosis
2 ○ Urinary tract disease
3 ○ Toxemia
4 ○ Anemia
5 ○ Immunizations given
6 ○ Tranquilizers given
7 ○ Gastroenteritis
8 ○ Rubella during first trimester
9 ○ Other febrile infections

29 PRENATAL CARE
0 ○ None
a GIVEN by:
1 ○ Hospital clinic
2 ○ Other clinic
3 ✓ Private physician
b MONTH of pregnancy in which care began:
4 ✓ 1st – 3rd
5 ○ 4th – 5th
6 ○ 6th
7 ○ 7th
8 ○ 8th
9 ○ 9th

30 NUMBER OF PRENATAL VISITS: 12

31 ANALGESICS DURING LABOR
0 ○ None
1 ✓ Narcotics
2 ○ Barbiturates
3 ✓ Tranquilizers
4 ✓ Antihistamines
5 ○ Inhalants
6 ○ Hypnosis
7 ○ "Natural childbirth"
8 ○ Other

32 LABOR
0 ○ Spontaneous
1 ✓ Induced
a METHOD of induction:
2 ○ Oxytocics
3 ✓ Other medicinal
4 ○ Artificial rupture of membranes
b METHOD of stimulation:
5 ○ Oxytocics
6 ○ Other medicinal
7 ○ Artificial rupture of membranes

33 HOURS BETWEEN RUPTURE OF MEMBRANES AND DELIVERY
1 ✓ Less than 1 hr.
2 ○ 1–7 hrs.
3 ○ 8–23 hrs.
4 ○ 24–47 hrs.
5 ○ 48 hrs. or more
6 ○ Unknown

34 LENGTH OF LABOR
a First stage (hours): 2
b Second stage (minutes): 20

REMARKS:

RESERVED FOR CPHA USE

CPHA 201-11-71 Printed in U.S.A.

Figure 12-2. 1971 Birth Abstract.

computer, is felt by CPHA to be a major current limitation. The second step may be overcome by moving to visual scanning or other direct-to-tape input device. The first step is more serious. Specialized supplements have been developed from time to time. Other than the Birth Abstract, these have not been popular, and none is currently available. Recent increases in the amount of information, such as items 47 and 49 of the 1970 form have brought protests from some participating hospitals.[1,7]

Processing of Information by CPHA

Case abstracts are forwarded to the offices of CPHA in batches of 100 until all discharges for a given month have been submitted. Once received by the commission, the information on the abstracts is key-punched and permanently stored on magnetic tape. Key punch operators are trained by the commission to detect certain minor errors in abstract form, and these are returned to the hospital for correction. In addition the commission has trained personnel on its staff who check input forms from hospitals beginning to use the services. Case abstracts are checked until such time as the error rate as detected by audit falls below 2 percent. These personnel, who have extensive familiarity with the information on the abstract sheets, are able to detect logical inconsistencies and coding errors. During the initial months of PAS membership, hospitals routinely enter all diagnoses in longhand as well as in ICDA code so that the coding may be checked by the commission. Extensive editing routines are built into the computer processing to detect mechanical errors and omissions. Sex and diagnosis, age and diagnosis, and several other comparisons are made automatically. The inspection and error detection routines, together with educational services which the commission offers to librarians, administrators and medical staff members of participating hospitals, are an important and often overlooked aspect of their activities. They provide assurance of at least minimum reliability of the information abstracted. Without this assurance, the output of the system would be valueless.

Computer processing of the information is generally of minimal complexity and limited to the preparation of specific totals and proportions. The data for each participating hospital are processed monthly and are accumulated and reprocessed for the half year. It is not possible to obtain sequential time series data (i.e., continuing values for a given statistic over several months or years) from the electronic operations. Computer data files are not kept chronologically for hospitals. Special requests can be made for analyses of means, medians, variances and frequency distributions which can be constructed within the data available for a given time period.

The limitations upon manipulation of the information may be the biggest drawback to the PAS system. Member hospitals are not offered the opportunity to alter the output except to obtain certain groupings of diagnosis or service. There is no possibility of data reduction through quality control techniques such as those described in chapter 10. The information is not kept in chronological order, except within relatively short periods. Since the CPHA deliberately avoids any judgment of quality, neither statistical nor judgmental indicators are used to isolate problem areas by mechanical means. No matter how flagrant the deviation, there is almost no error signal generation in PAS-MAP, either for individual cases or sample values. (The length-of-stay package, discussed below, is a striking exception to these statements. The output also "flags" cases lacking minimal admission laboratory work.)

Technical problems reduce the usefulness of the system in other ways. The six-month accumulation means that long-term and cyclic demand analyses described in chapter 3 are not directly available. The system is case-oriented, not patient-oriented, and does not lend itself to analysis of care of given individuals over a long time span.

Reports

The basic notion of PAS-MAP is a two-fold output, consisting of condensed tabulations of individual outputs on the one hand, and statistical summaries on the other. The individual case tabulations are listed on the C form (figure 12-3) and contain all the information on the case abstract in a highly coded form. They are in essence, organized printouts of the input data bank. The C forms are organized in various ways to permit systematic case review. Under the basic PAS plan they are compiled monthly by primary diagnosis and most important operation. Additional lists are prepared in order of patient number and of all deaths. Semiannually the lists are recompiled, cumulated and cross-tabulated by secondary and subsequent diagnoses and surgery to form the basic disease and surgical indexes required for medical records libraries. Under the MAP plan, additional lists are compiled quarterly by major service, covering patients included in the categories of the appropriate MAP report. The purpose of the C form lists is primarily to provide a single-case identification mechanism to supplement the statistical forms. Anomalies of care or points of interest are to be detected by subjective review of the statistical forms described below. The appropriate column of the C form can be scanned to pick out cases of interest, and they can be studied briefly from the abstract or identified for detailed review of the complete history. Alternatively, the C reports can be scanned without reference to the statistics to pick out cases of interest.

The data are used to calculate two basic statistical tabulations, the A form, which organizes discharges by medical specialty or service, and the B form which organizes discharges by forty-four categories of primary diagnosis. The two statistical tabulations are also supplied on a six-month basis, and the A form is

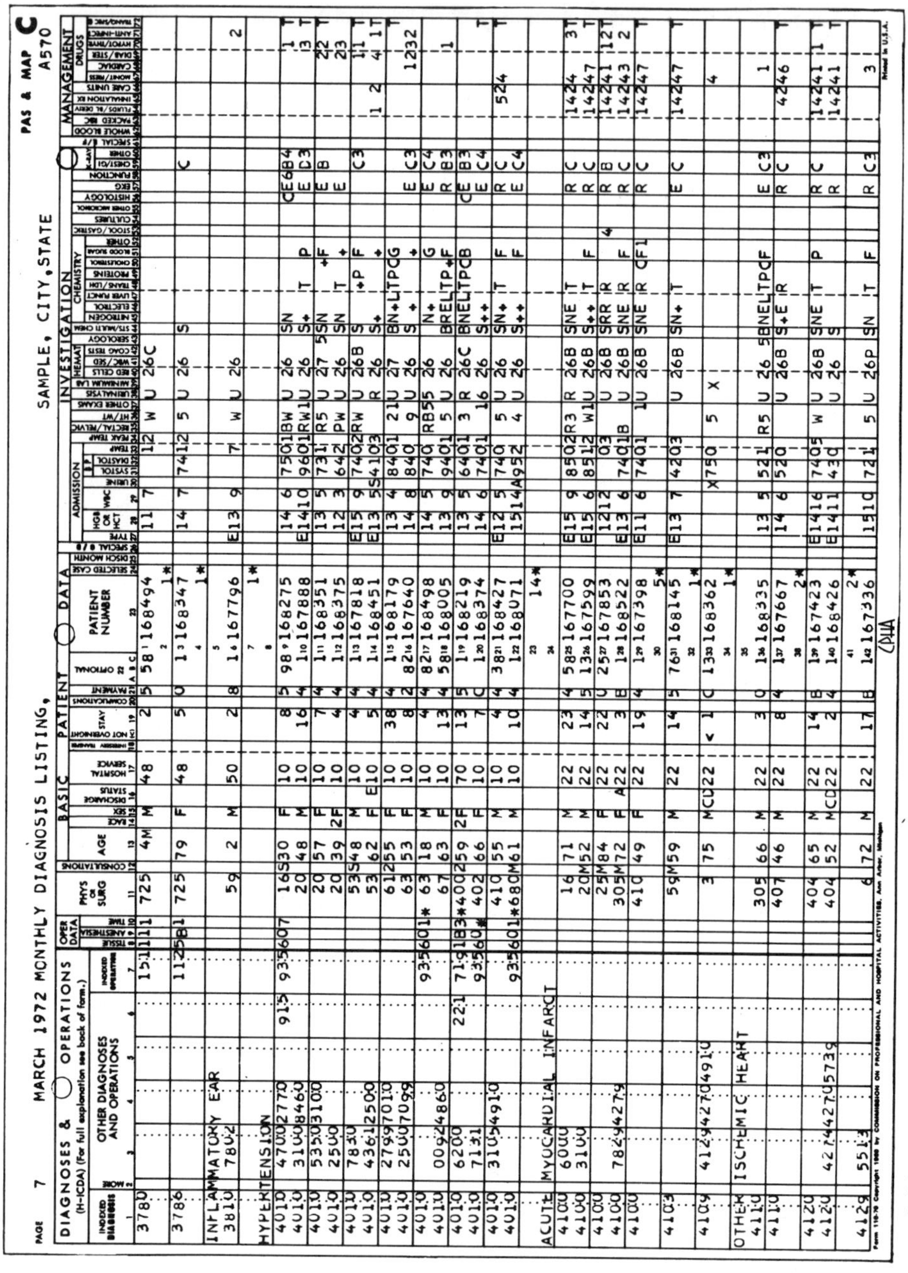

C FORM – CASE ABSTRACT LISTING (Front Side)

Used for PAS Monthly Listings and Semiannual Indexes, PAS-MAP Quarterly Reports, Length of Stay Package Quarterly Reports

Figure 12–3. Specimen Monthly Diagnosis Listing.

PAS — MAP

Each line on this form presents one patient's case abstract. Reports using this form, together with the sequence of patients for each, are listed in the tables below

Report				Primary Sequence	Secondary Sequence
PAS	Monthly	Diagnosis	Listings	final diagnosis explaining admission (col. 1)	physician (col. 11)
		Operation		most important operation (col. 7)	surgeon (col. 11)
		Death		final diagnosis explaining admission (col. 1)	physician (col. 11)
		Patient		patient number (col. 23)	
	Semiannual	Diagnosis	Indexes	diagnosis (col. 1)	physician (col. 11)
		Operation		operation (col. 7)	surgeon (col. 11)
		Physician		diagnosis (col. 1)	
		Surgeon		operation (col. 7)	

Report			Primary Sequence	Secondary Sequence
PAS–MAP Listings (Quarterly)	for all patients	PEDIATRIC MEDICINE	final diagnosis explaining admission (col. 1)	physician (col. 11)
		MEDICINE	final diagnosis explaining admission (col. 1)	physician (col. 11)
		SURGERY (BY DIAGNOSIS)	final diagnosis explaining admission (col. 1)	physician (col. 11)
		OBSTETRICS (BY DIAGNOSIS)	final diagnosis explaining admission (col. 1)	physician (col. 11)
		NEWBORN	standard AMA birth weight group (see col. 3)	final diagnosis explaining admission (col. 1)
	for all operated patients	CHILDREN (BY OPERATION)	most important operation (col. 7)	surgeon (col. 11)
		ADULTS (BY OPERATION)	most important operation (col. 7)	surgeon (col. 11)
		OBSTETRICS (BY OPERATION)	most important operation (col. 7)	surgeon (col. 11)

1. INDEXED DIAGNOSIS

Diagnoses are coded by *Hospital Adaptation of ICDA* (H-ICDA, CPHA, 1968).

In listings by Dx and physician, cases are in sequence by Dx in this column. This Dx is the **final Dx explaining admission** ("primary" Dx), except when the prefix ⌶ appears. For a cross-indexed entry, ⌶ indicates the Dx as secondary and P in col. 3 designates the primary Dx.

Explanations for the letters T and E appear under "3-6. OTHER DIAGNOSES AND OPERATIONS."

2. MORE

The symbol # prints in this column whenever the patient had more secondary diagnoses or operations than can be printed on one line. For such patients, all diagnoses and operations appear at the end of the Monthly Diagnosis and Operation Listings and quarterly PAS–MAP listings.

3-6. OTHER DIAGNOSES AND OPERATIONS

Diagnoses in addition to the one indexed in col. 1 and operations in addition to the one indexed in col. 7 appear in columns 3-6. (Dx codes contain 4 digits and thus are distinguished from the 3-digit operation codes.) If there are more diagnoses or operations than can be printed in these columns, the symbol # will appear in col. 2.

The letter P preceding a code in col. 3 or 6 indicates a "primary" diagnosis or operation.

Birth weights print in col. 3 for newborn, stillborn, and babies 1-7 days old on admission. Birth weights are distinguished from other codes by G which indicates grams (2750G) or by the slash (/) which separates pounds and ounces (5/11 = 5 lbs. 11 oz.).

External Cause of Injury Codes. An E prefixes an External Cause of Injury code. The E code relates to the immediately preceding Dx code (800.0 – 999.9).

Tumor Morphology Codes. A T prefixes a tumor morphology code from SNOP (*Systematized Nomenclature of Pathology*, College of American Pathologists, 1965). T codes appear only in semiannual reports.

7. INDEXED OPERATION

In listings by operation and surgeon, cases are in sequence by operation in this column. This operation is the **most important operation** ("primary" operation), except when the prefix ⌶ appears. For a cross-indexed entry, ⌶ indicates the operation as secondary and P in col. 6 designates the primary operation. An S in column 7 indicates a spontaneous delivery.

On PAS–MAP quarterly listings, the prefix "+" means that the patient is not counted as operated (see back of M form) and is excluded from the accompanying M form table. When such a patient has a spontaneous delivery S appears.

8. TISSUE for most important operation

Pathology report in chart
1. Diseased A
2. Diseased B
3. No disease
4. Not coded by pathologist

No pathology report
5. Tissue removed, no report
6. No tissue removed

Codes 1, 2 and 3 are assigned by the pathologist. "Diseased A" is tissue disease which generally requires surgical removal. "Diseased B" is tissue disease where surgical removal is not clearly indicated from the pathological findings alone.

This tissue code is printed only when the most important operation appears in col. 7. When secondary operations are cross indexed this column is blank. 23

9. ANESTHESIA for most important operation (or delivery)

0 None
1 Inhalation alone
2 Intravenous alone
3 Spinal alone
4 Saddle block alone
5 Epidural or caudal alone
6 Nerve or field block alone
7 Local alone
8 "Other" alone
B Inhalation and IV
G Inhalation and any other except IV
V IV and any other except inhalation
S Spinal and any other except IV or inhalation
R Any combination of codes 4-8

The anesthesia code is printed only when the most important operation appears in column 7. When secondary operations are cross indexed this column is blank. 22

10. TIME OF EARLIEST SURGERY OR TIME OF DELIVERY

The symbol # shows that the earliest operation began or delivery occurred within six hours of the patient's admission. If more than six hours elapsed, the day is indicated (0 = day of admission, 1 = next day, ... 9 = 9 or more days). 21

11. PHYSICIAN OR SURGEON

Code numbers are assigned by the hospital; names are known only to the hospital. On Dx and patient listings the attending physician's number appears. On operation listings the operating surgeon's number appears.

An asterisk (*) at the left of col. 11 indicates that the attending physician and the operating surgeon are two different people. On the physician and surgeon indexes the only numbers printed are of surgeons (or attending physicians) other than the indexed doctor. 2, 24, 27

12. CONSULTATIONS from

⌶ Same as responsible service (coded in col. 17)
M Internal Medicine
S Surgery
G OB Gyn
C Pediatrics
P Psychiatry
R Physical Medicine

The **number** of consulting services prints when there are consultations from more than one service. 14

13. AGE ON ADMISSION

Numbers represent **years** of **age** unless indicated as follows:

D. Days
M. Months
NB. Newborn
SB. Stillborn 3

14. RACE

Blank. White or not recorded
1. Nonwhite
2. Black
3. Asiatic
4. Special A (see MRL) 9

15. SEX

M. Male
F. Female
Blank. Not recorded 4

16. DISCHARGE STATUS

Discharged alive:
Blank. With approval
X. Against advice
T. Transferred to other hospital
E. Transferred to extended care facility
H. Transferred to home care program

Died:
A. Autopsy
D. No autopsy

*The following letters precede death code A or D where appropriate:

P. Postoperative death
O. Died in OR
C. Coroner's case 8

17. HOSPITAL SERVICE

2. Pediatric Medicine
10. General Medicine
22. Cardiology
38. Psychiatry
40. General Surgery
48. Ophthalmology
50. ENT
54. Dental
58. Orthopedics
62. Urology
70. Gynecology
74. Obstetrics
or {75. Abortion; 76. OB–Not Delivered; 77. OB–Delivered}
80. Newborn
89. Stillborn 13a

Letters following the numerical code designate the teaching status of the case:

W. Ward
T. Teaching
Blank. Private

For the meaning of any other codes, see MRL. 13b

18. INTERSERVICE TRANSFER

The symbol ⌶ prints in this column when the patient was transferred from one service to another within the hospital. 13c

19. STAY in days

< 1 = Not overnight
Y = Stay to the nearest year (for 1,000 days or more)
??? = Length of stay is not computable 5, 6

20. COMPLICATIONS

I. Hospital infection
C. Other hospital complication
B. Both 12

21. PAYMENT

Blank. Not recorded
0. U.S. Medicare or Canadian Provincial only

Letters in parentheses designate payment supplementing Medicare or Provincial.

1 (W) Workmen's compensation
2 (M) Medicaid
3 (G) Government agencies
4 (B) Blue Cross
5 (C) Commercial insurance
6 (V) Voluntary charities
7 (S) Special B (see MRL)
8 (P) Private 10

22. OPTIONAL (see MRL) 15

23. PATIENT NUMBER

Number assigned by hospital; names are known only to hospital. Asterisks indicate patient number was not recorded. 1

24. SELECTED CASE

X. Selected case (see MRL)
* Flags total count following each group of patients. 55

25. DISCHARGE MONTH

The first nine months are numbered, and the months of October, November, and December are O, N, and D. This column is blank on monthly listings. 6

26. SPECIAL C, D (see MRL)

C. Special C
D. Special D
B. Both 39

***27. TYPE OF ADMISSION**

E. Emergency } defined by
U. Urgent } hospital
T. Transferred from other hospital 11

‡28. ADMISSION HEMOGLOBIN OR HEMATOCRIT

The hospital elects one procedure to record for all patients. The admission hemoglobin is in grams per 100 ml, disregarding tenths. Hematocrit appears as percent. 29

‡29. ADMISSION WHITE BLOOD COUNT

The admission total white blood cell count is given in thousands. 30

‡30. ADMISSION URINE

X. No admission urinalysis
Blank. Negative findings
A. Albumin positive
S. Sugar positive
B. Both 31

‡31-32. ADMISSION BLOOD PRESSURE

The systolic blood pressure on admission appears in column 31 and the diastolic in column 32 according to the following codes:

9. 220 or over
8. 190–219
7. 160–189
6. 140–159
5. 120–139
4. 100–119
3. 90–99
2. 80–89
1. 50–79
0. 49 or less 42

‡33. ADMISSION TEMPERATURE

Code indicates degrees F (or 1/2 degrees C) of elevation above normal oral temperature.

X. Admission temperature not taken
0. 98.9 F or less (under 37.0 C)
1. 99.0–99.9 (37.0–.4)
2. 100.0–100.9 (37.5–.9)
3. 101.0–101.9 (38.0–.4)
4. 102.0–102.9 (38.5–.9)
5. 103.0–103.9 (39.0–.4)
6. 104.0–104.9 (39.5–.9)
7. 105.0 or more (40.0+) 43

34. PEAK TEMPERATURE

The same codes as used in col. 33 print here to show the highest temperature recorded for the patient. When the admission temperature (col. 33) was the highest recorded temperature, column 34 is blank. 43

35. RECTAL AND PELVIC EXAMINATIONS

R. Rectal
P. Pelvic
B. Both 33

36. HEIGHT, WEIGHT

H. Height recorded
W. Weight recorded
B. Both (if age under 20)

Index for patients 20 and older, based on U.S. adult median weight for sex and height:

1. Weight under 65% of U.S. median
2. 65–74%
3. 75–84%
4. 85–94%
5. 95–107%
6. 108–122%
7. 123–137%
8. 138–152%
9. Over 152% 18, 19, 20

37. OTHER EXAMINATIONS

1. Funduscopic
2. Tonometry
4. Skin tests
3, 5, 6, 7 = combinations (sum of codes) 33, 54

***38. URINALYSIS**

Blank. No urinalysis
U. Admission urinalysis only ‡
R. Repeat or routine done after admission
4. Bile, urobilinogen
5. Hormones
6. Calcium, minerals 31

39. MINIMUM LAB

Blank. Urinalysis plus Hgb or Hct at any time
X. Lab work not done
Not applicable for newborn 29, 31, 35

***40. HEMATOLOGY–RED CELLS**

1. Hemoglobin
2. Hematocrit
3. Red blood cells, indices
4. Reticulocytes, nucleated RBCs
5. Red cell abnormality
C. CBC = Hgb + RBC + WBC + differential 35

41. HEMATOLOGY–WHITE CELLS AND SEDIMENTATION RATE

1. Sedimentation rate
2. Total white blood cell count
4. Differential white blood cell count
3, 5, 6, 7 = combinations (sum of codes) 35

42. HEMATOLOGY–COAGULATION TESTS

P. Prothrombin time
C. Other coagulation tests
B. Both 35

***43. SEROLOGY**

Excludes serological test for syphilis (see column 44)

3. Special human antibodies
4. Bacterial antibodies
5. Rheumatoid factors
6. Heterophil
7. C reactive protein
8. Viral antibodies 52

44. STS AND MULTICHANNEL CHEMISTRY

S. Serological test for syphilis
M. Multichannel chemistry
B. Both 32

45-50. BLOOD CHEMISTRY tests done

N. NITROGEN DERIVATIVES 45
E. ELECTROLYTES, pH 45
L. LIVER FUNCTION 45
T. TRANSAMINASE LDH 45
P. PROTEINS, PROTEIN ELECTROPHORESIS 45
C. CHOLESTEROL, LIPIDS 45

In these columns a + sign denotes an abnormal result and R means the abnormal test was repeated. 47, 49

***51. BLOOD SUGAR**

F. Fasting, random
P. 2-hour postprandial
B. Both F and P
+ ≥ 150 mg% found in either of above
G. Glucose tolerance test done 46

52. OTHER BLOOD CHEMISTRY

1. Amylase, lipase, absorption tests
2. Serum iron
4. Toxicology
3, 5, 6, 7 • combinations (sum of codes) 54

53. STOOL AND GASTRIC EXAMINATIONS

1. Gastric analysis
2. Stool analysis
4. Stool for blood
3, 5, 6, 7 = combinations (sum of codes) 51

***54. CULTURE**

T. Throat or nose
U. Urine
H. Blood
C. Other 48

55. OTHER MICROBIOLOGY

1. Bacterial smear
2. Antibiogram
4. Parasitology
3, 5, 6, 7 = combinations (sum of codes) 50

***56. HISTOLOGY**

C. Cervical Papanicolaou
P. Other Papanicolaou
2. Cell block
F. Frozen section 53

57. EKG

E. Done
R. Repeated 34

***58. FUNCTION**

6. Thyroid
7. EEG
8. Kidney
9. Pulmonary 34

***59. X-RAY: CHEST, G.I.**

R. Routine (survey) chest
C. Diagnostic chest, respiratory
D. Digestive tract, gallbladder
B. Both C and D 44

***60. X-RAY: SKELETAL, OTHER**

3. Skeletal
4. Urogenital
5. Pleural & peritoneal cavities NOS
6. CNS & CNS spaces
7. Cardiovascular
8. External soft tissue 44

61. SPECIAL E, F (see MRL)

E. Special E
F. Special F
B. Both 39

62. WHOLE BLOOD

The number of whole blood transfusions, 500 ml each or less. 9 = 9 or more. 36a

63. PACKED RED BLOOD CELLS

The number of packed red blood cell transfusions. 9 = 9 or more. 36b

64. FLUIDS, PLASMA

1. Parenteral fluids
2. Plasma, blood derivatives
4. Rh immune globulin
3, 5, 6, 7 = combinations (sum of codes) 40

65. INHALATION THERAPY

1. IPPB
2. Other inhalation therapy
4. Oxygen
3, 5, 6, 7 = combinations (sum of codes) 40

66. CARE UNITS

1. Intensive care unit
2. Cardiac (coronary) care unit
4. Isolation
3, 5, 6, 7 = combinations (sum of codes) 39, 40

67. MONITOR/PRESSOR

1. Hypothermia
2. Vasopressors
4. Monitoring device
3, 5, 6, 7 = combinations (sum of codes) 37, 40

68. CARDIAC DRUGS

1. Cardiac regulating drugs
2. Anticoagulants
4. Vasodilators
3, 5, 6, 7 = combinations (sum of codes) 37

69. ANTIDIABETICS/STEROIDS

1. Steroids
2. Oral antidiabetics
4. Insulin
3, 5, 6, 7 = combinations (sum of codes) 37

70. HYPOTENSIVES/THYROID DP.UGS

1. Diuretics
2. Hypotensives (antihypertensives)
4. Thyroid/antithyroid
3, 5, 6, 7 = combinations (sum of codes) 37

71. ANTI-INFECTIVES

1. Sulfas
2. Antibiotics
4. Other anti-infectives
3, 5, 6, 7 = combinations (sum of codes) 38

72. TRANQUILIZERS, SPECIAL G

T. Tranquilizers
G. Special G (see MRL)
B. Both 38, 40

• **ASTERISKED ITEMS:** When more than one of the items listed for a column has been marked on a PAS Case Abstract, the applicable code nearest the bottom of the list is printed for that patient.

‡ **ADMISSION, PREOPERATIVE, PREDELIVERY FINDINGS:** Each finding is from the first test of its kind done during the ADMISSION PERIOD, which begins with the patient's admission to the hospital and ends at 11:59 p.m. of the following day, at the time of earliest surgery, or at the time of delivery, whichever comes first.

Note: On the monthly **PATIENT LISTING** only, the content of columns 26-72 is changed:

a. Hospital options from PAS Case Abstract items 57-63 print in columns 26-50.
b. The admission and discharge days and dates print in columns 52-72.
c. DUP prints in col. 23 for duplicated patient numbers or readmissions instead of a repeat of the preceding patient number.
d. No supplementary listing (see explanation for col. 2) is printed at the end of the Patient Listing or Death Listing.

Note: The **SHADED AREA** following each column's explanation shows the PAS Case Abstract item numbers for reference.

C FORM – CASE ABSTRACT LISTING (Reverse Side)

Figure 12-3. Specimen Monthly Diagnosis Listing, (Continued).

recomputed to show certain data as percentage rates and averages for a six-month interval.

Two tabulations are aimed specifically at information relating to the utilization of inpatient hospital care. The first, the D form, provides mean length of stay for each of several age categories by individual primary diagnosis and by groups of primary diagnosis and also for individual operations and groups of operations. In 1966 the Commission added a fifth set of reports, available as an extra cost option, called "The Length of Stay Package." These are reported on form S.

Subscribers to the Medical Audit Program, which is also an extra-cost option, receive two additional reports, M1 and M2, which present detailed statistical tallies of findings, investigations, and management of patients by primary diagnosis group and by operation group. One additional form, the perinatal study form P, summarizes information from both the mothers' and the infants' abstract, and the special birth abstract form, and presents findings in a one-line condensed summary for each patient. Statistical data from the perinatal study analyzing infant deaths, birthweight, and Apgar score are provided annually as well.

Review of all these forms in detail is beyond the scope of this book, and extensive information is available on the subject from the commission. Attention will be concentrated here on the five major statistical forms: A, B, M1, M2, and S.

Form A. The A form (figure 12-4) reports the number of discharges and the sum of their hospital days by each medical specialty service of the hospital. Service is either assigned by the hospital on the abstract form or can be assigned based on the primary diagnosis by a computer program of the Commission. It can be assigned automatically by the physician's specialty. It is also possible to report the number of teaching and the number of nonteaching discharges within each specialty service on this form. Age distributions into three groups, below fourteen, fourteen and over, and sixty-five and older, are provided for each service in terms of discharges and patient days. The number of deaths and the number of autopsies are given for each service, as are the number of patients having surgery in total and the number having surgery within six hours of admission. The number of emergency admissions, the number of consultations, and the number of patients discharged without the Joint Commission requirement for minimum laboratory are also given by service. Four major categories of expected source of payment are given by service in both number of discharges and a number of patient days. Subtotals are accumulated for the medical service generally, the surgical service generally, the gynecology service, the obstetrical service, and the number of newborns. Totals excluding newborn, and excluding both obstetrics and newborn, are calculated, as is a grand total. In one version of semiannual A report, numbers of patients are given as in the monthly reports. In the other, the number of patients column is replaced by a percentage of total patients, the sum of hospital days column is replaced by the average length of stay, and other rates and percents are calculated.

In addition to these data classified by service, gross summary data are given on the number of abstracts, the overall average length of stay, the number of patients in other payment sources combined, and an analysis of discharges in terms of still births, transfers, coroner's cases, and deaths within two days. The number of still births autopsied is reported, and the gross death rate and autopsy rate are calculated. A condensed length of stay analysis reports the number of patients not staying overnight and those staying one day, two days, and over thirty days.

In a moderate-sized hospital, there are commonly about 25 rows of service classifications and 24 columns of reports for each classification. There are thus 600 separate statistics in the main array, and 20 additional gross statistics reported at the bottom.

Form B. The B form (figure 12-5) is a condensed summary of data on management of care. The patients are classified by 44 disease categories. Some of the same information as the A form is reported by the new categories, but much of the report shows the number of patients whose records show a variety of selected measures of outcome, investigation, or therapy. In addition to these statistics, the foot of the report contains figures for the number of still births, the average hemoglobin or hematocrit recorded from the admission laboratory, the percentage of patients with consultation, the number of cases in each classification of report of surgical tissue, and the total number of patients either with or without the remaining items of diagnosis and therapy which appear on the patient abstract. In addition, a distribution is given of the number of patients receiving one unit, two units and more than nine units of whole blood together with the total number of units of blood administered.

There are forty-seven rows and twenty-seven columns in the main body of the report, together with 52 gross statistics reported in the lower section. There are thus a possibility of 1,321 separate statistics on the B report, although the nature of the use of various items of investigation and treatment is such that many cells in the right hand sections of the report will be blank in any given month or even six-month period.

Despite the presence of nearly 2,000 separate statistics on the A and B forms, many of the difficulties discussed by Lembcke and Myers still exist. It is doubtful that statistical quality controls could be effectively used at this level of specificity, even if the PAS program limitations permitted it. These analyses assume a basic process which is unchanging. Many of the A and B statistics are aggregates of several processes, with changing mixes. The B categories, for example, include both medical and surgical treatment of the same disease. Length of stay and use of services would not be expected to be the same in both

A FORM – DISCHARGE ANALYSIS

Used for PAS Monthly, Semiannual, and Annual Reports

DISCHARGE ANALYSIS B — PROFESSIONAL ACTIVITY STUDY — COMMISSION ON PROFESSIONAL AND HOSPITAL ACTIVITIES — **B**

Ar70 — MARCH 1972 — SAMPLE — CITY, STATE — A570

CPHA

#	PATIENT GROUP BY FINAL DIAGNOSIS EXPLAINING ADMISSION	H-ICDA‡	TOTAL PATIENTS (2)	AVG STAY (EXCL DEATHS) (3)	MEDIAN STAY (EXCL DEATHS) (4)	PATIENTS NOT STAYING OVERNIGHT (EXCL DEATHS) (5)	% MALES (6)	PATIENTS 13 YEARS AND YOUNGER (7)	PATIENTS 65 YEARS AND OLDER (8)	DEATHS (9)	HOSPITAL COMPLICATIONS: INFECTIONS (10)	HOSPITAL COMPLICATIONS: OTHER (11)	% PTS WITH CONSUL (12)
1	Infective	001–136	34	4.7	4	2	44	17	4				12
2	Malignant Neoplasms	140–209	27	18.0	14		37	1	8	5			56
3	Other Neoplasms	210–239	16	7.3	5		25	2	3				25
4	Diabetes Mellitus	250	14	8.9	8		29		4				7
5	Other Endocrine	240–246; 251–258	2	6.5	6								50
6	Nutritional, Metabolic	260–279	1	2.0	2		100	1					
7	Hematologic	280–289	8	4.1	2		25	2					25
8	Mental	290–319	8	5.4	4		63						63
9	Other Nervous System	320–358	27	9.6	8		59	3	2				33
10	Eye	360–379	12	6.1	6		42	3	5				
11	Ear	380–389	1	2.0	2		100	1					
12	Hypertension	400–405	14	10.1	7		36		1				36
13	Acute Myocardial Infarction	410	7	18.4	19		57		4	2			57
14	Other Heart	390–398; 411–429	44	11.5	8		73		25	4			23
15	Cerebrovascular	430–438	15	15.0	17		33		6	6			60
16	Other Vascular	440–458	15	10.3	10		33		6	1			47
17	Acute URI	460–465	3	5.0	7		33	2					33
18	Pneumonia & Bronchitis	480–491	27	10.1	9		52	9	3			1	33
19	Hypertrophy of T & A	500	21	2.2	2		52	17				1	
20	Other Resp	470; 492–493; 501–519	10	6.0	4		70	1	3				20
21	Dental	520–526	4	2.8	3		50						25
22	Peptic Ulcer	531–534	21	11.4	10		62		3			1	43
23	Other Upper GI	527–530; 535–537	5	5.4	5		40	1					
24	Appendix	540–543	7	6.9	5		86	1					29
25	Hernia	550–553	37	6.6	6	1	70	6	6				14
26	Cholecystitis & Calculus	574–575	19	10.6	9		32		2	1			32
27	Other GI	560–573; 576–577	31	11.7	8		39	2	5	2	1	1	55
28	Genitourinary	580–607	46	8.5	5		70	6	9				28
29	Breast	610–611	10	3.2	3		10	1					
30	Female Genital	612–629	29	6.7	3						1		57
31	MATERNITY: Comp of Pregnancy	630–639	25	3.0	2	5							16
32	MATERNITY: Abortions	640–646	8	2.8	3								75
33	MATERNITY: Normal Delivery	650	75	4.7	5								4
34	MATERNITY: Complicated Delivery	651–661	41	6.1	5						1		22
35	MATERNITY: Comp of Puerperium	670–678											
36	Skin	680–709	5	6.2	5		60	1					20
37	Musculoskeletal	710–739	45	9.7	8		69		1				27
38	Congenital Anomalies	740–759	12	3.5	2		58	9		1			17
39	Diseases of Infancy	772–778											
40	Symptoms, Signs	780–797	20	9.4	7		70	5	2			1	35
41	Fractures	800–829	27	11.3	8		48	1	6				26
42	Other Trauma	830–959	50	8.4	5		80	8	3	2			32
43	Adverse Effects	960–999	10	9.8	9	1	80	2	3				40
44	Special Conditions	Y00–Y17											
45	Newborn	Y20–Y29	111	7.0	5		56	111					19
46													
47	Grand Total		943	7.9	5	9	45	213	114	24	3	5	26
48	Total, except Newborn		832	8.0	6	9	44	102	114	24	3	5	27
49	Total, except Newborn, Maternity		683	8.8	6	4	53	102	114	24	2	5	30

INVESTIGATION: PATIENTS WHOSE RECORDS SHOW

#	PATIENT GROUP	MINIMUM LAB NOT MET (13)	NO URINE TEST (14)	NO HEMATOLOGY (15)	NO ADMISSION BLOOD PRESSURE (16)	EKG (17)	BLOOD CHEMISTRY: SUGAR (18)	BLOOD CHEMISTRY: NITROGEN DERIV (19)	BLOOD CHEMISTRY: LIVER FUNCTION (20)	X-RAY: CHEST (EXCL ROUTINE) (21)	X-RAY: SKELETAL (22)	DIAG RADIO-ISOTOPES (23)
1	Infective	2	1	1	16	1	6	6	2	8		
2	Malignant Neoplasms				1	7	16	19	5	22	6	3
3	Other Neoplasms				2	3	7	6		10	3	2
4	Diabetes Mellitus					5	14	9	2	6	1	
5	Other Endocrine						2	2	1	2		
6	Nutritional, Metabolic				1							
7	Hematologic				2	2	2	2	1	5		1
8	Mental					1	6	4	1	4	3	2
9	Other Nervous System				2	1	17	15	2	18	12	3
10	Eye				3		1	1	1	6		
11	Ear				1							
12	Hypertension					11	12	12	3	10	5	
13	Acute Myocardial Infarction	1	1	1	1	6	3	6		6		
14	Other Heart	1				43	31	38	9	40	6	
15	Cerebrovascular	1	1		1	6	15	13	1	11	4	2
16	Other Vascular					4	8	8	2	9	1	
17	Acute URI				2			1	1	2	1	
18	Pneumonia & Bronchitis	2	1	1	9	11	13	15	5	26	1	
19	Hypertrophy of T & A				15	1	1	1		2		
20	Other Resp				1	3	6	5	2	9	1	
21	Dental									2		
22	Peptic Ulcer	1	1		1	5	9	9	2	15		
23	Other Upper GI				1	3	3	3		4	2	
24	Appendix					1		1		3		
25	Hernia	1	1		6	7	6	9	2	28	1	2
26	Cholecystitis & Calculus					4	7	7	7	17	1	
27	Other GI	1			2	11	18	19	9	24		
28	Genitourinary				5	16	25	38	4	32	2	1
29	Breast						2	1		2		
30	Female Genital					3	11	6	2	27	1	
31	Comp of Pregnancy	3	1	3				1		2	1	
32	Abortions						1			5		
33	Normal Delivery	3	3	1	4		4	1	1	2	4	
34	Complicated Delivery	2	2	1	2		2	2		7	5	
35	Comp of Puerperium											
36	Skin				1	1	1	2		2		
37	Musculoskeletal				1	4	17	18	2	28	22	1
38	Congenital Anomalies				7		1	1		5	2	
39	Diseases of Infancy											
40	Symptoms, Signs	1	1		1	7	6	12	3	13	5	1
41	Fractures				1	4	7	8	2	20	21	
42	Other Trauma	5	3	2	6	6	13	17	3	28	36	2
43	Adverse Effects					1	2		2	3	1	
44	Special Conditions											
45	Newborn		109	104			1		18	3	1	
46												
47	Grand Total	24	125	114	95	178	296	318	95	468	149	20
48	Total, except Newborn	24	16	10	95	178	295	318	77	465	148	20
49	Total, except Newborn, Maternity	16	10	5	89	178	288	314	76	449	138	20

MANAGEMENT

#	PATIENT GROUP	DIAG ENDOSCOPY (24)	CULTURE (25)	ANTIBIOGRAMS (26)	PATIENTS GIVEN: ANTIBIOTICS (27)	PATIENTS GIVEN: OTHER ANTI-INFECTIVES (28)	PATIENTS GIVEN: ANTI-DIABETICS (29)	PATIENTS GIVEN: DIURETICS (30)	PATIENTS GIVEN: RADIATION THERAPY (31)	PATIENTS: TRANSFUSED (32)	PATIENTS: OPERATED (33)	PATIENTS: ICU – CCU (34)
1	Infective	3	15	9	10		1	2			3	
2	Malignant Neoplasms		6	2	12	1		4	7	8	14	2
3	Other Neoplasms	2	2		7		1	1		1	15	1
4	Diabetes Mellitus		2	2	3		14					1
5	Other Endocrine						1				1	
6	Nutritional, Metabolic											
7	Hematologic		1	1	4					2	3	
8	Mental				1						1	1
9	Other Nervous System		2	1	2	2					10	
10	Eye				1			1			12	
11	Ear				1							
12	Hypertension	1			1	1	4	6			1	2
13	Acute Myocardial Infarction				3	1		1				6
14	Other Heart		7	4	7	3	11	28				13
15	Cerebrovascular		3	2	5	1	3	6		1	5	5
16	Other Vascular		1	1	6			3		1	6	1
17	Acute URI	1	1	1	1						2	
18	Pneumonia & Bronchitis	2	14	10	23		3				4	4
19	Hypertrophy of T & A				3						21	
20	Other Resp		2		6		1				2	
21	Dental				1						4	
22	Peptic Ulcer		3	3	5	1	2	1		5	7	4
23	Other Upper GI		1	1				1				
24	Appendix		2	2	4						6	
25	Hernia		1		8			1			32	1
26	Cholecystitis & Calculus		4	2	7		2				16	1
27	Other GI	5	5	2	10	3	1	4		4	6	3
28	Genitourinary	7	28	17	19	13	4	1		1	33	1
29	Breast						1				10	
30	Female Genital	2	4	3	6	1	2	1		2	25	1
31	Comp of Pregnancy					1		1		2	5	
32	Abortions						1			1	8	
33	Normal Delivery		4	1	7	4		5			9	1
34	Complicated Delivery		3	2	4	2		4		7	30	
35	Comp of Puerperium											
36	Skin		2	1	3	1					1	
37	Musculoskeletal	1	3		6	1	1			2	35	1
38	Congenital Anomalies	1	1	1	1						11	
39	Diseases of Infancy											
40	Symptoms, Signs		3	3	7	2		1		2	4	4
41	Fractures		4	2	11			2		1	21	3
42	Other Trauma		2	2	19	2		1		4	14	10
43	Adverse Effects		2	2	3						1	3
44	Special Conditions											
45	Newborn		2	2	2					1	1	
46												
47	Grand Total	25	130	79	219	40	53	75	7	45	379	69
48	Total, except Newborn	25	128	77	217	40	53	75	7	44	378	69
49	Total, except Newborn, Maternity	25	121	74	206	33	52	65	7	34	326	68

35 Total Abstracts	947
36 Stillborn	4
37 Average Hgb or Hct (Excl newborn)	13.4
38 STS	681

TISSUE OF MOST IMPORTANT OPERATION: NO TISSUE REMOVED (39)	PATHOLOGY REPORT IN CHART: DISEASED A (40)	DISEASED B (41)	NO DISEASE (42)	NOT CODED BY PATHOLOGIST (43)	TISSUE REMOVED, NO REPORT (44)	PATIENTS WITH HISTOLOGY: CERVICAL PAP (45)	OTHER PAP (46)	CELL BLOCK (47)	FROZEN SECTION (48)	MULTI-CHANNEL CHEMISTRY (49)
147	163	1	66		2	7	7	7	9	32

PATIENTS WITH X-RAYS: ROUTINE (SURVEY) CHEST (50)	GI (51)	GU (52)	PLEURAL & PERIT CAVITIES (53)	CNS & CNS SPACES (54)	CARDIO-VASCULAR (55)	EXTERNAL SOFT TISSUE (56)
	130	78	34	26	11	

MANAGEMENT: PATIENTS WHOSE RECORDS SHOW USE OF: TRANQUILIZERS (57)	CANCER CHEMOTHERAPY (58)	HYPOTHERMIA (59)	MONITORS (60)	CARDIAC CARE UNIT (61)	PARENTERAL FLUIDS (62)	PLASMA, BLOOD DERIV (63)	RH IMMUNE GLOBULIN (64)	PATIENTS TRANSFUSED (INCLUDES PACKED RBC): 1 UNIT (65)	2 UNITS (66)	9 OR MORE UNITS (67)
268	3		34	33	174		9	12	15	

Anesthesia	ANY ANESTHESIA (68)	INHAL ONLY (69)	INHAL + IV (70)	SPINAL ONLY (71)	SADDLE BLK (72)	LOCAL ONLY (73)	NO ANESTH (74)
a. Related to Delivery	84					14	9
b. For other Patients	342	40	271	2	1	22	

PATIENTS WITH FUNCTION TESTS: THYROID (75)	EEG (76)	KIDNEY (77)	PULMONARY (78)	SPECIAL C (79)	SPECIAL D (80)	SPECIAL E (81)	SPECIAL F (82)	SPECIAL G (83)
23	25		3					

PATIENTS WITH: PARASITOLOGY (84)	BACTERIAL SMEAR (85)	THROAT CULTURE (86)	URINE CULTURE (87)	PHYSICAL MEDICINE PATIENTS: DIAGNOSTIC TESTS (88)	PT (89)	OT (90)	OTHER (91)	ISOLATION (92)	OXYGEN (93)	IPPB (94)	OTHER INHAL THERAPY (95)	UNITS OF BLOOD GIVEN: WHOLE BLOOD (96)	PACKED RBC (97)
11	119	11	55		1			31	59	39	7	108	11

✱ Figure exceeds space provided

‡Hospital Adaptation of ICDA, Commission on Professional and Hospital Activities, 1968

B FORM — DISCHARGE ANALYSIS

Used for PAS Monthly, Semiannual, and Annual Reports

Figure 12-5. B Form – Discharge Analysis.

PAS — MAP

Each line on this form presents one patient's case abstract. Reports using this form, together with the sequence of patients for each, are listed in the tables below.

Report				Primary Sequence	Secondary Sequence
PAS	Monthly	Diagnosis	Listings	final diagnosis explaining admission (col. 1)	physician (col. 11)
		Operation		most important operation (col. 7)	surgeon (col. 11)
		Death		final diagnosis explaining admission (col. 1)	physician (col. 11)
		Patient		patient number (col. 23)	
	Semiannual	Diagnosis	Indexes	diagnosis (col. 1)	physician (col. 11)
		Operation		operation (col. 7)	surgeon (col. 11)
		Physician		diagnosis (col. 1)	
		Surgeon		operation (col. 7)	

Report			Primary Sequence	Secondary Sequence
PAS–MAP Listings (Quarterly)	for all patients	PEDIATRIC MEDICINE	final diagnosis explaining admission (col. 1)	physician (col. 11)
		MEDICINE	final diagnosis explaining admission (col. 1)	physician (col. 11)
		SURGERY (BY DIAGNOSIS)	final diagnosis explaining admission (col. 1)	physician (col. 11)
		OBSTETRICS (BY DIAGNOSIS)	final diagnosis explaining admission (col. 1)	physician (col. 11)
		NEWBORN	standard AMA birth weight group (see col. 3)	final diagnosis explaining admission (col. 1)
	for all operated patients	CHILDREN (BY OPERATION)	most important operation (col. 7)	surgeon (col. 11)
		ADULTS (BY OPERATION)	most important operation (col. 7)	surgeon (col. 11)
		OBSTETRICS (BY OPERATION)	most important operation (col. 7)	surgeon (col. 11)

1. INDEXED DIAGNOSIS

Diagnoses are coded by *Hospital Adaptation of ICDA* (H-ICDA, CPHA, 1968).

In listings by Dx and physician, cases are in sequence by Dx in this column. This Dx is the **final Dx explaining admission** ("primary" Dx), except when the prefix ⌑ appears. For a cross-indexed entry, ⌑ indicates the Dx as secondary and P in col. 3 designates the primary Dx.

Explanations for the letters T and E appear under "3-6 OTHER DIAGNOSES AND OPERATIONS."

2. MORE

The symbol # prints in this column whenever the patient had more secondary diagnoses or operations than can be printed on one line. For such patients, all diagnoses and operations appear at the end of the Monthly Diagnosis and Operation Listings and quarterly PAS–MAP listings.

3-6. OTHER DIAGNOSES AND OPERATIONS

Diagnoses in addition to the one indexed in col. 1 and operations in addition to the one indexed in col. 7 appear in columns 3-6. (Dx codes contain 4 digits and thus are distinguished from the 3-digit operation codes.) If there are more diagnoses or operations than can be printed in these columns, the symbol # will appear in col. 2.

The letter P preceding a code in col. 3 or 6 indicates a "primary" diagnosis or operation.

Birth weights print in col. 3 for newborn, stillborn, and babies 1-7 days old on admission. Birth weights are distinguished from other codes by G which indicates grams (2750G) or by the slash (/) which separates pounds and ounces (5/11 = 5 lbs. 11 oz.).

External Cause of Injury Codes. An E prefixes an External Cause of Injury code. The E code relates to the immediately preceding Dx code (800.0 – 999.9).

Tumor Morphology Codes. A T prefixes a tumor morphology code from SNOP (*Systematized Nomenclature of Pathology*, College of American Pathologists, 1965). T codes appear only in semiannual reports.

7. INDEXED OPERATION

In listings by operation and surgeon, cases are in sequence by operation in this column. This operation is the **most important operation** ("primary" operation), except when the prefix ⌑ appears. For a cross-indexed entry, ⌑ indicates the operation as secondary and P in col. 6 designates the primary operation. An S in column 7 indicates a spontaneous delivery.

On PAS–MAP quarterly listings, the prefix "+" means that the patient is not counted as operated (see back of M form) and is excluded from the accompanying M form table. When such a patient has a spontaneous delivery S appears.

8. TISSUE for most important operation

Pathology report in chart
1. Diseased A
2. Diseased B
3. No disease
4. Not coded by pathologist

No pathology report
5. Tissue removed, no report
6. No tissue removed

Codes 1, 2 and 3 are assigned by the pathologist. "Diseased A" is tissue disease which generally requires surgical removal. "Diseased B" is tissue disease where surgical removal is not clearly indicated from the pathological findings alone.

This tissue code is printed only when the most important operation appears in col. 7. When secondary operations are cross indexed this column is blank. 23

9. ANESTHESIA for most important operation (or delivery)

- 0 None
- 1 Inhalation alone
- 2 Intravenous alone
- 3 Spinal alone
- 4 Saddle block alone
- 5 Epidural or caudal alone
- 6 Nerve or field block alone
- 7 Local alone
- 8 "Other" alone
- B Inhalation and IV
- G Inhalation and any other except IV
- V IV and any other except inhalation
- S Spinal and any other except IV or inhalation
- R Any combination of codes 4-8

The anesthesia code is printed only when the most important operation appears in column 7. When secondary operations are cross indexed this column is blank. 22

10. TIME OF EARLIEST SURGERY OR TIME OF DELIVERY

The symbol # shows that the earliest operation began or delivery occurred within six hours of the patient's admission. If more than six hours elapsed, the day is indicated (0 = day of admission, 1 = next day, ... 9 = 9 or more days). 21

11. PHYSICIAN OR SURGEON

Code numbers are assigned by the hospital; names are known only to the hospital. On Dx and patient listings the attending physician's number appears. On operation listings the operating surgeon's number appears.

An asterisk (✱) at the left of col. 11 indicates that the attending physician and the operating surgeon are two different people. On the physician and surgeon indexes the only numbers printed are of surgeons (or attending physicians) other than the indexed doctor. 2, 24, 27

12. CONSULTATIONS from

- ⌑ Same as responsible service (coded in col. 17)
- M Internal Medicine
- S Surgery
- G OB Gyn
- C Pediatrics
- P Psychiatry
- R Physical Medicine

The **number** of consulting services prints when there are consultations from more than one service. 14

13. AGE ON ADMISSION

Numbers represent **years** of age unless indicated as follows:

D. Days; M. Months; NB. Newborn; SB. Stillborn 3

14. RACE

Blank. White or not recorded; 1. Nonwhite; 2. Black; 3. Asiatic; 4. Special A (see MRL) 9

15. SEX

M. Male; F. Female; Blank. Not recorded 4

16. DISCHARGE STATUS

Discharged alive:
- Blank. With approval
- X. Against advice
- T. Transferred to other hospital
- E. Transferred to extended care facility
- H. Transferred to home care program

Died:
- A. Autopsy
- D. No autopsy

*The following letters precede death code A or D where appropriate:
- P. Postoperative death
- O. Died in OR
- C. Coroner's case 8

17. HOSPITAL SERVICE

2. Pediatric Medicine	50. ENT	74. Obstetrics
10. General Medicine	54. Dental	or 75. Abortion
22. Cardiology	58. Orthopedics	or 76. OB–Not Delivered
38. Psychiatry	62. Urology	or 77. OB–Delivered
40. General Surgery	70. Gynecology	80. Newborn
48. Ophthalmology		89. Stillborn

13a

Letters following the numerical code designate the teaching status of the case.

W. Ward; T. Teaching; Blank. Private

For the meaning of any other codes, see MRL. 13b

18. INTERSERVICE TRANSFER

The symbol ⌑ prints in this column when the patient was transferred from one service to another within the hospital. 13c

19. STAY in days

- < 1 = Not overnight
- Y = Stay to the nearest year (for 1,000 days or more)
- ??? = Length of stay is not computable 5, 6

20. COMPLICATIONS

I. Hospital infection; C. Other hospital complication; B. Both 12

21. PAYMENT

Blank. Not recorded
0. U.S. Medicare or Canadian Provincial only

Letters in parentheses designate payment supplementing Medicare or Provincial.

1 (W) Workmen's compensation	5 (C) Commercial insurance
2 (M) Medicaid	6 (V) Voluntary charities
3 (G) Government agencies	7 (S) Special B (see MRL)
4 (B) Blue Cross	8 (P) Private

10

22. OPTIONAL (see MRL) 15

23. PATIENT NUMBER

Number assigned by hospital; names are known only to hospital. Asterisks indicate patient number was not recorded. 1

24. SELECTED CASE

- X Selected case (see MRL)
- ✱ Flags total count following each group of patients 55

25. DISCHARGE MONTH

The first nine months are numbered, and the months of October, November, and December are O, N, and D. This column is blank on monthly listings. 6

26. SPECIAL C, D (see MRL)

C. Special C; D. Special D; B. Both 39

***27. TYPE OF ADMISSION**

E. Emergency, U. Urgent (defined by hospital); T. Transferred from other hospital 11

‡28. ADMISSION HEMOGLOBIN OR HEMATOCRIT

The hospital elects one procedure to record for all patients. The admission hemoglobin is in grams per 100 ml, disregarding tenths. Hematocrit appears as percent. 29

‡29. ADMISSION WHITE BLOOD COUNT

The admission total white blood cell count is given in thousands. 30

‡30. ADMISSION URINE

- X. No admission urinalysis
- Blank. Negative findings
- A. Albumin positive
- S. Sugar positive
- B. Both 31

‡31-32. ADMISSION BLOOD PRESSURE

The systolic blood pressure on admission appears in column 31 and the diastolic in column 32 according to the following codes:

9. 220 or over	5. 120–139	2. 80–89
8. 190–219	4. 100–119	1. 50–79
7. 160–189	3. 90–99	0. 49 or less
6. 140–159		

42

‡33. ADMISSION TEMPERATURE

Code indicates degrees F (or 1/2 degrees C) of elevation above normal oral temperature.

X. Admission temperature not taken

0. 98.9 F or less (under 37.0 C)	4. 102.0–102.9 (38.5–.9)
1. 99.0–99.9 (37.0–.4)	5. 103.0–103.9 (39.0–.4)
2. 100.0–100.9 (37.5–.9)	6. 104.0–104.9 (39.5–.9)
3. 101.0–101.9 (38.0–.4)	7. 105.0 or more (40.0+)

43

34. PEAK TEMPERATURE

The same codes as used in col. 33 print here to show the highest temperature recorded for the patient. When the admission temperature (col. 33) was the highest recorded temperature, column 34 is blank. 43

35. RECTAL AND PELVIC EXAMINATIONS

R. Rectal; P. Pelvic; B. Both 33

36. HEIGHT, WEIGHT

H. Height recorded; W. Weight recorded; B. Both (if age under 20)

Index for patients 20 and older, based on U.S. adult median weight for sex and height:

1. Weight under 65% of U.S. median

2. 65–74%	5. 95–107%	8. 138–152%
3. 75–84%	6. 108–122%	9. Over 152%
4. 85–94%	7. 123–137%	

18, 19, 20

37. OTHER EXAMINATIONS

1. Funduscopic; 2. Tonometry; 4. Skin tests — 3, 5, 6, 7 = combinations (sum of codes) 33, 54

***38. URINALYSIS**

- Blank. No urinalysis
- U. Admission urinalysis only ‡
- R. Repeat or routine done after admission
- 4. Bile, urobilinogen
- 5. Hormones
- 6. Calcium, minerals 31

39. MINIMUM LAB

- Blank. Urinalysis plus Hgb or Hct at any time
- X. Lab work not done

Not applicable for newborn 29, 31, 35

***40. HEMATOLOGY–RED CELLS**

- 1. Hemoglobin
- 2. Hematocrit
- 3. Red blood cells, indices
- 4. Reticulocytes, nucleated RBCs
- 5. Red cell abnormality
- C. CBC = Hgb + RBC + WBC + differential 35

41. HEMATOLOGY–WHITE CELLS AND SEDIMENTATION RATE

1. Sedimentation rate; 2. Total white blood cell count; 4. Differential white blood cell count — 3, 5, 6, 7 = combinations (sum of codes) 35

42. HEMATOLOGY–COAGULATION TESTS

P. Prothrombin time; C. Other coagulation tests; B. Both 35

***43. SEROLOGY**

Excludes serological test for syphilis (see column 44).

- 3. Special human antibodies
- 4. Bacterial antibodies
- 5. Rheumatoid factors
- 6. Heterophil
- 7. C-reactive protein
- 8. Viral antibodies 52

44. STS AND MULTICHANNEL CHEMISTRY

S. Serological test for syphilis; M. Multichannel chemistry; B. Both 32

45-50. BLOOD CHEMISTRY tests done

N. NITROGEN DERIVATIVES	45
E. ELECTROLYTES, pH	45
L. LIVER FUNCTION	45
T. TRANSAMINASE LDH	45
P. PROTEINS, PROTEIN ELECTROPHORESIS	45
C. CHOLESTEROL, LIPIDS	45

In these columns a + sign denotes an abnormal result and R means the abnormal test was repeated. 47, 49

***51. BLOOD SUGAR**

- F. Fasting, random
- P. 2-hour postprandial
- B. Both F and P
- +. ≥ 150 mg% found in either of above
- G. Glucose tolerance test done 46

52. OTHER BLOOD CHEMISTRY

1. Amylase, lipase, absorption tests; 2. Serum iron; 4. Toxicology — 3, 5, 6, 7 = combinations (sum of codes) 54

53. STOOL AND GASTRIC EXAMINATIONS

1. Gastric analysis; 2. Stool analysis; 4. Stool for blood — 3, 5, 6, 7 = combinations (sum of codes) 51

***54. CULTURE**

T. Throat or nose; U. Urine; H. Blood; C. Other 48

55. OTHER MICROBIOLOGY

1. Bacterial smear; 2. Antibiogram; 4. Parasitology — 3, 5, 6, 7 = combinations (sum of codes) 50

***56. HISTOLOGY**

C. Cervical Papanicolaou; P. Other Papanicolaou; 2. Cell block; F. Frozen section 53

57. EKG

E. Done; R. Repeated 34

***58. FUNCTION**

6. Thyroid; 7. EEG; 8. Kidney; 9. Pulmonary 34

***59. X-RAY: CHEST, G.I.**

- R. Routine (survey) chest
- C. Diagnostic chest, respiratory
- D. Digestive tract, gallbladder
- B. Both C and D 44

***60. X-RAY: SKELETAL, OTHER**

- 3. Skeletal
- 4. Urogenital
- 5. Pleural & peritoneal cavities NOS
- 6. CNS & CNS spaces
- 7. Cardiovascular
- 8. External soft tissue 44

61. SPECIAL E, F (see MRL)

E. Special E; F. Special F; B. Both 39

62. WHOLE BLOOD

The number of whole blood transfusions, 500 ml each or less. 9 = 9 or more. 36a

63. PACKED RED BLOOD CELLS

The number of packed red blood cell transfusions. 9 = 9 or more. 36b

64. FLUIDS, PLASMA

1. Parenteral fluids; 2. Plasma, blood derivatives; 4. Rh immune globulin — 3, 5, 6, 7 = combinations (sum of codes) 40

65. INHALATION THERAPY

1. IPPB; 2. Other inhalation therapy; 4. Oxygen — 3, 5, 6, 7 = combinations (sum of codes) 40

66. CARE UNITS

1. Intensive care unit; 2. Cardiac (coronary) care unit; 4. Isolation — 3, 5, 6, 7 = combinations (sum of codes) 39, 40

67. MONITOR/PRESSOR

1. Hypothermia; 2. Vasopressors; 4. Monitoring device — 3, 5, 6, 7 = combinations (sum of codes) 37, 40

68. CARDIAC DRUGS

1. Cardiac regulating drugs; 2. Anticoagulants; 4. Vasodilators — 3, 5, 6, 7 = combinations (sum of codes) 37

69. ANTIDIABETICS/STEROIDS

1. Steroids; 2. Oral antidiabetics; 4. Insulin — 3, 5, 6, 7 = combinations (sum of codes) 37

70. HYPOTENSIVES/THYROID DRUGS

1. Diuretics; 2. Hypotensives (antihypertensives); 4. Thyroid/antithyroid — 3, 5, 6, 7 = combinations (sum of codes) 37

71. ANTI-INFECTIVES

1. Sulfas; 2. Antibiotics; 4. Other anti-infectives — 3, 5, 6, 7 = combinations (sum of codes) 38

72. TRANQUILIZERS, SPECIAL G

T. Tranquilizers; G. Special G (see MRL); B. Both 38, 40

* **ASTERISKED ITEMS:** When more than one of the items listed for a column has been marked on a PAS Case Abstract, the applicable code nearest the bottom of the list is printed for that patient.

‡ **ADMISSION, PREOPERATIVE, PREDELIVERY FINDINGS:** Each finding is from the first test of its kind done during the ADMISSION PERIOD, which begins with the patient's admission to the hospital and ends at 11:59 p.m. of the following day, at the time of earliest surgery, or at the time of delivery, whichever comes first.

Note: On the monthly **PATIENT LISTING** only, the content of columns 26-72 is changed:

a. Hospital options from PAS Case Abstract items 57-63 print in columns 26-50.
b. The admission and discharge days and dates print in columns 52-72.
c. DUP prints in col. 23 for duplicated patient numbers or readmissions instead of a repeat of the preceding patient number.
d. No supplementary listing (see explanation for col. 2) is printed at the end of the Patient Listing or Death Listing.

Note: The **SHADED AREA** following each column's explanation shows the PAS Case Abstract item numbers for reference.

C FORM – CASE ABSTRACT LISTING (Reverse Side)

Figure 12-5. B Form – Discharge Analysis, (Continued).

methods of treatment. Some of the most interesting statistics on the A and B reports are in the lower sections and are not categorized at all. Such statistics would have large variances, relative to their means, and would not be likely to be useful in detecting variations in quality. A number of the most clinically revealing statistics about diagnosis and treatment are not reported on the A and B forms at all. In summary, it seems that these forms are too incomplete and too grossly aggregated to make a substantial contribution to a quality review system.

The Medical Audit Report. The two-page medical audit program report M1 and M2 (figures 12-6 and 12-7) substantially refines information about the investigation and treatment of patients grouped by diagnosis, both by categorizing patients by service and also by increasing the number of categories of diagnosis. In addition, a number of specific statistics of considerable interest in both quality and utilization control are calculated which do not appear on the A and B reports. The reports are prepared quarterly, with one report for each of the four major clinical services: medicine, surgery, pediatrics and obstetrics. A fifth report is devoted specifically to the analysis of newborns, categorized by birth weight. Revised basic patient lists are prepared on the C form, giving a one-line coded presentation of the case abstract for each patient included in each category or row of the M report. In addition to the five reports by major service and for newborns, three additional sets of the M forms are prepared for adult surgery, pediatric surgery, and obstetrical surgery which categorized the patients according to their most important operation. Seventy-two disease categories are used as opposed to 44 in the B report, while a number of rows actually presented on any one table is reduced by dividing the report up into the specific clinical services.

Use of Information

The increased specificity and improved format of the M report should greatly aid in the process of conducting a medical audit. A number of specific items of information are present in the M form which permit rapid scanning for deviant values or a relatively easy establishment of either policy or statistical control limits for their review. Among these are a number of columns indicating failure to obtain minimal laboratory workup. Several columns record the number of exceptions to the policy that patients should have temperature, blood pressure, white blood count, urinalysis and hematocrit or hemoglobin recorded on admission, and if not on admission, certainly before discharge. It can be a simple matter to establish either a policy that all cases appearing in this column be reviewed by a medical audit committee, or that the number of occurrences in this column for certain services be treated as a random variable with a low mean, and that all cases be investigated by the committee whenever the value of the variable exceeds a certain preestablished limit calculated as indicated in chapter 10.

Similar approaches can be used with some of the comparative statistics. These variables deal with the percentage of patients having intravenous fluids but no previous electrolyte determination (excluding surgical patients), antibiotics but no antibiogram, transfusions with a low hematocrit or hemoglobin, and transfusions with a high hematocrit or hemoglobin. They can be handled as time series statistics where the percentages given are treated as fractions defective, and the means and standard deviations are calculated in the manner suggested in chapter 10. A similar technique could be applied to the follow-up of admission urinary findings. It would be assumed, however, that under good conditions of quality control the number of patients appearing in these boxes would be small and the control limits could be established on the basis that the distribution followed a Poisson process.

A number of items of potential use in utilization review appear in the M report which are not on preceding reports. Among these are information about mean and median lengths of stay and also information for the 75th and 90th percentiles of length of stay. Also included is an analysis of the variation of the number of admissions and the number of discharges by day of the week. The effect of day of admission on the length of stay is also included, and with it a test of statistical significance of the variation. This test is conducted in the manner suggested in chapter 3.

Relating to the utilization of services, the M report contains a "variety index," which is calculated for each patient by taking the unweighted sum of all of the investigational activities entered into the case abstract. The index values are reported for both "teaching" and "nonteaching" patients. The average index for the service is weighted by the diagnostic distribution. Unfortunately, the value of these statistics in control of utilization or quality is uncertain. The reliability of the index, which is based on the presence of certain tests but not the number of tests, is unknown. The M report can be used to survey other specific groups of patients in addition to those of a single service. Data for a given disease, say diabetes, can be displayed for several doctors, or several age groups, or even for several hospitals. Requests for regional comparisons of this kind are becoming more frequent, according to the Commission. This flexibility opens a number of opportunities of a research nature, as well.

Substantial information about the demand for hospital services can also be developed from the M report. Although the amount of manual work involved in this may be excessive for analyzing demand on a routine basis, the availability of the report would substantially speed any specific studies aimed at the analysis of demand. Demands for various diagnostic services and for a variety of treatment services are given in the M report. These are usually not in terms of the total units of service demanded, but rather in terms of the number of demands for one or more units of the service. The column values present the number of

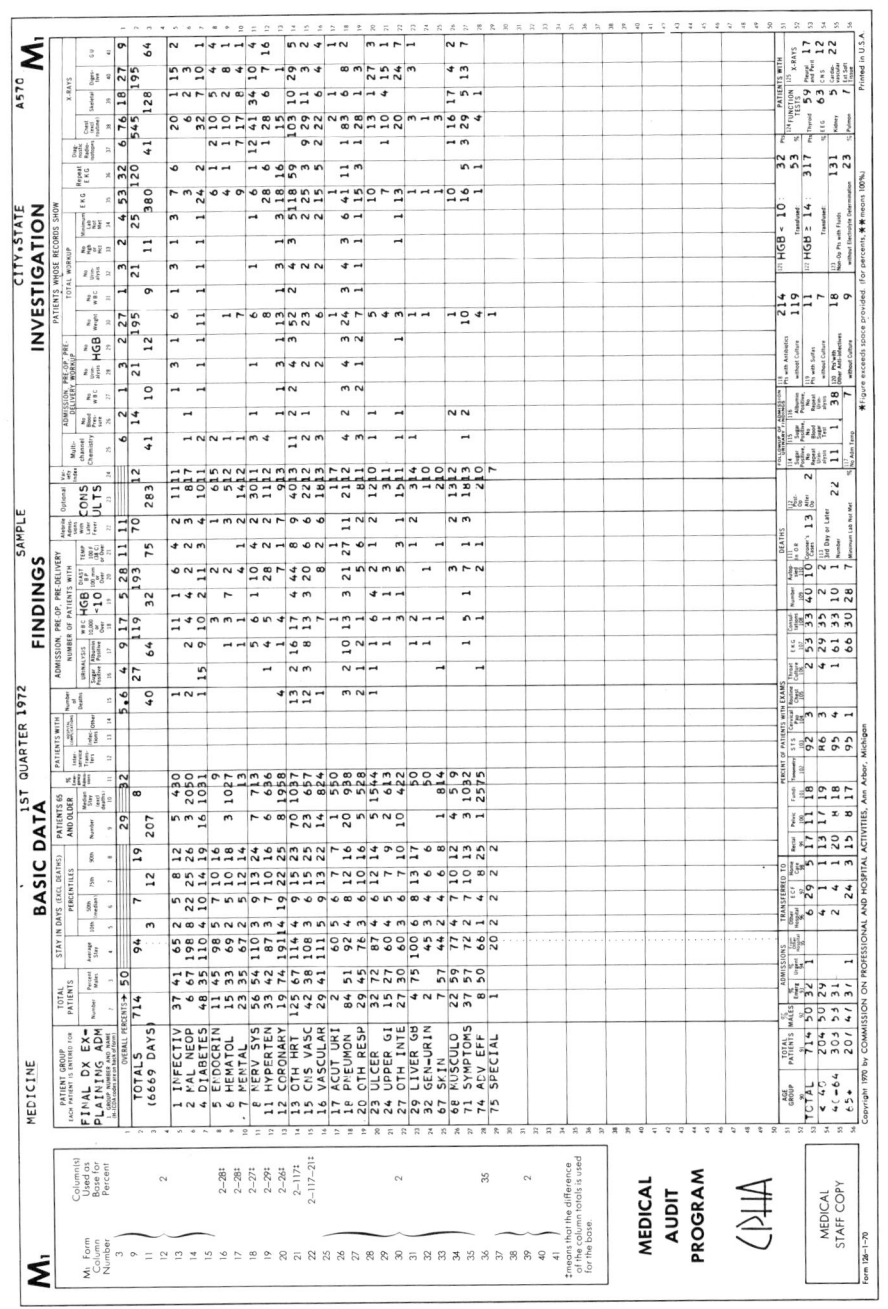

Figure 12-6. M1 Form — Basic Data, Findings, Investigation.

The PAS-MAP reports are prepared for each calendar quarter. They display the medical practice of the hospital to assist the medical staff in evaluating the quality of medical care. The reports for each of the four major clinical services, and for newborn, are prepared from the PAS Case Abstracts. Arrangements can be made with CPHA if special PAS-MAP reports are desired.

The assignment of a patient to the different PAS-MAP reports is governed by the hospital service of the patient. Hospital service for any given patient is specified as follows.

1) The Medical Record Librarian may enter a service code on the abstract.
2) If no service code was entered, the CPHA computer will assign service by attending physician if such an arrangement has been made with CPHA.
3) Otherwise, the CPHA computer will assign service on the basis of final diagnosis explaining admission and most important operation.

Each discharged patient is included in only one of the five reports by diagnosis. Each operated patient is also included in one of the three reports by operation. The following table includes the service code range for each diagnosis report.

Title	Patient Group	Sequence of M Forms and Primary Sequence of Listings	Secondary Sequence of Listings
Summary of Services	All patients (both percents and totals are displayed).	Major Clinical Service (no listings)	
Pediatric Medicine	Pediatric Service (codes 1-9) and Medical Service patients of pediatric age (defined by hospital).	Final Diagnosis Explaining Admission	Attending Physician
Medicine	Medical Service (10-39) patients except those assigned to Pediatric Medicine.	Final Diagnosis Explaining Admission	Attending Physician
Surgery (By Diagnosis)	Surgical Service (40-69) Patients. Gynecology Service (70-73) patients appear here or in the Obstetrics reports. See your Medical Record Librarian.	Final Diagnosis Explaining Admission	Attending Physician
Obstetrics (By Diagnosis)	Obstetrics Service (74-79) Patients. Gynecology Service (70-73) patients appear here or in the Surgery reports.	Final Diagnosis Explaining Admission	Attending Physician
Newborn	All hospital births (Liveborn and Stillborn).	Standard AMA Birth Weight Group	Final Diagnosis Explaining Admission
Children (By Operation)	All operated patients (see list on M2 form for exclusions) of pediatric age (defined by hospital) except those on the Obstetrics Service.	Most Important Operation	Operating Surgeon
Adults (By Operation)	All other operated patients except those on the Obstetrics Service.	Most Important Operation	Operating Surgeon
Obstetrics (By Operation)	All operated patients on Obstetrics Service.	Most Important Operation	Operating Surgeon

The notes below explain the content of the columns and boxes of the M report when the headings are not self-explanatory. The number to the right of the column or box title indicates the column of the C form where you can find the patients included in the statistic on the M form. When particular codes apply, they follow the column references, separated by a colon.

Column or Box		C Form Column: Code
	STAY IN DAYS excluding deaths PERCENTILES (5-8) Percentiles include only those patients discharged alive with approval or transferred. The meaning of percentiles can be illustrated by an example. If the 50th percentile (median) is 8 days, 50 percent of the patients stayed 8 days or less.	19
	PATIENTS 65 AND OLDER (9, 10)	
9.	**NUMBER OF PATIENTS**	13
10.	**MEDIAN STAY excluding deaths** Half of the patients 65 years old and older who were discharged alive with approval or transferred stayed this number of days or less.	19
12.	**INTERSERVICE TRANSFERS** Patients transferred from one service to another.	18: ¤
	PATIENTS WITH HOSPITAL COMPLICATIONS (13, 14) A hospital complication is defined as any condition which occurs after the patient's admission to the hospital and which modifies the course of the patient's illness or the medical care required.	
13.	**INFECTIONS** Patients for whom Hospital Infection (item 12, code 4) was marked on the case abstract.	20: I or B
14.	**OTHER** Patients for whom Other Hospital Complication (item 12, code 5) was marked on the case abstract.	20: C or B
	ADMISSION, PRE-OP, PRE-DELIVERY FINDINGS (16-21) Each finding is from the first test of its kind done during the admission period, which begins with the patient's admission to the hospital and ends at 11:59 p.m. of the following day, at the time of earliest surgery, or at the time of delivery, whichever comes first.	
17.	**URINALYSIS–ALBUMIN POSITIVE** A trace of albumin is not recorded as a positive finding.	30: A or B
22.	**AFEBRILE ADMISSIONS WITH LATER FEVER** Number of patients whose admission temperature was 99.9 F (37.9 C) or less, but whose peak temperature was 101.0 F (38.5 C) or more.	33, 34
23.	**OPTIONAL** See MRL. The same optional information appears here as in column 21 of Discharge Analysis A.	
24.	**VARIETY INDEX** The per-patient average number of different kinds of laboratory tests and diagnostic x-rays. For each patient, 63 classes of procedures may be recorded. These are PAS Case Abstract items 29-31, 34, 35, 44-46, 48, 50-54, and H-ICDA codes 93.0-95.7, 97.0, 99.7.	37-43, 45-60
25.	**MULTICHANNEL CHEMISTRY** Patients for whom multiple blood chemistry tests were performed by an automated multichannel analyzer.	4-: M or B
	TOTAL WORKUP (30-34) Patients who did not have the listed types of tests at any time during their hospital stay.	
34.	**MINIMUM LAB NOT MET** Patients, excluding babies born in the hospital, for whom minimum laboratory work (urinalysis and hemoglobin or hematocrit) was not done.	39: X
36.	**REPEAT EKG** Patients who had more than one electrocardiogram recorded.	57: R
37.	**DIAGNOSTIC RADIOISOTOPES (H-ICDA 94.6, 94.7)**	
93, 94.	**PERCENT EMERGENCY AND URGENT ADMISSIONS** "Emergency Admission" and "Urgent Admission" are defined by the hospital.	27: E or U
97.	**EXTENDED CARE FACILITY**	16: E
100.	**PERCENT OF FEMALE PATIENTS WITH PELVIC EXAMS**	15: F 35: P or B
103.	**SEROLOGICAL TEST FOR SYPHILIS**	44: S or B
104.	**PERCENT OF FEMALE PATIENTS WITH CERVICAL PAP SMEAR**	15: F 56: C
105.	**ROUTINE (survey) CHEST** Percent of patients for whom a chest x-ray (any size film) was done routinely as required by hospital policy. Excludes specifically ordered chest x-rays found in column 38.	59: R
	DEATHS (109-113)	
112.	**POST-OPERATIVE** Patients for whom Post-operative Death (PAS abstract item 8, code 8) was marked. Post-operative Death is defined by the hospital.	16: PA or PD
	AFTER OPERATION Operated patients who died in the hospital (see "Procedures NOT counted as operations" on back of M2 form for exclusions).	16: A or D
113.	**THIRD DAY OR LATER**	16: A or D 19: 3 or more
	MINIMUM LAB NOT MET Percent of deaths, excluding babies born in the hospital, without minimum laboratory work (urinalysis and hemoglobin or hematocrit).	39: X
115.	**FOLLOWUP OF ADMISSION URINARY FINDINGS–SUGAR POSITIVE, NO BLOOD SUGAR TEST** Patients with glycosuria on admission who did not have any kind of blood sugar test.	30: S or B 51: Blank
118.	**PATIENTS TREATED WITH ANTIBIOTICS** Number of these treated with antibiotics without antibiogram or culture.	71: 2,3,6,7 54: Blank 55: Blank, 1,4,5
121.	**PATIENTS WITH ADMISSION HEMOGLOBIN less than 10 grams/100 ml OR ADMISSION HEMATOCRIT less than 30 percent** (depending on which the hospital records).	28
	Percent of these patients transfused with whole blood or packed red cells.	62, 63
122.	**PATIENTS WITH ADMISSION HEMOGLOBIN of 14 grams/100 ml or more OR ADMISSION HEMATOCRIT 42 percent or more** (depending on which the hospital records).	28
	Percent of these patients transfused with whole blood or packed red cells.	62, 63
123.	**NONOPERATED PATIENTS RECEIVING PARENTERAL FLUIDS** (see "Procedures NOT counted as operations" on back of M2 form for exclusions).	64: 1,3,5,7
	Percent of these patients without electrolyte determination.	46: Blank

OPERATION GROUPS WITH H-ICDA CODE RANGES

Group Number and Name	H-ICDA Code Range
101. Central nervous system	01.0-03.9
102. Peripheral and sympathetic nerves	04.0-05.9
103. Thyroidectomy	06.1-06.2
104. Other endocrine	06.0; 06.3-07.9
105. Lens extraction	12.4-12.6
106. Other eye	08.0-12.3; 12.7-16.9
107. Ear	17.0-19.9
108. Tonsillectomy, adenoidectomy	23.1-23.3
109. Nose, larynx, trachea, and other pharynx	20.0-23.0; 23.4-23.9
110. Bronchus, lung, chest	24.0-26.9
111. Heart, intrathoracic blood vessels	30.0-33.9
112. Excision and ligation of varicose veins	36.5
113. Other peripheral and intra-abdominal blood vessels	34.0-36.4; 36.6-36.9
114. Hemic and lymphatic	37.0-38.9
115. Total mastectomy	39.2-39.5
116. Other breast	39.0-39.1; 39.6-39.9
117. Dental	40.0-40.9
118. Salivary glands, oral cavity, tongue	41.0-42.9
119. Gastrectomy	44.3-44.5
120. Other stomach, duodenum, and esophagus	43.0-44.2; 44.6-45.9
121. Appendectomy	49.1
122. Hemorrhoidectomy	51.3
123. Other intestinal tract	46.0-49.0; 49.2-51.2; 51.4-51.9
124. Cholecystectomy	53.5
125. Other biliary tract; pancreas	52.0-53.4; 53.6-54.9
126. Inguinal hernia	57.0-57.1
127. Other hernia, abdominal wall, peritoneum	55.0-56.9; 57.2-57.9
128. Prostatectomy	65.1-65.5
129. Circumcision	68.2
130. Other genitourinary	60.0-65.0; 65.6-68.1; 68.3-68.9
131. Ovary and fallopian tube	69.0-70.9
132. Hysterectomy	71.0-71.5
133. Diagnostic dilation and curettage of uterus	71.9
134. Other uterus; cervix	71.6-71.8; 72.0-72.9
135. Vagina, vulva, perineum	73.0-74.9
136. Artificial rupture of membranes	76.0
137. Outlet and low forceps, episiotomy	76.3-76.6; 76.9
138. Breech extraction	77.0-77.2
139. Cesarean section	78.0-78.9
140. Dilation and curettage after delivery or abortion	79.1-79.2
141. Other obstetrical procedures	75.0-75.9; 76.1-76.2; 76.7-76.8; 77.3-77.9; 79.0; 79.3-79.9; 99.8
142. Reduction of fracture	82.0-82.9
143. Excision of intervertebral cartilage	83.4
144. Other orthopedic procedures	80.0-81.9; 83.0-83.3; 83.5-88.5
145. Skin, subcutaneous tissue	89.0-90.9
146. Diagnostic endoscopy	91.0-92-9
147. Radiography	93.0-95.7
148. Other miscellaneous nonsurgical procedures	96.0-99.7; 99.9

M1

DIAGNOSIS GROUPS WITH H-ICDA CODE RANGES

Group Number and Name	H-ICDA Code Range
1. Infective	001-136
2. Malignant neoplasm	140-209
3. Other neoplasm	210-239
4. Diabetes mellitus	250
5. Endocrine, nutritional and metabolic	240-246; 251-279
6. Hematologic	280-289
7. Mental	290-319
8. Nervous System	320-358
9. Eye	360-379
10. Ear	380-389
11. Hypertension	400-405
12. Acute myocardial infarction	410
13. Other heart	390-398; 411-429
14. Heart	390-429
15. Cerebrovascular	430-438
16. Other vascular	440-458
17. Acute URI	460-465
18. Pneumonia and bronchitis	480-491
19. Hypertrophy of tonsils & adenoids	500
20. Other respiratory	470; 492-493; 501-519
21. Respiratory	460-493; 501-519
22. Dental	520-526
23. Peptic ulcer	531-534
24. Mouth, other upper gastrointestinal	527-530; 535-537
25. Appendix	540-543
26. Hernia	550-553
27. Other intestine and peritoneum	560-569
28. Cholecystitis and calculus	574-575
29. Liver, pancreas and other gallbladder	570-573; 576-577
30. Urinary	580-599
31. Male genital	600-607
32. Genitourinary	580-607
33. Breast	610-611
34. Cervicitis	620
35. Uterovaginal prolapse	623
36. Metrorrhagia	626.6
37. Other menstrual	626.0-626.5; 626.7-626.9
38. Other gynecological	612-616; 621-622; 624-625; 627-629
39. Female genital	612-629
40. Infection of pregnancy	630
41. Ectopic pregnancy	631
42. Hemorrhage of pregnancy	632 except 632.3
43. Threatened abortion	632.3
44. False labor	634.8
45. Acute toxemia of pregnancy	637
46. Other toxemia of pregnancy	638-639
47. Other complications of pregnancy	634.0-634.7; 634.9; 635
48. Complications of pregnancy	630-639
49. Abortion	640-646
50. Normal delivery	650
Delivery with complications:	
51. Placenta previa	651.0-651.1
52. Premature separation of placenta	651.2-651.3
53. Retained placenta	652
54. Other postpartum hemorrhage	653
55. Fetopelvic disproportion	655
56. Breech presentation	656.0
57. Uterine inertia	657.1-657.2
58. First degree laceration	658.0
59. Second and third degree laceration	658.1-658.3
60. Other obstetrical trauma	658.9-660.9
61. Premature rupture of membranes	661.0
62. Previous cesarean section	661.3
63. Umbilical cord complications	661.5-661.7
64. Other complications	651.4-651.9; 654; 656.1-657.0; 657.3-657.9; 661.1-661.2; 661.4; 661.8-661.9
65. Delivery	650-661
66. Complications of puerperium	670-678
67. Skin and subcutaneous tissue	680-709
68. Musculoskeletal	710-739
69. Congenital anomalies	740-759
70. Diseases peculiar to newborn infants	772-778
71. Signs, symptoms and ill-defined conditions	780-797
72. Fractures	800-829
73. Other trauma	830-959
74. Adverse effects	960-999
75. Special conditions	Y00-Y17
76. Newborn	Y20-Y29
77. Other	001-136; 240-607; 680-778

Figure 12–6. M1 Form – Basic Data, Findings, Investigation, (Continued).

M_2 MEDICINE INVESTIGATION (cont) 1ST QUARTER 1972 SAMPLE MANAGEMENT CITY,STATE A570

Group Number (same as column 1) 42	Total Patients (same as column 2) 43	Patients with Blood Chemistry: Blood Sugar 44	Nitrogen Derivatives 45	Electrolytes, pH 46	Liver Function 47	Transaminase, LDH 48	Proteins, Protein electrophoresis 49	Cholesterol, Lipids 50	Abnormal Results (Col 45-50): Found 51	Tests not Repeated 52	Patients with Other Tests: Bacteriology 53	Frozen Section or Cell Block 54	Any Papanicolaou 55	Gastric, Stool 56	All Operated Patients: Number of Patients 57	Percent Operated First 2 Days: Within 6 hrs 58	After 6 hrs 59	Tissue of Most Important Operation: Tissues Coded 60	Diseased A 61	Diseased B 62	No Disease 63	% of Patients with Consultations 64
PERCENTS →		70	71	37	13	30	14	13	35	73	19	2	3	5	9	3	51	25	93		7	33
	714	498	504	267	94	217	97	96	452	329	136	11	21	39	61			15	14		1	
1	37	19	18	7	8	11	7	2	28	16	7	1	1	2	4		75	3	3			27
2	6	6	6	2	2	3	3	1	6	6	3	1	1	1	2			2	2			83
4	48	48	33	16	5	9	6	6	27	17	7		2	1	1			1	1			21
5	11	10	9	6	2	3	4	7	5	5	2				1							45
6	15	5	6	4	5	5	2	1	8	6	2		1	3	1		**	1	1			33
7	23	18	17	6	2	4	2	3	7	7	2				3		67					52
8	56	42	34	9	3	4	5	5	10	10	2		1		11		45	1	1			41
11	33	29	31	16	4	13	6	7	31	27	1		1									27
12	19	7	17	17		16		5	23	13	2			1	1							42
13	125	81	100	81	22	80	18	26	142	87	19			5	2	50						25
15	42	40	37	24	3	4	7	7	36	28	4			2	10	10	40					38
16	29	21	23	9	5	8	4	5	16	14	7	1	1		7		71	1	1			55
17	2	1	2		1	2	1		1	1	1				1							50
18	84	56	55	24	10	22	12	8	37	29	48	6	8	2	5		40	2	2			20
20	29	17	15	10	5	7	5	4	10	7	9				2		**	1	1			28
23	32	17	18	8	1	5	1	2	9	7	2			13								28
24	15	11	10	2	1	1			8	8	1		1	1								20
27	27	19	21	2	1	2	1	2	8	8	3		2	4								44
29	4	3	3	2	3	2	2	1	6	6												50
32	2	2	2	1					2	2					1		**	1	1			50
67	7	4	4			1	1	1	3	2	2											29
68	22	18	16	4	1	2	4	2	3	3	2	1	1		2		50	1	1			41
71	37	22	25	14	9	10	5	1	19	16	9	1	1	4	7		71	1			1	46
74	8	2	2	3	1	3	1		7	4	1											38
75	1																					

Group Number 42	Blood Transfusions (includes whole blood and packed RBC): Total Patients 65	Patients with 1 Unit 66	Patients with 2 Units 67	Units: Total 68	% Packed RBC 69	Patients Given: Plasma, Blood Derivatives 70	Parenteral Fluids 71	Care in ICU or CCU 72	Oxygen 73	Inhalation Therapy 74	Radiation Therapy 75	Patients Given Drugs: Oral Antidiabetics 76	Hormones: Insulin 77	Thyroid, Antithyroid 78	Steroid 79	Hypotensives 80	Diuretics 81	Vasopressors 82	Vasodilators 83	Cardiac Regulators 84	Anticoagulants 85	Sulfas 86	Antibiotics 87	Other Anti-infectives 88	Tranquilizers 89
PERCENTS →	3	15	20		23		20	14	17	9		10	7	2	7	9	19		11	20	7	2	30	3	37
	20	3	4	60			140	103	120	61	1	68	47	16	48	61	136	2	82	142	47	11	214	18	264
1							6	1				3			2	3	2			1			12	1	12
2	4	1	1	11	36		1		2		1				4		3			3			3		3
4							5	1	3	4		20	34		3	6	8		3	13			12		16
5												1		4	3		2	1					4	1	3
6	4		1	11	55		2		1	1						2	1		1	2	1		3		5
7							3	2							2								4		16
8							4	3	2	1		2	1		5	1	1		6	1	1	2	5	1	23
11							1	2	1	1		4	1		2	17	15		2	4		1	2	1	12
12	1	1		1			16	18	16			1			1		1		4	7	15	1	7		13
13	2			6	33		35	41	52	5		16	5	1	4	13	71	1	32	78	17	4	31	5	60
15	1			4			20	12	3	2		2	3		3	7	8		20	7	2	1	12		8
16							2	1	3	1		1		1		2	8		8	5	10		10	2	7
17																							1		
18	1	1		1			15	6	21	35		9	1	5	7	5	7		2	12	1		73		27
20							6	2	6	8		3	1	4	3		2		1	4			17	1	11
23	5		1	20	10		7	3	2	1		3					2		1	4			3	1	11
24							1			1		1				1	1								5
27	1		1	2			1								1	2	2			1		1	1	1	9
29							3	1															2		2
32																1									
67													1		2								2		
68							1					1		1	5	1	2					1	1		4
71	1			4			7	7	5	1		1							2				7	4	12
74							4	3	3						1								2		4
75																									1

Group	126 SPECIAL
C	
D	
E	
F	
G	

127 BLOOD SUGAR

Fasting, Random	440
2-Hour Postprandial	58
≥ 150 mg %	95
Non-diabetic ≥ 150 mg %: Number	29
Non-diabetic ≥ 150 mg %: Without GTT	26

128 OTHER TESTS

Skin	27
Toxicology	8

129 SPECIAL CARE

CCU	74
Isolation	14

130 OPERATED PTS OVER 40

PATIENTS:	43
No Chest X-ray	4
No EKG	22
No Blood Sugar	7
No Nitrogen Deriv	8

131 DIASTOLIC BP ≥ 100mm

PATIENTS:	193
No Diagnosis of Hypertension	138
No Diuretics	133
No Hypotensives	149

132 DIURETICS

PATIENTS:	136
No Blood Pressure	2
No Weight	51
No Urinalysis	2
No Electrolyte Determination	56

133 ANTICOAGULANTS

PATIENTS:	47
No Pro Time	3
No Coag Test	10
Low Hgb/Hct	1

134 OTHER THERAPY

IPPB	59
Hypothermia	
Rh Immune Globulin	
PT	10
OT	

135 Packed RBC Patients as % of All Patients Transfused: 30

136 DATA BY DAY OF ADMISSION AND DISCHARGE

	All Pts	Mon	Tues	Wed	Thurs	Fri	Sat	Sun
Average Stay by Day of Admission (Excl 31+ Stays)	88	94	88	77	83	96	84	87
Is average stay significantly different from (All Pts)								
% Admitted on		15	14	13	13	19	12	13
% Discharged on		12	16	13	15	18	18	8

ANALYSIS BY TEACHING STATUS 137	Total Patients 138	Median Stay (Excl Deaths) 139	Variety Index 140	Multichannel Chemistry 141	Min Lab Not Met 142
				%	%
				%	%
ALL PTS	714	7	12	6 %	4 %

Form 126-2-70 Copyright 1970 by COMMISSION ON PROFESSIONAL AND HOSPITAL ACTIVITIES, Ann Arbor, Michigan

*Figure exceeds space provided. (For percents, ** means 100%.)

M_2

M_2 Form Column Number	Column(s) Used as Base for Percent
44–50	43
51	45 to 50#
52	51
53–57	43
58	57
59	57
60	57
61	60
62	60
63	60
64	43
65	43
66	65
67	65
69	68
70–89	43

#means that the sum of the column totals is used for the base.

MEDICAL AUDIT PROGRAM

MEDICAL STAFF COPY

Printed in U.S.A.

M_2 FORM – INVESTIGATION, MANAGEMENT

Used for PAS-MAP Quarterly Reports

Figure 12-7. M2 Form – Investigation Management.

Procedures NOT counted as operations:

1) Procedures which are coded primarily for indexing purposes:

H-ICDA code	
32.7	Closed chest cardiac massage
32.8	Electric defibrillation and countershock
38.0	Bone marrow aspiration
70.7	Insufflation of fallopian tube
81.6	Traction or fixation without manipulation for reduction
91.0	Otoscopy } for removal of foreign body
91.1	Rhinoscopy } for removal of foreign body
91.2	Laryngoscopy and tracheoscopy } without effect upon tissue or lesion
91.5	Endoscopy of colon and rectum } without effect upon tissue or lesion
91.7	Colposcopy } without effect upon tissue or lesion
91.8	Other endoscopy
91.9	Fiber optic examination, any site
93.2	Radiography of nasolacrimal ducts and nasal sinuses
93.3	Bronchography
93.4	Cholecystography and cholangiography
93.5	Intravenous pyelography (IVP)
93.7	Cystography
93.8	Nephrotomography
94.1	Mammography
94.2	Hysterography
94.5	Other contrast radiography
94.6	Radioisotope scanning examination
94.7	Other radioisotope examination
94.8	Ultrasonic radiography
94.9	Other radiography
96.0	Superficial radiation therapy
96.1	Deep radiation therapy
96.2	Supervoltage or megavoltage irradiation
96.3	Particle irradiation from electrical source
96.5	Radioactive isotope therapy
96.6	Chemotherapy } for cancer
96.8	Hormone therapy } for cancer
96.9	Other therapy } for cancer
97.0-97.9	Physical Medicine and Rehabilitation
98.0-98.9	Osteopathic manipulative therapy
99.0	Electroshock therapy
99.1	Insulin shock therapy
99.2	Psychotherapy
99.3	Exchange transfusion
99.6	Hyperbaric oxygenation
99.7	Spinal puncture
99.8	Medical induction of labor
99.9	Other nonsurgical procedures

2) The routine procedures to assist delivery:

H-ICDA code	
76.0	Surgical induction of labor
76.1	External version
76.3-76.6	Outlet and low forceps delivery with and without episiotomy
76.9	Episiotomy

3) Circumcision, H-ICDA 68.2, for newborn

M2

1970 ○

1971 ○

1st Quarter ○

2nd Quarter ○

3rd Quarter ○

4th Quarter ○

PAS-MAP

All patients { SUMMARY OF SERVICES ○

All patients {
- PEDIATRIC MEDICINE ○
- MEDICINE ○
- SURGERY (BY DIAGNOSIS) ○
- OBSTETRICS (BY DIAGNOSIS) ○
- NEWBORN ○

All operated patients {
- CHILDREN (BY OPERATION) ○
- ADULTS (BY OPERATION) ○
- OBSTETRICS (BY OPERATION) ○

The notes below explain the content of the columns and boxes of the M report when the headings are not self-explanatory.

The number to the right of the column or box title indicates the column of the C form where you can find the patients included in the statistic on the M form. When particular codes apply, they follow the column references, separated by a colon.

Column or Box — C Form Column: Code

44. PATIENTS WITH BLOOD CHEMISTRY (44-50) BLOOD SUGAR test (any) 51

51. ABNORMAL RESULTS—FOUND 45-50: + or R
Number of *tests* among those displayed in columns 45-50 with abnormal results

52. ABNORMAL RESULTS—TESTS NOT REPEATED 45-50: +
Number of tests (column 51) not repeated

53. MICROBIOLOGY 54, 55: 1-3, 5-7
Patients who had one or more of: bacterial smear, culture, antibiogram

54. FROZEN SECTION OR CELL BLOCK 56: 2 or F
Patients who had a frozen section, a cell block, or both

55. ANY PAPANICOLAOU (cervical or other) 56: C or P

56. GASTRIC analysis, STOOL analysis 53

ALL OPERATED PATIENTS (57-63)
See list at left for exclusions.

60. TISSUE OF MOST IMPORTANT OPERATION CODED by pathologist 8: 1-3

61. DISEASED A (generally requiring surgical removal) 8:1

62. DISEASED B (diseased, but surgical removal not clearly indicated from pathological findings alone) 8:2

63. NO DISEASE 8:3

68. TOTAL UNITS 62, 63
The symbol "+" means that at least one patient had 9 or more *units* of whole blood or packed cells

72. CARE IN ICU OR CCU 66: 1-3, 5-7
Patients treated in an intensive care unit, cardiac (coronary) care unit, or both

73. PATIENTS GIVEN OXYGEN 65: 4-7
Excludes routine oxygen during anesthesia or in recovery room

74. INHALATION THERAPY 65: 1-3, 5-7
Patients treated with intermittent positive pressure breathing apparatus or other inhalation therapy

75. RADIATION THERAPY (H-ICDA 96.0-96.5)

126. SPECIAL C, D, E, F, G 26, 61, 72
Optional data. See MRL.

127. BLOOD SUGAR—NON-DIABETIC ≥ 150 mg % 51
Patients without a recorded diagnosis of diabetes mellitus (H-ICDA 250.0-250.9) who had a blood sugar of 150 mg % or more

WITHOUT GLUCOSE TOLERANCE TEST 51: +
Number of these non-diabetic patients who did not have a glucose tolerance test

130. OPERATED PATIENTS OVER 40
Patients 40 years old or older who were operated (see list at left for exclusions).

Number of these patients who had no:

Chest x-ray (any)	59: Blank or D
EKG	57: Blank
Blood sugar (any)	51: Blank
Nitrogen derivatives (BUN, NPN, etc.)	45: Blank

131. DIASTOLIC BLOOD PRESSURE ≥ 100 mm 32: 4-9
Patients with an admission diastolic blood pressure of 100 mm or more (see column 20 on M₁ form).

Number of these patients who had no:

Diagnosis of hypertension (H-ICDA 400.0-405.0)	
Diuretics	70: Blank, 2, 4, 6
Hypotensives	70: Blank, 1, 4, 5

132. DIURETICS 70: 1, 3, 5, 7
Patients treated with diuretics (see column 81).

Number of these patients who had no:

Blood pressure recorded on admission	31, 32: Blank
Weight recorded	36: Blank or H
Urinalysis	38: Blank
Electrolyte determination	46: Blank

133. ANTICOAGULANTS 68: 2, 3, 6, 7
Patients treated with anticoagulants (see column 85).

Number of these patients who had no:

Prothrombin time	42: Blank or C
Other coagulation test	42: Blank or P

Number of these patients who had low Hemoglobin (<10 gm%) or hematocrit (<30%) 28

134. OTHER THERAPY
Patients with

Intermittent positive pressure breathing apparatus	65: 1, 3, 5, 7
Hypothermia	67: 1, 3, 5, 7
Rh immune globulin	64: 4-7
Physical therapy (H-ICDA 97.1)	
Occupational therapy (H-ICDA 97.3)	

135. PACKED R B C PATIENTS AS PERCENT OF ALL PATIENTS TRANSFUSED 62, 63

$$\frac{\text{Number of patients given packed cells}}{\text{Number of patients given whole blood, packed cells, or both}} \times 100$$

136. DATA BY DAY OF ADMISSION AND DISCHARGE
Patients with stays of 31 days or more are excluded from all computations.

Line 53—
Average stay of all patients discharged during the period of this report followed by the average stay of patients admitted each day of the week. The digit to the right of the dotted line indicates tenths of a day.

Line 54—
If the difference between the stay of patients admitted on any given day of the week and the all-patient average is statistically significant (at the 5% level), "Yes" prints. A significance test is not done for fewer than 10 patients.

Lines 55, 56—
Percent of patients admitted and discharged on each day of the week.

137-142. ANALYSIS BY TEACHING STATUS 17
Patients are grouped by teaching status (such as ward, teaching private, and private) if the hospital has arranged to record this information. Otherwise, all patients are shown on one line.
For definitions see notes for columns 6, 24, 25, and 34 on M₁ form.

Figure 12–7. M2 Form – Investigation Management, (Continued).

patients demanding any service in a given quarter. For many services it should be possible to refer to the attached C report list to identify the records of patients demanding service. By sampling from those patients who demanded service a mean value of the number of units per patient could be calculated to the necessary degree of accuracy, either by service or by diagnosis. It may also be possible to view the time series of one or both of the investigational indexes as an approximation of the growth of diagnostic services required per patient discharge.

The number of urgent patients admitted is reported on the M form, as is the number of emergency patients admitted and the number of emergency operations performed within six hours of admission. These data are given both by service and by procedure and by diagnosis. If this information is accurately recorded in the medical record and thus accurately reported on the M form, it becomes a measure of an important segment of hospital demand. In addition to providing measures of the percentage of demand in these two categories, the patients falling into the categories are identified for further study by sampling or otherwise.

The Length-of-Stay Package

The use of statistical techniques in PAS-MAP has increased in recent years. In addition to tests of significance of length of stay versus the day of week of admission, the commission has developed statistical analysis for the measurement of changes in the variety index. Standard deviations of the index by a diagnostic category and operative category were calculated by the Commission, and a nomograph for testing the significance of the difference of individual hospitals from pool data was presented to subscribing hospitals in 1964.[18] The most statistically sophisticated program that the commission has developed to date is the length-of-stay analysis which is reported on form S (figure 12-8). Using data from several million discharges and most subscribing hospitals, the commission creates a matrix of 3,660 cells which categorized discharges as follow: (a) final diagnosis causing hospitalization—183 diagnostic groups; (b) the patient age in five groups—0-19, 20-34, 35-49, 50-64, and 65 and older—(c) whether operated or not operated; (d) whether there were or were not secondary diagnoses.[19] For each cell in which cases occurred the mean, variance and 5th, 10th, 50th, 75th, 90th, 95th, and 99th percentiles of the length-of-stay distribution were calculated. Patients who died were excluded from the calculations. These sets of statistics comprise a master table against which the achievement of small groups of patients can be compared and the comparison tested for statistical significance. The work is updated periodically, and the basic data is published in summarized form.[20]

A program has been constructed which will accept sets of discharges, allocate

PAGE 1 1ST QUARTER 1972 MEDICINE

PAS LENGTH OF STAY STUDY
MAP DATA

SAMPLE, CITY, STATE

A570

BASE DATA
9.0 million patient discharges during the period JAN 70–DEC 70 from 1127 short-term general PAS hospitals in UNITED STATES

1. **PATIENT GROUP**
   (For patients grouped by diagnosis or operation, H-ICDA codes are shown in this column.)
2. **TOTAL PATIENTS**
   Excludes patients (in reports "BY OPERATION") if all the procedure codes are among those listed on the back of this form as not constituting operations.
3. **TOTAL PATIENTS STUDIED**
   Excludes deaths; patients with age not recorded; patients with date of admission or discharge misrecorded; and patients who stayed 100 or more days (although these patients are counted in column 3. (See back of form for more detail.) Also excludes patients (in reports "BY OPERATION") if the primary procedure recorded on the PAS Case Abstract does not constitute an operation.
4. **AVERAGE STAY**
   The average stay of patients counted in column 3.
5. **AVERAGE STAY FOR MATCHING PATIENTS**
   The average stay of patients in the BASE DATA with characteristics similar to patients counted in column 3. (See back of form for more detail.)
6. **DIFFERENCE**
   The difference between the average stays shown in columns 4 and 5.
7. **IS DIFFERENCE SIGNIFICANT?**
   "YES" means that the stay pattern for the patient group studied differs, in a statistically significant way, from the pattern for the matching patients. (The computer gives each patient a tag showing whether he stayed a longer or a shorter time than half his matching patients. If the proportion of patients tagged as staying longer or as staying shorter is unusually high for the number of patients in the group, the computer prints "YES". Testing is done at the 5% level of significance.)
8. **SHORT STAY PATIENTS**
   Number of patients who stayed a shorter time than 95% of the matching patients (under the 5th percentile).
9. **LONG STAY PATIENTS**
   Number of patients who stayed longer than 90% of the matching patients (over the 90th percentile). Includes patients staying 100 or more days.

	FINAL DX EXPLAINING ADMISSION	TOTAL PATIENTS	TOTAL PATIENTS STUDIED	AVERAGE STAY	AVERAGE STAY FOR MATCHING PATIENTS	DIFFERENCE	IS DIFFERENCE SIGNIFICANT?	SHORT STAY PATIENTS	LONG STAY PATIENTS
		2	3	4	5	6	7	8	9
1	INFECTIVE 001–136	37	36	6.5	8.4	−1.9		2	4
2	MALIGNANT NEOPLASM 140–209	6	4	19.8	13.5	+6.3			5
4	DIABETES MELLITUS 250	48	47	11.0	11.2	−0.2		1	1
5	ENDOCRINE, NUTRITION, METABCL 240–246, 251–279	11	11	9.8	7.8	+2.0			2
6	HEMATOLOGIC 280–289	15	15	6.9	8.3	−1.4			
7	MENTAL 290–319	23	23	6.7	12.0	−5.3		2	
8	NERVOUS SYSTEM 320–358	56	56	11.0	9.2	+1.8	YES		8
11	HYPERTENSION 400–405	33	33	8.7	9.1	−0.4		1	3
12	ACUTE MYOCARDIAL INFARCTION 410	19	15	19.1	22.0	−2.9			
13	OTHER HEART 390–398, 411–429	125	112	11.4	12.8	−1.4		2	7
15	CEREBROVASCULAR 430–438	42	30	10.8	17.5	−6.7		1	
16	OTHER VASCULAR 440–458	29	28	11.1	13.6	−2.5			1
17	ACUTE UPPER RESP INFECTION 460–465	2	2	6.0	8.7	−2.7			
18	PNEUMONIA AND BRONCHITIS 480–491	84	81	9.2	10.3	−1.1		1	5
20	OTHER RESPIRATORY 470, 492–493, 501–519	29	27	7.6	9.1	−1.5			2
23	PEPTIC ULCER 531–534	32	31	8.7	7.9	+0.8		.2	5

Form 140.71 Copyright 1970 by COMMISSION ON PROFESSIONAL AND HOSPITAL ACTIVITIES, Ann Arbor, Michigan Printed in U.S.A.

S FORM — LENGTH OF STAY COMPARISON   Used for Length of Stay Quarterly Reports

Figure 12-8. S Form — Length of Stay Comparison.

them to the appropriate cells of the original matrix, construct a table comparing median length of stays in the cells of the sample set with the corresponding cells from the master table, construct the weighted median for each set, and indicate the significance of the difference as tested by the fraction of sample patients above the pool median. In addition, a second program will compare individual cases in the sample set with a preestablished percentile of the appropriate master table's cell and will print on a C report form the abstract for any case which is outside the preestablished limits. Hospitals subscribing to the length-of-stay package routinely receive reports of length of stay for their patients in total, and by physician, and by service with the corresponding master table mean stay and an indication of significance and deviation at the 5 percent confidence level. In addition, the S report shows the number of patients in the hospital set for each category which exceed the 90th or fail to reach the fifth percentile of the master set distribution for their cell. If a hospital exactly matched the master table distribution, an average of 15 percent of their patients would appear in these two categories. Review of the deviation from this level can provide an indication as to the change in shape of their length of stay distribution as compared to the master table. In addition, printed values on the C report facilitate utilization review of individual cases following the procedure usually used in the medical audit.

Use of PAS Data

The experience of hospitals participating in PAS-MAP is difficult to assess collectively. Undoubtedly differences in the strength and kind of motivation that led hospitals to join affect the amount of use they make of the information. In addition, those hospitals which are known by the Commission to be particularly active users generally supply substantial refinement and study of the output data by administrative, medical, or medical records personnel. This includes the preparation of selected summary or representative statistics, or the careful and detailed review of reports to identify situations or cases of particular interest to medical staff committees. It would appear that further refinement of the statistics in this manner is of great value in increasing the efficiency of committee activity and in relieving the staff of work which is to them often tedious and unrewarding.

Extensive special studies are possible using the data available from PAS. One such study by Stapleton and Zwerneman compared the quality of private medical care among certified specialist physicians, noncertified physicians, and patients on a nursing unit which was used for teaching purposes by the intern and resident staff. Using data essentially taken from the M form, the researchers established a variety of tables comparing patients grouped according to the categories of physicians. Differences in the results were tested by chi square.[21]

As previously noted, a number of significant differences did appear which tended to indicate generally that the patients of noncertified physicians received less thorough workups than those of certified physicians or house staff members.

Limitations of PAS-MAP Data

PAS alone has a number of mechanical limitations which are relieved by the use of the combined PAS-MAP output forms. The statistics in the A and B reports are too grossly aggregated, and a number of important indices are not statistically reported. The B report is not organized by service and thus inhibits a plan of searching for quality variation which might be logically related to the hospital organization. These difficulties are to a large extent overcome by the inclusion of the M report. Some other limitations remain, however. For the most part, these are inherent in the basic constraints of the system. The system does not provide for continuity of care to individual patients; that is, it is not normally easy to compare subsequent admissions of the same patient. It covers only inpatient care, and the limitation of abstracting effort means that the values of many tests or the number of repetitions of tests and therapeutic activities must be omitted. There are also some problems with using the discharge as the base for statistics. It is not normally convenient to reconstruct census-based data. Even such elementary questions as the average census of the hospital can be approximated only with some months' delay. (It is necessary for all patients who are in the hospital on the day of interest to have been discharged before the census can be measured.) The lack of either judgmental or statistical quality standards means that all possible statistics must be reported. With a few exceptions, they are all given equal weight on the reporting form. As can be seen from the examples, this leads to a voluminous and formidable set of numbers. It is rare that any one reader will be interested in all of these numbers or even any substantial fraction of them at any one reading. The coded nature of the output on some of the forms, particularly the indexes and lists on form C, facilitates scanning and case selection, but appears to make case review from the abstract more difficult.[a]

Suggestions for the improvement of PAS-MAP within the context of a manually-prepared case abstract generally center around increased flexibility of both input and output documents. As noted above, Comiskey has suggested departmentally-oriented forms for both abstract and output with additional combined output sheets for certain items of general interest.[22] A student proposal for modifying PAS to meet the needs of all Connecticut hospitals proposed: (a) adding data on the patient's address, (b) identifying the institu-

---

[a]CPHA maintains that it has the capability of printing the abstract in English text, but prefers to use the condensed format because of its comparative possibilities (personal correspondence, Dr. Slee).

tions to which and from which transfer occurred, (c) using a constant patient number regardless of the hospital of admission within Connecticut, and (d) a constant doctor number to be added to the input form. Any monthly reports received by the hospitals would be the same as the current PAS-MAP format, but a few summary reports would be included to permit staff executive committees, administrators, and trustees to maintain current reports of critical indicators. An example of one of these is shown in figure 12-9. The report is organized to give current data by service and to give total data for the present month, past month and previous twelve months combined. In addition, provision was made for showing the state average achievement on the indicator.[23]

Output forms showing state aggregated data and historic trends of indices, such as proposed for Connecticut hospitals, require a substantial change in the computer system so that such data are routinely available on disk or other relatively rapid access storage device. The proposed system for Connecticut envisaged such a random access storage file and proposed to make further use of it by permitting extensive special studies both of groups of hospitals and of time series analysis of specific statistics selected by individual hospitals. Flexibility of this sort would facilitate both quality control and planning activities in member hospitals. It would also permit easy establishment of hospital service areas and extensive use of the information for regional and statewide planning purposes. Pooled data on the quality of medical care should be of substantial use to the state's Regional Medical Program which could use it both to isolate problems in the quality of care and to measure its own progress against these. It is estimated that for the thirty-five hospitals in Connecticut, approximately 30,000,000 characters of storage would be required for a five-year random access record. If relatively slow access times are accepted, automated storage is now both feasible and economically within reach for a small state or region. Such a system may soon be practical on a national level from the view point of the size of the storage problem. However, the data would still have to be reported regionally. The national report's usefulness would be substantially reduced with less than 100 percent cooperation.

Research is currently being undertaken to place large parts of the medical record directly on the computer. To the extent that this is achieved, the limitations imposed by the preparation of manual abstracts would be eliminated. At that time it will be possible to take many of the statistics defined by PAS and translate them to built-in quality of care controls. Thus programs could routinely remind the physician that minimum laboratory work had not been ordered on his patient rather than relying on detection of this failure some days or weeks after the fact. Other statistics, such as the percentage of normal tissue removed for specified operations, could be drawn from the computer on request or could be routinely programmed for publication monthly in convenient and specifically designed output forms.

The creation and use of computer-accessible data banks on a permanent basis

QUALITY OF CARE REPORT

INDICATORS	State Average (%)	Present Month (%)	Past Month (%)	Previous 12 Months (%)	MED (%)	SURG (%)	OB-GYN (%)	PED (%)	Other (%)
Admitting Lab:									
No admitting laboratory tests									
No urinalysis									
No hemoglobin or hematocrit									
Blood Use:									
Single unit transfusions									
Transfusion reactions									
Pathology:									
Tissue requiring removal									
Tissue removal justifiable									
No tissue disease									
No tissue reported									
Autopsy and Mortality:									
Autopsy rate									
Death rate									
Anesthesia death rate									
Post-op death rate									
Infant mortality rate									
Perinatal death rate									
Maternal mortality rate									
Consultations:									
General rate									
Primary C-section rate									
Sterilization rate									
Procedures which interrupted known or suspected pregnancies*									
Other:									
Post-op infection rate									
Primary C-section rate									
C-section rate									
Therapeutic abortion rate									
Sterilizations									
Complications rate									
Prematurity rate									

*Absolute numbers

Figure 12-9. Quality of Care Report.

represents a fundamental change in approach from that which PAS-MAP has used so far. It will increase the cost of the service by a substantial amount, and the justification of the increased cost must come from increased use of the information. The opportunities lie in both planning and control, but the greatest immediate returns seem to lie with control, particularly control of utilization. An experimental system exploring the opportunities in computerized data storage is described in the following chapter.

Additional Readings

Commission on Professional and Hospital Activities, 1968 Green Road, Ann Arbor, Michigan 48105. The Commission has a variety of descriptive literature on its services and reports of analysis of its data.

Donabedian, A. "Evaluating The Quality of Medical Care," *Milbank Memorial Fund Quarterly*, pt. 2, July 1966.

Donabedian, A. *A Guide to Medical Care Administration*, vol. 2, American Public Health Association, Washington, D.C., 1969.

13 Advanced Information Systems for Hospital Planning and Control

Characteristics of a Comprehensive Information System

The future development of the use of quantitative techniques for planning and control is inevitably linked with the development and use of computer applications in hospitals. As of the early 1970s, these uses, while impressive in themselves, remained far short of an integrated hospital information system. Computer applications in any enterprise follow a pattern of three stages. Elementary applications replace clerks in the production chores of management—pay checks, account statements, inventory lists, etc. The second level of application is to recurring process decisions—scheduling, quality control, inventory reorder decision, etc. The third stage applies the computer to nonrecurring decisions. These are principally planning decisions. Applications begin with forecasting and include the development of models to find the optimum size of facilities and design of processes. Ultimately, this stage reaches an interactive level where the computer becomes an extension of the manager's brain, proposing alternatives, analyzing and criticizing them, and learning from its past activities.

During the 1960s, hospitals made partial but incomplete achievements in the first area, scattered and fragmentary efforts in the second, and only experimental forays into the third. "Business office" functions are the easiest to transfer to the computer, and by 1970 many applications had been made. These handle varying portions of activities in different hospitals, but generally they process basic accounting information including generation of patient accounts, records of quantity and dollar value of sales, payrolls and personnel records, inventory records, and records of supplies utilization. The systematic collection of a great deal of information about resources and outputs is a by-product of these production systems.

The first common hospital applications were generally to payroll and accounts receivable preparation. Initially, hospitals purchased or leased computers for these tasks, and many hospitals still operate their own computer equipment for this purpose. Later, however, the advantages of sharing equipment, programs, and computer operating personnel among several hospitals led to various forms of cooperative systems. The simplest of these is the *service bureau* concept, where a hospital purchases services, including some programming, from a commercial vendor. Other schemes were developed which included cooperative management of the computer service, and the development of skilled programming teams capable of serving hospitals' unique problems. These systems have been sponsored by Blue Cross plans, religious orders, and corporations owned and operated by hospitals. Their advantages lie in the economics of computer services:

1. Larger machines have a higher total cost, but also a much larger processing capability, so that their cost per unit of computation is lower
2. Larger machines are more flexible. They can handle a wider variety of problems. They can be programmed more cheaply
3. Many hospital problems are similar. Basic programming for inpatient accounts, for example, is essentially the same in any hospital, although details may vary. Programming skills are scarce and expensive, and they can be shared as well as hardware

Centralized systems have a valuable by-product as well. They tend to produce comparable interhospital and regional data which are of management interest.

The information processing associated with medical records and medical care remains a major production function in the hospital which so far has not been computerized at an economical level. Prototype machines for replacing the paper work functions of the medical records, such as the transmission of medical orders and the recording of notes on diagnosis and treatment, have been developed by several computer manufacturers and proven as technically feasible. Their costs, however, have not been comparable to manual costs. The prototypes generally rely upon cathode ray tube display and light pen or other high speed input device. These require a highly structured set of program routines and subroutines. The input/output device itself is of very high cost. It must be supported by an expensive investment in software development and a very large, high-speed computer system with large storage capability.

Achievements at the second level of computer utilization, application to recurring management decisions, are occurring steadily. Considerable research effort is being devoted to the development of models for staffing, scheduling, and reordering. By 1969, several commercial companies were selling package processes for specific tasks such as nurse scheduling or inpatient bed scheduling. The general area of control systems on quality, utilization and efficiency is also a part of second level applications. The application such as PAS and HAS described in chapters 11 and 12 are early examples of computer use at this level. The advantages of centralized, rather than individual hospital computers, apply to these activities as well as production applications.

These models of recurring decision-making processes have slightly different computer hardware and software requirements than do business office functions. The "memory" functions of the computer tend to be less important than the "logic" functions. Calculations become more numerous so that ease of programming and computing speed are more necessary. They also have different interactions with human operators. A paycheck or patient charge printer repeats a previously established routine hundreds of times without change or interruption. A nurse scheduling program runs two or three times a day and provides guidelines to a human supervisor. Conditions change between each run, requiring new input of information. Convenient transmission of information to and from the point of use—the nursing floor or the admitting office, for example—becomes more desirable, so that questions of remote terminals arise. The computers best suited for this work are the large "general purpose" machines which are more common in universities than in hospitals. Machines of this size are expensive in themselves, but they carry with them extensive software costs as well. Hospitals will probably find it necessary to group together to afford the kind of hardware and software that is required.

This trend is continued into the third level, nonrecurring decisions. Here the human decision maker is even more dominant. He designs the model, selects the solution technique, and calls into play one or more of the mathematical algorithms which will aid his thinking. As we have seen in the preceding chapters, these range from regression and analysis of variance to mathematical programming, simulation, and present value analysis. The software for these tasks is in libraries of statistical and operations research programs. Universities maintain such libraries and so do the large computer manufacturers, but they are clearly out of reach of individual hospitals.

All of these factors seem to indicate the eventual centralization of computer services, either around cooperative arrangements among hospitals and related agencies or around the capabilities of commercial firms. Exactly what hardware will reside in the hospital of the future is probably subject to change as the years go by. There is a good chance that much work will be done locally, but large parts will be done through centralized services. Not only do the hardware and software considerations encourage this conclusion. The need for certain shared data, such as the residence and hospitalization patterns necessary for relevance index calculations press in the same direction. Developments in computer technology are reinforcing this trend to centralization. It is now quite feasible and in some cases economically practical to use computer facilities at great distances. Technology has advanced to the point where the information user can interact directly and instantly with the computer through input/output devices whose performance is quite independent of whether the central processing unit is nearby or far away. Such capability of instantaneous direct interaction between user and computer is called *on line, real time* computer use. It has already found practical industrial application in airline scheduling and banking.

The development of comprehensive hospital management information systems will parallel the technical and economic computer capability for second and third stage applications, but it will also reflect the general pressures of a social and political nature toward centralized planning, stricter cost control, and more comprehensive institutional services. The evolution of information systems will be in a piecework fashion, with gaps and weaknesses caused by unsolved technical problems. The biggest technical gap in the foreseeable future is that caused by the lack of computerized medical record information. It can be partially filled by computerizing abstracted information in the manner pioneered by PAS, and by using information collected from other sources. Other areas where the practical system will fall short of the ideal will occur and will have to be met by similar efforts to estimate or to reconstruct the missing information. The outline of the general information system for hospital management is now relatively clear, however. It will include the following components:

1. Basic measures of resource utilization and output will be generated essentially as a by-product of computerized accounting processes, with standardized definitions and calculating routines
2. Data on demand and utilization will be accumulated regionally on small geographic areas permitting the routine calculation of service specific relevance and commitment indices
3. Data on the quality and utilization of medical care will be obtained from an abstracting process very similar to the present PAS system. This will be manual until the record itself is computerized. It may remain a manual process, at least in part, some time after that
4. Additional information on the state of the demand upon the system, and the quality of performance will be input to the computer at frequent intervals (daily or more often). This information will be used in staffing, scheduling, inventory reorder and quality control models, to advise middle management of hospitals in a variety of areas
5. There will be provisions to include specialized data of various kinds pertinent to specific planning or control problems. This will include special sampling studies and opinion surveys. Computer routines will facilitate analysis, while data collection will be largely manual
6. Data banks of historical information in output, resource consumption, quality and other statistics of interest will be available on either magnetic tape or disk storage. These data will be organized to facilitate either routine or special computer analysis. They will include comparative information among hospitals and regional compilations
7. Computer programs will be available for most analytic tasks. These will include general programs for multiple regression and analysis of variance, statistical quality control, simulation, and mathematical programming. They will also include routines for constructing graphs and visual display. Specialized programs will be developed for handling recurring decisions such as inpatient scheduling and nurse staffing
8. There will be provision for both routine and specialized output. Routine outputs will be highly differentiated and oriented to the needs of

individual hospitals and departments. They will stress error signals and tend to suppress normal findings. Reports will be oriented towards management action rather than data display, since the original data will be on file and special reports can draw upon the files as needed

Substantial costs are involved in the development of such systems. These costs will not be justified solely by the substitution of mechanical for human calculating manpower. That level of justification—the number of clerk positions eliminated in the business office and related monetary returns on the computer investment—will never be sufficient to cover the total information system costs. The major justification will come instead from improved decision-making. Better planning of service requirements, more equitable and efficient resource allocation, and better control of quality and utilization of services will be the major returns on the expenditure. When the computerized medical record becomes cost feasible, the justification will lie in error reduction and quality improvement and in the reduction of time requirements of highly trained professionals like doctors and nurses. While all of these benefits could be reduced to tangible monetary terms, it is not likely that they will be. Computer development and investment decisions will be nonmonetary cost benefit decisions which will be unusually demanding in terms of management judgment.

No regional data system exists today with the kind of integrated data files and program capability reflected in these criteria. However, some effort is being made in this direction. One example of the advanced efforts is the Connecticut Utilization and Patient Information System (CUPIS). This system went into operation in 1971, in a form including much of the information necessary for demand analysis and analysis of the quality of patient care. Eight hospitals in Connecticut (of thirty-five eligible) participated by 1972. Accounting procedures and other components which are necessary can presumably be added to the system as it evolves. The CUPIS system is particularly worthy of study because of its integration with a highly sophisticated, computer-oriented statistical quality control procedure, called Basic Utilization Review Program (BURP). CUPIS and BURP are reviewed here as a prototype of systems to come.

The CUPIS Data Base

Organization for CUPIS

The state of Connecticut has some advantages in terms of size and resources which give it unusual opportunities to develop a comprehensive management information system.[1] The state is relatively small and is served by only thirty-five acute general hospitals, all of which are voluntary not-for-profit organizations and long-standing members of the Connecticut Hospital Association. In addition, there is only a single Blue Cross Plan in the state. This circumstance, of a relatively small group with generally cohesive interests, was augmented by the resources of the Yale University School of Medicine and Program in Hospital Administration. As a result, the state was one of the first to establish a standardized cost-accounting system. The Connecticut Hospital Association first provided standardized departmental cost reports for member hospitals a number of years ago. Several hospitals were also members of PAS, and thus familiarity was gained with the combined use of accounting data and patient record data for planning and control purposes. A survey of the possibilities of statewide, uniform patient statistical data was undertaken by graduate students in the Yale Program in Hospital Administration in 1967 at the request of the Connecticut Hospital Association.[2] Following completion of this study, a developmental project was undertaken by the Connecticut Regional Medical Program, with an advisory committee composed of representatives of Connecticut Blue Cross Association, Connecticut Hospital Association, the State Medical Society, the State Health Department and Yale University, School of Medicine and the newly established medical school at the University of Connecticut. The proposal established a target date of January 1, 1970 for an operating computerized data reduction system. The data input is a modified version of the PAS case abstract, with limited charge data added to medical record abstracts. The system will:

1. Generate indices of institutional performance and effectiveness based on the same patient summary information
2. Provide the data base for a two-phase Utilization Review Screening system for the various institutions in the state
3. Produce planning data based on patient services rendered in various institutions
4. Elaborate data to serve as the basis on which the institution-centered Regional Medical Program's operating programs can be evaluated.
5. Serve as a data bank for other research in the delivery of institutional medical care[3]

Elements 1 and 2 received most of the early emphasis.[4] Developmental costs of the system have been sponsored by federal grant through the Regional Medical Program. Operating costs are to be transferred gradually to the hospitals who will pay on a per discharge basis.

The Characteristics of Input

Input to CUPIS-BURP is to be obtained from three basic sources: an admission record, financial activities, and a discharge case abstract. The system as working accommodates any form of admission record, allowing the hospitals flexibility. Case abstracts follow PAS lines generally, but are at present less detailed. Considerable hospital individualization can be accommodated, in the design and extension of the abstract. The long-range goal of an automated life medical record will require unique identity of patients and doctors throughout the state. This problem is technically soluble, but present important political and social ramifications which have not yet been resolved. Financial records on individual patients can be accepted in either paper copy or computer tape form.

Data Storage and Output

The goals of CUPIS require on line, real time retrieval of large quantities of information collected over several years and many hospitals, doctors, and patients. This implies very large storage capability and remote terminal operation. Other goals stress data reduction and the reporting only of significant information in a format usable for individual hospitals whose needs may differ. These require large computing capability.

A variety of reports are available on routine and special bases. Routine reports are organized to the needs of individual departments and medical services within the hospital. They will include reference to past performance of the statistics shown and identification of deviant or unusual situations. Indexes of cases will be supplied in a manner similar to PAS. One of the principal outputs of CUPIS will be the data required for BURP. Special reports are planned with data tabulations, time series analysis and forecasts, and multivariate analysis both on a cross-sectional and a time series basis. The package of routine and special reports is expected to include equivalents or substitutes for all the reports of PAS-MAP, including the length-of-stay-package. Reports reflecting the historical and geographic dimensions of CUPIS data represent additional capability, not presently found in PAS-MAP. These ambitions require extensive printing capability in terms both of total volume and of format flexibility. The retrieval of information in real time also implies direct computer access from numerous remote sites.

System Hardware

The combination of the storage, calculating, and output requirements dictates the selection of computer hardware. The machine must have capability of very large storage files which can be searched for information specified by any of the dimensions outlined above. The ability to search historically through the file in short enough time to permit response to direct inquiry means that the files must be mechanically arranged so that they can be searched quickly in spite of their size. The ability to use relatively complex programs for statistical quality control and multivariate analysis purposes requires that the computer must have a large core storage and high computational speed. The requirement for specialized output creates a need for a highly sophisticated, user-oriented language to permit efficient communication between users and the machine. The combination of these characteristics is found only in the largest commercial computers available in the early 1970s. While the hardware planned for the project is not as large as that required for capture of the complete medical record, it is larger than what would be contemplated by even the most ambitious single hospital for its own data processing purposes. The nature of computer capability is such that it is estimated that the processing of data from the CUPIS files will require only 10 percent of the capability of the machine selected. The additional capability may be used to meet other data processing needs of the sponsoring organizations to defray the cost of the equipment. The same computer may be used to compile other data of interest in a comprehensive information system, such as data on cost and resources.

Participating hospitals and agencies will have limited direct communication with the computer through a teletype network already established by Connecticut Blue Cross. While the teletype is not a suitable device for the transmission or receipt of large quantities of data, it is feasible for a limited amount of work. The abstracts of the medical record and other bulk data will be mailed to a central point for input into the computer by card punch or optical scanning device. Most output reports will be generated by a high speed printer at the site and later mailed to the user.

BURP—A Sophisticated Quality and Utilization Monitor System

One of the purposes of CUPIS is to bring a higher degree of control to the utilization of hospital resources in Connecticut and to the quality of medical care. To achieve this end, work was begun on an elaborate case by case monitoring system of discharge patient records. This effort is called the Basic Utilization Review Program.[5] It was based upon the opportunities which appeared to exist in combining two earlier streams of research in utilization control with the CUPIS data bank. BURP depends first upon the use of large capability, high speed computers to apply statistical quality control techniques to medical abstracts. This application was demonstrated by Leighton and Headley of CPHA in the development of the length-of-stay-package described in the previous chapter.[6] The second component is the utility of criteria based, retrospective medical review to identify cases where either the quality of medical care or the appropriateness of use of hospital resources is inferior to authoritative expectations. Lembcke demonstrated the usefulness of criteria based review to the question of overall quality of care.[7] The application of criteria based review to utilization review and control was demonstrated by Payne, Fitzpatrick, and Riedel.[8]

Criteria-based analysis of either quality or utilization requires a comparison of the management of each individual case against relatively specific criteria which deal with elements occurring throughout the hospital stay. Each record must be reviewed carefully and extensively. The review is usually by physicians, and in any case doctors must make the final decision. The process is thus extremely costly. It is totally impractical to contemplate reviewing more than the small fraction of the hospital discharges in this way. Furthermore, particularly after the review process has been used long enough to encourage compliance with the criteria, very few deviant cases will be detected. The combination of high cost and low yield show the usefulness of some cheaper preselection mechanism which will reduce the total number of cases to be reviewed while at the same time increasing the probability of finding cases of interest. BURP supplies such a screening mechanism by statistical quality control techniques. The cases identified as deviant can be subjected to criteria review. Those judged to have differed from the criteria provide the basis for improved process control by education or other manner. The others, not different from criteria, represent false positives.

The quality control techniques in BURP treat length of stay and dollar volume of ancillary services as variables measures, and use the central limit theorem to identify deviant cases. In order to do this, it is necessary to find a suitable process for the underlying probability distribution. Such a process is said to be statistically "well-behaved," meaning principally that it is unimodal. Such processes frequently occur in organizations or in nature. They might be expected to occur in medical care within very narrowly defined groups of patients, who had the same physiological and psychological characteristics and the same disease process. Leighton and Headley showed the utility of assuming that patients grouped by age, sex, diagnosis, complication, and surgery generated a well-behaved statistical process. If the process is well-behaved, the central limit theorem can be applied with much smaller sample size than would be necessary otherwise. It is the application of the theorem that permits understanding type 1 and type 2 errors associated with any given control limit.

The BURP procedure includes a special on-line program called "Autogroup" for the identification and selection of well-behaved patient groups. The method used regards hospital care as a set of mutually exclusive statistical processes. Each discharge record is assigned to exactly one process, and the medical data associated with that record are regarded as one observation from that process. An acceptance region is defined for each process. Records whose observed statistics lie outside the acceptance boundaries are screened out as deviant cases and referred to a medical screening for study against criteria. This is the general function of a statistical quality control program of any sort. In addition to this function, BURP also monitors the stability of each process.

"With time, medical knowledge grows and public priorities change. As a result, treatments and medical policies change. It is expected that such changes will gradually distort [the] originally defined processes. It is necessary to detect such changes and readjust the processes accordingly."[9] The statistical analysis can be used for this detection and readjustment activity. Using the central limit theorem, means of subsamples and the deviation of subsamples from their means within each process can be followed over time. Gradual shifts within each process as well as sudden deviations from the process can be identified from control charts. These changes can be the result of either of two causes. They may represent a change in the practice of medicine which is not acceptable to the criteria and which would presumably be corrected by user hospitals and their medical staffs. Alternatively, they may represent a medically acceptable change in the process which reflects the loss of the well-behaved characteristic. Autogroup is being constructed to permit adjustments in the definition of processes as the need for these becomes apparent. This need becomes clear when either the means or standard deviations of recent samples differ significantly from those of earlier ones, when an unexpected number of unexplainable deviations remain after criterion review, or perhaps when medical advice indicates that a new treatment process has gained recognition. As the need occurs, it is necessary for the Autogroup operator to study the frequency distribution of cases within the process and within similar processes which might be constructed by altering the age, diagnosis, or treatment parameters. The operator strives to keep each process well-behaved, but at the same time strives to minimize the number of processes necessary to reach that goal. The larger the number of processes, the longer the average waiting time will be to collect a meaningful subsample in each process.

In order to do this job of redefining the processes efficiently, the Autogroup operator should be able to issue direct queries to the data bank about the control charts and the underlying frequency distributions for each of the processes. This can be done when the data bank is kept on-line to the computer and the operator can recover the information he needs quickly. An entire set of computer commands must be established to permit the operator to investigate various processes, modify them by trial and error and restore the system to an operating state. These commands are part of the computer software necessary to implement the BURP system. Like CUPIS, BURP requires a medium to large size computer and a large quantity of programming skill. It is thus never likely to be feasible on a single hospital computer.

A schematic diagram of the BURP is shown in figure 13-1. To date, two utilization variables have been selected and trial programs have been established for computer screening. The first variable is the length of stay within the hospital. Deviant cases would be those which had an unusually long or an unusually short stay when compared to the process to which they were assigned. A second variable, the dollar volume of ancillary services per day of stay, has

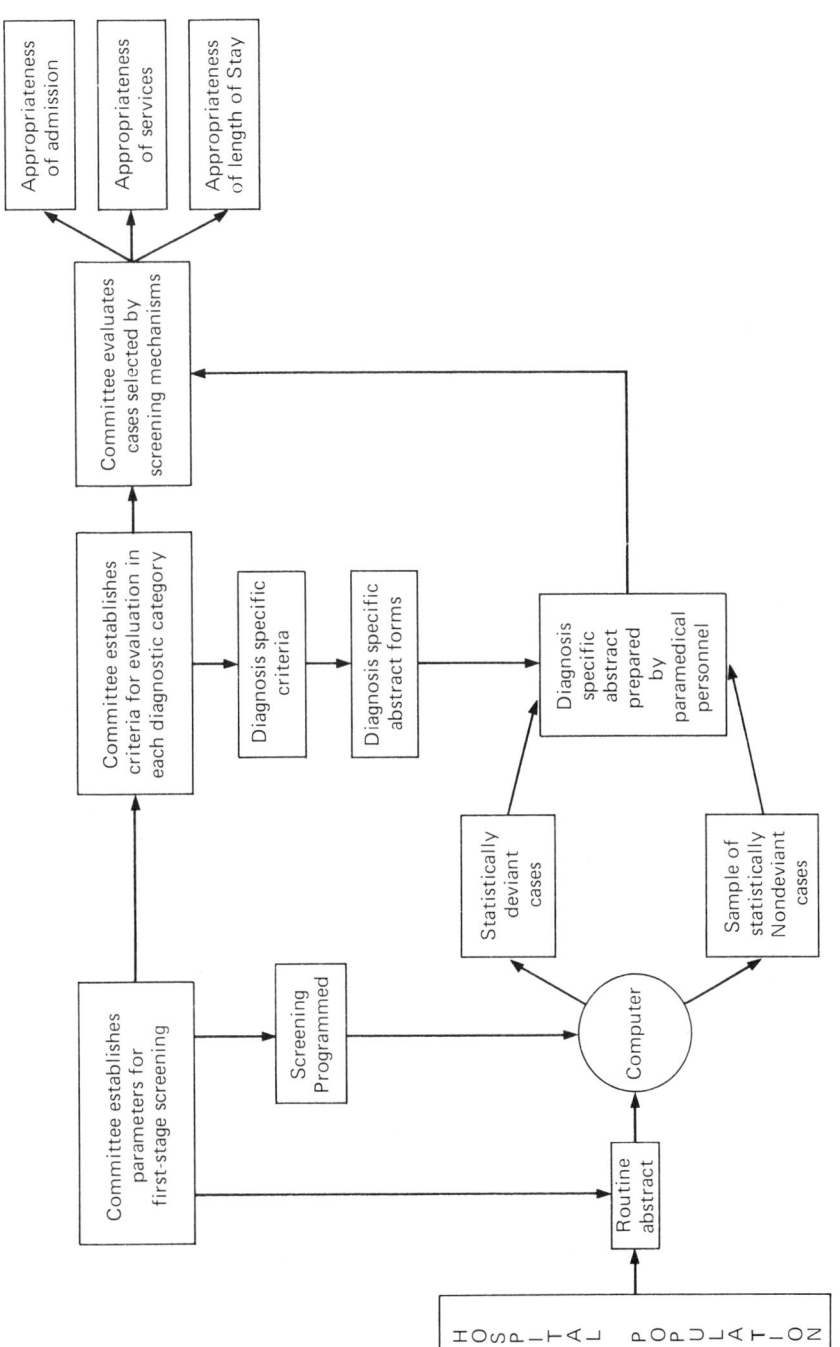

Figure 13-1. BURP Model. Source: Reproduced with the permission of Dr. Donald C. Riedel, Professor of Public Health (Medical Care), Yale School of Medicine.

also been tested. While this variable is a relatively crude aggregate, it does serve to indicate a different aspect of the use of hospital services from simply occupying a patient bed. Early experience with it as a detector of cases of interest has been encouraging.

BURP is an interesting example of systematic interaction between human and machine resources, as figure 13-1 shows. The machine component handles the entire mechanism of screening and presumably presents to the screening committee groups of cases which are particularly likely to be rewarding in terms of deviation from criteria or unusual medical interest. The screening committee can use these cases for medical education, to justify unexpectedly high charges against insurance through third party payment, or in rare cases, to discipline physicians. The screening process keeps the cost in terms of physician man hours to a minimum for a given level of control. The Autogroup operator acts as a super control, primarily upon the machine component. He has routine data on the state of the control system and is able by the definition of new groups to maintain its efficiency. In doing this, he relies upon another component of the machine services, the software packages necessary to study the frequency distributions of various processes and alter processes. These are shown on the figure as the initialization module. He also has capability of setting the control boundaries which determine the number of cases referred to the screening committee and the expected size of type 1 and type 2 errors. He has the assistance and guidance of an initialization committee which presumably is not independent of the screening committee and has a number of medical members. This committee can guide the operator in the definition of new groups and other activities regarding the system which are necessary.

Work has only begun in exploring the full usefulness of BURP. By 1972, screening processes and criteria had been applied to thirty diagnoses. In addition, work is proceeding on the development of additional diagnostic categories. It is unlikely that the system will ever reach 100 percent coverage of hospital admissions. The frequency of various diagnoses is by no means uniform. A few diagnoses account for a large percentage of hospital use, and control of these is obviously important. Conversely, a large number of diagnoses even collectively account for only a small fraction of hospital use. Most of these would have to be treated as one or more statistical processes. The sample size within some of these processes, even for a group of thirty-five hospitals, will be too small to be meaningful.

The system can be expanded in other ways, however. One of these is to establish concurrent rather than retrospective review. Under concurrent review schemes, each patient would be assigned to a process upon admission. The screening mechanism could identify deviant situations as soon as a sufficient number of patient days had been accumulated in the current subsample to place it outside the established control limit. In this way, occurrence of some unusual long stays might be detected early and prevented by immediate review and discharge. To take this step means the modification of the CUPIS system so that information is input on the patient's admission rather than discharge and updated whenever changes occur which alter the assignment of the patient to a given process. There is strong interest in this possibility, and investigation of its practicality is underway.

Another route for the expansion of CUPIS and BURP is to extended care facilities. Even crude concurrent review might prove useful in controlling length of stay in this area. The group in Connecticut has also proposed extending CUPIS and BURP to the outpatient situation. This involves an entirely new effort at data collection and computerization. Another group at Yale has developed case summary and evaluation sheets for ambulatory care which might serve as a basis for computerized abstract.[10] Among other difficulties, new terminal points of episodes of ambulatory care must be defined to serve as equivalents to admission and discharge. The Yale group has proposed finding the point in treatment when the patient is instructed to return only if necessary as the discharge equivalent and the point where the patient seeks a change in this status as the admission equivalent. Various other kinds of quality and utilization control processes suggest themselves as possible from the combination of the BURP model and the CUPIS data bank. These various attributes-type measures of medical care—complications, infectious, unexpected surgical pathology, etc.— might be treated statistically according to the BURP processes, for example. But these opportunities remain to be developed.

Towards A Working Comprehensive Information System

The total Connecticut information system should be defined to include not only CUPIS and BURP, but also the manual cost allocation system and the utilization and census data for geographic areas. The program is ambitious and presses to the limit of both current hospital regionalization and current information processing technology. Its proposals and achievements suggest the nature of the eventual comprehensive system. Clearly, all those aspects currently envisioned for CUPIS and BURP, including data on outpatient care and care in facilities other than acute general hospitals, are to be included. This aspect of the information system might be called its *breadth*. Breadth is of primary interest to agencies larger than single hospitals whose responsibilities include financing the total system and reducing variation in the availability and use of services. HMO's have substantial interest in breadth. To the extent that hospitals move in that direction, so will they. Otherwise, to the individual hospital, breadth may be less important per se than because it greatly increases the power of the information service purchased for a given expenditure. Larger data collection efforts, more analysis, and bigger computers can be afforded than would be possible if the system had fewer members. A broad system serving the planning needs of the state of Connecticut develops the data necessary for planning in each operating unit as a second product. The responsibility and cost of identifying population density functions for the use of each individual facility, of collecting and forecasting population data, and of developing multivariate models for forecasting many kinds of population-based demand may be shared with other institutions. The cost of the kinds of forecasts described in chapters 1 to 5 can be reduced at the same time the reliability and utility of the forecast are improved.

The *depth* of an information system may be defined as the extent to which it meets the needs for planning and control information within an individual institution. Substantial amounts of work remain to be done on this dimension as well. Only two measures of resources are currently proposed in the Connecticut system. CUPIS has capability of identifying physician manpower through the use of the AMA registrations. The cost accounting system measures the dollar value of resources consumed by various departments of participating hospitals. These systems must be broadened to include direct man hours by department and measures of demand or output for each of the services of the institutions. The inclusion of this information will permit estimation of unit cost on a department basis, and will open up opportunities for analyzing and improving scheduling and staffing opportunities and the optimal use of capital investment. These forms of data are required for the routine use of various optimization models described in chapters 6 through 9. The vital question of what specific services are economically justifiable for each hospital within the state is one of those which must be studied with these data. The opportunities do not become apparent until the unit costs of each service in each hospital are calculated and presented by the information system. This step apparently involves the input of descriptive data on demand—resources and output of each department in each institution together with the computerization of the dollar cost calculations. Other elements of the depth of the system include the measure and control of service quality other than medicine as well as the measurement of human resources. These areas involve entirely new data collection efforts of the type described in chapter 11 and the computerization of the information for rapid and effective analysis.

There is ultimately another stage to the comprehensive information system which begins when some of the immediate problems of depth and breadth have been overcome, and large sections of the total information are available for processing and consideration. This is a stage where policy questions for individual hospitals and the group of Connecticut hospitals can be studied in such a way that tentative answers can be formulated and the impact of these answers upon the individual units and the state as a whole can be forecast directly. This is the third and final stage of computer utilization. The effect of policy questions on the location and size of certain facilities, the value of scheduling alternatives and capital investment, the desirability of improvements in control of utilization, the impact of alterations in reimbursements of payment plans and possibly even of changes in coverage of insurance contracts are among the many questions which will eventually be studied in this way. Although Connecticut is certainly one of the national leaders in this area, it is clear that they have a great distance to go, both with technical and organizational problems. The rest of us, by and large, have scarcely begun.

Notes

Notes

Chapter 1
Introduction

1. Substantial research in a variety of disciplines supports the notions outlined here. For a review of much of this, with bibliographies, see the Health Services Research Study Project, published by the *Milbank Memorial Fund Quarterly*, July 1966, part 2, and October 1966, part 2. The papers by P.J. Feldstein, "Research on the Demand for Health Services" and I.M. Rosenstock, "Why People Use Health Services," are particularly relevant.

Chapter 3
Forecasting by Multivariate Analysis and Techniques for Forecasting Variation

1. Ezekiel and K.A. Fox, *Methods of Correlation and Regression Analysis*, John Wiley and Sons, New York, 1965, contains a thorough and reasonably nontechnical discussion of the subject.

2. Survey data of this kind is reported by U.S. National Center for Health Statistics, Data from the National Health Survey, series 10, USPHS, DHEW, Washington, publ. no. 1000, various dates.

3. For examples of multiple regression models from survey data, see G.C. Wirick and R. Barlow, "The Economic and Social Determinants of the Demand for Health Services," *Economics of Health and Medical Care*, Bureau of Public Health Economics, Ann Arbor, 1964, pp. 95-125; G.C. Wirick, "A Multiple Equation Model of the Demand for Health Care" *Health Services Research*, Winter 1966, American Hospital Association, Chicago; P.J. Feldstein, "The Demand for Medical Care," chapter 4 in *The Report of the Commission on the Cost of Medical Care*, vol. I, pp. 57-76, American Medical Association, Chicago, 1964.

4. U.S. National Center for Health Statistics, *Computer Simulation of Hospital Discharges*, U.S. Dept. of Health, Education & Welfare, PHS Publication 1000, series 2, no. 13, Government Printing Office, Washington, D.C., 1966.

5. G.D. Rosenthal, "The Demand for General Hospital Facilities," American Hospital Association, Chicago, 1964, Hospital Monograph Series 14, and "Factors Affecting the Utilization of Short-term General Hospitals," *American Journal of Public Health*, November 1965, pp. 1734-40. Rosenthal's results for 1950 and 1960 data of the same nature show wide variations. For example, the patient day model has five significant independent variables for each year. However, only two of these are the same (see p. 35). Similar difficulties are shown by the admissions model.

6. R.L. Cardwell, M.G. Reid, and M. Shain, "Hospital Utilization in a Major Metropolitan Area," Hospital Planning Council for Metropolitan Chicago, 1964. Available from University Microfilms, Inc., Ann Arbor, Michigan as Hospital Management Document no. 282, reel 1.19.

7. Henri L. Beenhakker, "Multiple Correlation—A Technique for the Prediction of Hospital Beds," *Operations Research*, 1963, pp. 824-39.

8. NCHS, series 2, no. 13.

9. NCHS, series 10.

10. Feldstein and German, "Predicting Hospital Utilization: An Evaluation of Three Approaches," *Inquiry*, vol. 2, no. 1, June 1965.

11. Ibid., p. 35.

12. R.G. Brown, *Statistical Forecasting for Inventory Control*, McGraw-Hill, New York, 1959, p. 45 ff.

13. S. Heda, "Evaluation of Exponential Smoothing Models for Short Term Hospital Forecasting," work in process, University of Michigan, Program and Bureau of Hospital Administration.

14. M.S. Blumberg, "DPF Concept Helps Predict Bed Needs," *Modern Hospital*, December 1961, p. 75. See J.P. Young, "A Queueing Theory Approach to the Control of Hospital Inpatient Census," doctoral dissertation, The Johns Hopkins University, Baltimore, 1962.

Chapter 4
Determining Population Service Areas and Calculating Use Rates

1. E. Poland and P.A. Lembcke, "Delineation of Hospital Service Districts—Methodology and Statistical Appendices" (multilith), Community Studies, Inc., Kansas City, 1962, p. 1.

2. Ibid.

3. Joint Committee on the AHA and PHS on Areawide Planning of Hospitals and Related Health Facilities, *Report*, USPHS, Div. of Hospital and Medical Facilities, Publication No. 855, Wash., D.C. (1961), p. 56.

4. Poland and Lembcke, "Delineation of Hospital Service Districts." The method apparently existed for many years before Poland and Lembcke wrote it out in unusual detail. Their work, cited above, is the only recent and complete description of the method. I have abstracted from it in this discussion, and removed some of the calculations involving population groups usually only a few hundred persons in number.

5. U.S. Bureau of Census, ADMATCH program. Descriptive literature and programs available from the Bureau.

6. Ibid., pp. 29-35.

7. U.S. Post Office Department, *Directory of Post Offices*, POD Publication 26, revised annually, Washington, D.C.

8. See Poland and Lembcke, "Hospital Service," pp. 98-100.

9. I am indebted to Robert M. Sigmond for the labeling of these two indices, based upon his experience as director of the Allegheny County, Pennsylvania, Health Facilities Planning Council (personal communication).

10. Commission on Hospital Care, *Hospital Care in the United States*, Commonwealth Fund and Harvard University Press, Cambridge, 1947, pp. 289-301.

11. D.L. Drosness, and S.W. Lubin, "Planning can be based on patient travel," *Modern Hospital* 106, no. 4 (April 1966): 92-94.

12. See Walter M. Burnett, "Determinants of Hospital Utilization: A Case Study," State University of Iowa, doctoral dissertation, 1965. Available from University Microfilms, Inc., Ann Arbor, no. 65-6677.

13. R.L. Morrill and R. Earickson, "Hospital Variation and Patient Travel Distances," *Inquiry* 5, no. 4 (December 1968): 26 ff.

14. R.L. Morrill and R. Earickson, "Variations in the Character and Use of Chicago Area Hospitals," *Health Services Research*, 3, no. 3 (Fall 1968). 24 ff.

15. *Sales Management: The Magazine of Marketing*, "Survey of Buying Power," published annually (June) by Sales Management, New York.

16. Population Studies Center, University of Michigan, in cooperation with the State Resource Planning Division, Michigan Department of Commerce, "Michigan Population, 1960 to 1980," Michigan Department of Commerce, Lansing, 1966, p. 16 ff.

17. "California Population Resources in Relation to the Problem of Health Facility Planning," Hospital Utilization Research Project, California Department of Health, Berkeley, paper no. 5, 1964. Available from University Microfilms, Inc., Ann Arbor, as Hospital Management Document AR0017, reel 1.51.

18. "Health Care for Lenawee County: A Plan for Action," Bureau of Hospital Administration, University of Michigan, Ann Arbor, 1966, pp. 58-62.

19. I. Hess, D.C. Riedel, and T.B. Fitzpatrick, *Probability Sampling of Hospitals and Patients*, Bureau of Hospital Administration, University of Michigan, Ann Arbor, 1961, p. 23.

Chapter 5
Demand Forecasts in Specialized Situations

1. R.I. Lee and L.W. Jones, *The Fundamentals of Good Medical Care*, University of Chicago Press, Chicago, 1933.

2. U.S. National Center for Health Statistics, *Fertility Measurement*, USPHS publication 1000, series 4, no. 1. Annual data are published in "The Natality Volume," *Vital Statistics of the United States*, with advance reports in *Monthly Vital Statistics Report*, by the Division of Vital Statistics, USNCHS.

3. USPHS, Division of Hospital and Medical Facilities, "Procedures for Areawide Planning," publication 930-B-3, Washington, D.C. pp. 22-27.

4. Professional Activity Study, electronic data processing services provided by the Commission on Professional and Hospital Activities, Ann Arbor, Michigan.

5. F.E. Browning, "The Record in Hospital Bed Utilization" in *Utilization Review*, American Medical Association, Chicago, 1965.

6. J.G. Zimmer, "An Evaluation of Observer Variability in a Hospital Bed Utilization Study," *Medical Care* 5, no. 4, (1967): 221-33.

7. ———, and E.W. Groomes, "An Observer Reliability Study of Physicians' and Nurses' Decisions in Utilization Review of Chronic Care Facilities," *Medical Care* 7, no. 1 (1969), pp. 14-20.

8. Kerr L. White, "Estimating Needs for Progressive Patient Care Facilities in a University Hospital," available from University Microfilms Incorporated, Ann Arbor, as Hospital Management Document no. 288, reel 1.19.

9. R.A. Preston, K.L. White, E.J. Strachan, and H.B. Wells, "Patient Care Classification as a Basis for Estimating Graded Inpatient Facilities," *Journal of Chronic Diseases* 17, no. 9, (1964), pp. 761-72.

10. "The Progressive Patient Care Hospital; Estimating Bed Needs," USPHS publication no. 930-C-2, Washington, D.C., 1963.

11. R.J. Connor, "Hospital Inpatient Classification System," doctoral dissertation, Johns Hopkins University, Baltimore, 1960; see J.P. Young, "A Method for Allocation of Nursing Personnel to Meet Inpatient Care Needs," available from University Microfilms, Inc., Hospital Management Studies Document no. 29, reel 12.

12. J.R. Griffith, L.E. Weeks, *The McPherson Experiment: Expanding Community Hospital Services*, Bureau of Hospital Administration, University of Michigan, Ann Arbor, 1967, ch. 9, M. Sturdavant and H.C. Mickey, "An Experiment in Minimal Care," *Hospitals, JAHA*, February 16, 1966, pp. 72-78 et seq. March 1, March 16.

13. Preston, "Patient Care Classification," Weeks and Griffith, *Progressive Patient Care an Anthology*, Bureau of Hospital Administration, University of Michigan, Ann Arbor, 1964, and R.I. Walker, "Evaluation of Minimal Care Center," *Hospitals, JAHA*, July 1964, pp. 75-78.

14. U.S. Public Health Service, Division of Hospital and Medical Facilities "The Progressive Patient Care Hospital: Estimating Bed Needs," PHS Publication No. 930-C-2, Wash., D.C. (1963).

15. Griffith, *McPherson Experiment*, ch. 11.

16. Norman C. Dalkey, *The Delphi Method: An Experimental Study of Group Opinion*, RAND Corp., RM-5888-PR., June 1969; N.C. Dalkey and Olaf Helmer, "An Experimental Application of the Delphi Method to the Use of Experts," *Management Sciences*, 9 (1963): 458-67. See also other papers by these authors, available from the RAND Corp.

17. T.J. Gordon and O. Helmer, *Report on a Long Range Forecasting Study*, RAND Corp., P-29-82, September 1964.

18. Alan Sheldon, unpublished work, "Recent Use of the Delphian: Future Medical Care and Medical Education," Harvard Medical School, Boston, Massachusetts.

19. A.D. Bender, A.E. Strack, et al., "Delphic Study Examines Developments in Medicine," *Futures*, June 1969, p. 301.

20. John W. Williamson, "Prognostic Epidemiology: Concept and Product," unpublished paper, The Johns Hopkins University School of Hygiene and Public Health, 1971.

Chapter 6
Total Value Analysis

1. See E.H. Bowman and R.B. Fetter, *Analysis for Production and Operations Management*, R.D. Irwin, Homewood, Illinois, 1967.

2. See R.M. Bramblett, "Optimal Quantities for Hospital Supply Groupings" in H. Smalley and J. Freeman, *Hospital Industrial Engineering*, Reinhold, New York, 1966, pp. 294-98. Bramblett solves the order quantity problem under conditions of stochastic demand.

Chapter 7
Queueing and Simulation Models for Resource Allocation

1. See Jeanne W. Palmer, "Measuring Bed Needs for General Hospitals: Historical Review of Opinions with Annotated Bibliography," USPHS, Washington, D.C., 1956, mimeo.

2. Commission on Hospital Care, *Hospital Care in the United States*, Commonwealth Fund and Harvard University Press, Cambridge, 1947, p. 285.

3. Joint Commission of the American Hospital Association and U.S. Public Health Service, *Areawide Planning for Hospitals and Related Health Facilities*, HEW PHS, Publication 855, Washington, D.C., 1961, p. 25.

4. J.D. Thompson, O.W. Avant, and E.D. Spiker, "How Queueing Theory Works for the Hospital," *Modern Hospital*, March 1960.

5. J.D. Thompson, et al., Yale Studies of Hospital Function and Design, unpublished compilation of papers in USPHS Grant W-53, 1959.

6. J.D. Thompson, et al., "Predicting Requirements for Maternity Facilities," *Hospitals*, February 16, 1963.

7. Ibid.

8. Joel Kavet, "The Application of Computer Simulation Techniques to the Surgical Subsystem," unpublished master's essay, Yale University, 1967.

9. E.H. Bowman, and R.B. Fetter, *Analysis for Production and Operations Management*, 3rd Ed., R.D. Irwin, Homewood, Ill., 1967, p. 425.

10. J.P. Young, "Stabilization of Inpatient Bed Occupancy Through Control of Admissions," *Hospitals*, JAHA, October 1, 1965, pp. 41-48.

11. R.G. Dunn, "Predicting the Availability of Beds for Scheduling Elective Admissions," unpublished master's essay, University of Michigan, 1967, and "Scheduling Elective Admissions," *Health Services Research*, 2, no. 2 (1967): 181-215.

12. G.P. Briggs, Jr., "Inpatient Admissions Scheduling: Application to a Nursing Service," unpublished Ph.D. dissertation, University of Michigan, Ann Arbor, 1971.

Chapter 8
PERT and Mathematical Programming Models

1. J. Blickstein, "How to Put PERT into Marketing," *Printer's Ink*, October 23, 1964, pp. 27-29.

2. C. Heinzel, "PERT Technique Can Aid in Annual Report Preparation," *Public Relations Journal*, April 1964, pp. 11-14.

3. Carl Heyel, *Encyclopedia of Management*, Reinhold Publishing Corp., New York, 1964, p. 687 ff.

4. Ibid.

5. W.J. Baumol, *Economic Theory and Operations Analysis*, 2nd Ed., Prentice Hall, Englewood Cliffs, New Jersey, 1965. Chapters 5 and 6 offer a good discussion for the nonmathematically oriented student.

6. W.L. Dowling, "A Linear Programming Approach to the Analysis of Hospital Production," unpublished doctoral dissertation, University of Michigan, Ann Arbor, 1970. I am indebted to Dr. Dowling for permission to use the example.

7. R. Earickson, "The Case for Decentralizing Cook County Hospitals: Some Applications of Linear Optimization in Hospital Planning," 1968, available from University Microfilms, Inc., Ann Arbor as Hospital Management Document AR2102; also K.S. Park and J.R. Freeman, "Community Health Resource Allocation with Linear Programming Methods," University of Florida Health Systems Research Division, 1969, available from University Microfilms, Inc., Ann Arbor, as Hospital Management Document MN2040.

8. H. Wolfe and J. Young, "Staffing the Nursing Unit—Part I, Controlled Variable Staffing; Part II, The Multiple Assignment Technique," *Nursing Research*, 14, no. 3: 244-53 and no. 4: 299-303 (1965). Also H. Wolfe, *Multiple Assignment Model for Staffing Nursing Units*, doctoral dissertation, The Johns Hopkins University, Baltimore, 1964.

9. J.R. Freeman, "Quantitative Criteria for Hospital Inpatient Nursing Unit Design," unpublished doctoral dissertation, Georgia Institute of Technology, 1967. Available from University Microfilms, Inc., as Hospital Management Document NU 3003.

10. J.C. Balintfy, "Menu Planning by Computer," *Communications of the ACM*, 7, no. 4, April 1964, and Balintfy and E.C. Nebel, "Experiment with Computer Assisted Menu Planning," *Hospitals*, 40, no. 12 (June 16): 1966.

11. J.R. Griffith, L.E. Weeks, J.H. Sullivan, *The McPherson Experiment: Expanding Community Hospital Service*, University of Michigan, Bureau of Hospital Administration, Ann Arbor, Michigan, 1967, chapter 11.

12. S.M. Weir, "Variable Nurse Staffing in a Progressive Patient Care Hospital," unpublished master's thesis, University of Michigan, 1968. Available from University Microfilms as Hospital Management Document NU 2025.

13. M.D. Shanks, and D.A. Kennedy, *The Theory and Practice of Nursing Service Administration*, McGraw-Hill, New York, 1965.

14. See F.L. George and R.P. Kuehn, *Patterns of Patient Care*, Macmillan Company, New York, 1955; also F.G. Abdellah and E. Levine, *Effect of Nurse Staffing on Patient Satisfaction*, American Hospital Association, Hospital Monograph Series, no. 4, Chicago, 1958.

15. Commission on Administrative Services in Hospitals, 4777 Sunset Boulevard, Los Angeles, California, various reports.

16. See for example the MEDINET service of the General Electric Company, Watertown, Masschusetts, "Nursing Staff Allocation," 1969.

17. D.M. Warner, "A Two Phase Model for Scheduling Nursing Personnel in a Hospital," unpublished doctoral dissertation, Tulane University, 1971.

Chapter 9
Evaluating Capital Investment Opportunities

1. H. Smalley and J. Freeman, *Hospital Industrial Engineering*, Reinhold, New York, 1966, chapter 23.

2. This model can be extended to isolate warehousing and inventory costs if these are significant. Under conditions of batch processing or delivery, these are the same as the term in the inventory model,

$$Q(W + 1/2\,Ip)$$

where

Q = order quantity or bath size

I = interest rate

W = warehousing cost per item per year

p = price, or unit cost of manufacture (this can be estimated, if necessary).

In continuous manufacturing, the inventory may usually be expected to be nearly constant. The annual cost of warehousing and interest on the inventory can be estimated as $S(W + Ip)$ where S is the average stock level. These refinements are rarely critical in decision.

3. D.P. Rice and B.S. Cooper, "The Economic Value of Human Life," *American Journal of Public Health*, 57, no. 11 (November 1967), pp. 1954 ff.

4. *Historical Statistics of the U.S.*, Department of Commerce, series X330-342, p. 656, Government Printing Office, Washington, D.C., 1960.

5. Rice and Cooper, "Value of Human Life," attach values to life over age 65 by ignoring consumption of health and other services and apparently treating pensions and social security as earnings, but even so the present value of life of males fall 50 percent in five years before and after 65.

6. See H.M. and R.A. Somers, *Medicare and the Hospitals*, Brookings Institution, Washington, 1967, chapters 8 and 9.

Chapter 10
Nature and Application of Control Systems in Hospitals

1. See W.M. Hancock, "Managerial Use of Computer Data," *Journal of Methods Time Measurements*, 12, no. 4 (September-October, 1967).

2. A.J. Duncan, *Quality Control in Industrial Statistics*, 3rd Ed., R.D. Irwin, Homewood, Ill., 1965.

Chapter 11
Examples of Hospital Control Systems

1. B.S. Georgopoulis and F.C. Mann, *The Community General Hospital*, MacMillan, New York, 1962.

2. R.L. Brummet, E.G. Flanholtz, and W.C. Pyle, "Human Resources Myopia," *Monthly Labor Review*, January 1969, pp. 29-30.

3. R. Likert, *The Human Organization, Its Management and Value*, McGraw-Hill, New York, 1967, chapter 5.

4. R.W. Revans, "Morale and Effectiveness in General Hospitals," in McLachlan (ed), *Problems and Progress in Medical Care*, Oxford University Press, for the Nuffield Provincial Hospitals Trust, 1964.

5. R.H. Roy, *The Administrative Process*, The Johns Hopkins Press, Baltimore, 1958, pp. 1-25.

6. Community Systems Foundation, Ann Arbor, Michigan, maintains up-to-date work standards in these and other areas, and provides engineering services for their use in many parts of the United States.

7. *Chart of Accounts for Hospitals*, AHA, Chicago, Illinois, 1966.

8. H.D. Sanders, "An Analysis of the Nature of Certain Hospital Statistics, through Analysis of HAS Grouped Statistics," master's thesis, University of

Michigan, 1967, Available from University Microfilms, Inc., Ann Arbor as Hospital Management Document MN2017.

9. Ibid., pp. 74-78.

10. Bureau of Hospital Administration, University of Michigan. The work is supported by the National Center for Health Services Research and Development, grant number HS-00228.

11. Ibid., 1971 Progress Report.

12. USPHS, *How to Study Nursing Activities in a Patient Unit*, Rev. Ed., publication no. 370, Government Printing Office, Washington, D.C., 1964.

13. J.E. Williams and B. Donaldson, "SCORE: A Management Evaluation Program for Dietary Departments," *Journal of the American Dietetic Association*, April 1969, p. 283 ff.

14. B.W. Steinhauer, F. Cox, G. Stobie, and E. Quinn, "A Method of Hospital Infection Surveillance Incorporating the Use of the Computer," *Henry Ford Hospital Medical Journal*, Detroit, 15, no. 2, pp. 137-47.

15. Commission for Administrative Services in Hospitals, "A Quality Control Plan for the Housekeeping Department," Los Angeles, 1965. Available from University Microfilms, Inc., as Hospital Management Document HU 0018.

16. ———. "A Quality Control Plan for the Dietary Department," Los Angeles, 1965, available from University Microfilms, Inc., Ann Arbor, as Hospital Management Document DI0013.

17. L.W. Lewis, V. Carozza, et al., "Defining Clinical Content Graduate Nursing Programs, Medical-Surgical Nursing," Western Interstate Commission for Higher Education, Boulder, Colorado, 1967, p. 6.

18. American Nurses' Association, "Functions, Standards, and Qualifications for Practice," New York, 1963, p. 12.

19. M.K. Aydelotte, M.E. Tennor, et al., *An Investigation of the Relation between Nursing Activity and Patient Welfare*, State University of Iowa, 1960.

20. Ibid., p. 43 ff.

21. P.J. Verohnick, "Decubitous Ulcer Observations Measured Objectively," *Nursing Research*, 10 (Fall 1961): 211-214, reported in F.G. Abdellah and E. Levine, *Better Patient Care Through Nursing Research*, MacMillan Company, New York, 1965, pp. 505 ff.

22. R.W. Revans, "Morale and Effectiveness in General Hospitals," in McLachlan (ed), *Problems and Progress in Medical Care*, Oxford University Press, for the Nuffield Provincial Hospitals Trust, 1964.

23. Georgopoulos and Mann, *Community General Hospital*.

24. F.G. Abdellah, and E. Levine, *Patients and Personnel Speak*, United States Public Health Service, publication no. 527, Government Printing Office, Washington, 1964.

25. ———, "Quests for Quality: A Self-Evaluation Guide to Patient Care," National League for Nursing, New York, 1966.

26. The Commission for Administrative Services in Hospitals, "Quality

Control Plan for Nursing Service," available from University Microfilms, Inc., as Hospital Management Document NU1054.

27. R. Jelinek, R. Smith, et al., "Study of Nursing Unit Management," in progress, Bureau of Hospital Administration, University of Michigan, Ann Arbor, Michigan.

28. J.J. Hoopes, "Determination of the Statistical Reliability of the CASH Quality Control Checksheet for Patient Charts," unpublished master's thesis, University of Michigan, Program in Hospital Administration, 1967, Ann Arbor.

29. R. Jelinek, F. Munson and R. Smith, *SUM An Organizational Approach to Improved Patient Care*, W.K. Kellogg Foundation, Battle Creek, Mich., 1971.

30. R.L. Smith, "Analysis of the CASH-type Nursing Quality Instrument," unpublished paper, Bureau of Hospital Administration, University of Michigan, 1972.

31. R.L. Smith and B.L. Horn, personal communication.

Chapter 12
Measuring the Quality of the Medical Care Process

1. P.A. Lembcke, "Evolution of the Medical Audit," *JAMA* 199 (February 20, 1967): 545 ff.

2. K.S. Klicka, "Control of the Quality of Medical Care," chapter 6 in C.W. Eisele (ed.), *The Medical Staff in the Modern Hospital*, McGraw-Hill, New York, 1966.

3. A. Donabedian, "Evaluating the Quality of Medical Care," *Milbank Memorial Fund Quarterly*, pt. 2, July 1966, p. 190.

4. M.C. Sheps, "Approaches to the Quality of Hospital Care," *Public Health Reports*, 70 (September 1955): 877-86.

5. *Joint Commission on Accreditation of Hospitals*, Chicago, issued periodically.

6. M.T. MacEachern, *Hospital Organization and Management*, 3rd Ed., The Physicians' Record Co., Chicago, 1957, p. 243.

7. E.A. Johnson and L. Vivaldo, *A Method for the Qualitative Analysis of Hospital Performance*, Graduate Program in Hospital Administration, The University of Chicago, Chicago, 1960.

8. P.A. Lembcke, "Medical Auditing by Scientific Methods," *JAMA*, 162, no. 7 (October 13, 1956).

9. R.S. Myers, "Hospital Statistics Don't Tell the Truth," *Modern Hospital*, 83 (July 1954): 53-54.

10. George E. Parker, "The Value of Certain Objective and Subjective Measures of Medical Care in Hospitals," master's essay for Yale University, 1963, UMI Hospital Management Document, MD0020, reel 1.47.

11. C.W. Eisele, V.N. Slee, R.G. Hoffman, "Can the Practice of Internal

Medicine Be Evaluated?" *Annals of Internal Medicine* 44, no. 1 (January 1956): 144-60.

12. V.N. Slee, "CPHA Experience in Measuring Quality," a paper presented before the American Public Health Association Program Area Committee on Medical Care Administration, New York, November 11-12, 1966.

13. V.N. Slee, personal correspondence.

14. John A. Comiskey, "A Comparative Appraisal between an Internal Program and an External Program of Processing Medical Record Data," master's thesis, Program in Hospital Administration, University of Michigan, Ann Arbor, 1963. Also, see examples for maternity, tuberculosis, and mental illness, in *Hospital Discharge Data*, Report of the Conference on Hospital Discharge Abstracts Systems, J.H. Mornaghan and K.L. White, eds. Supplement to *Medical Care*, 8, no. 4, 1970.

15. B.G. Rowe, P.A. Bonner, and W.D. Harkins, "A Proposal for Centralized Computerized System of Medical Statistics for Connecticut Hospitals," project for the Program in Hospital Administration, Yale University, 1967.

16. V.N. Slee, personal correspondence.

17. Ibid.

18. Commission on Professional and Hospital Activities, "Measuring Laboratory and X-ray Utilization," *The Record*, 2, no. 9, December 1964.

19. E. Leighton and P. Headly, "Computer Analysis of Length of Stay," *Hospital Progress*, April 1968, pp. 67-70.

20. *Length of Stay in PAS Hospitals*, Commission on Professional and Hospital Activities, Ann Arbor, Michigan, October 1971.

21. J.F. Stapleton, and J.A. Zwerneman, "The Influence of an Intern-Resident Staff on the Quality of Private Patient Care," *Journal of the American Medical Association*, 194, no. 8 (November 22, 1965): 877-82.

22. Comiskey, "Medical Record Data."

23. Rowe, Bonner, and Hawkins, "Medical Statistics for Connecticut Hospitals."

Chapter 13
Advanced Information Systems for Hospital Planning and Control

1. The material in this chapter is developed from proposals and project documents of the CUPISS and BURP projects which were released to the author by the project directors, Professor John D. Thompson and Associate Professor Donald C. Riedel of Yale University. I am also indebted to Mr. R.R. Morrisse for comments and corrections.

2. B.G. Rowe, P.A. Bonner, and W.D. Harkins, "A Proposal for a Centralized Computerized System of Medical Statistics for Connecticut Hospitals,"

student paper, Department of Epidemiology and Public Health, Yale University, School of Medicine, 1967.

3. CUPIS proposal documents, Connecticut Regional Medical Program, 1968.

4. R.F. Morrisse, J.D. Thompson, and D.C. Riedel, unpublished paper presented at the Association of Health Records meeting, April 1971.

5. Significant components of BURP were developed with the support of the Community Health Service, HSMHA, contract HSM-110-69-89, Dr. Donald C. Riedel, principal investigator.

6. Leighton and Headly, "Length of Stay."

7. P.A. Lembcke, "Medical Auditing by Scientific Methods," *Journal of the American Medical Association*, 162, October 13, 1956, p. 646; and O.G. Johnson, *A Medical Audit Report*, School of Public Health, University of California, Los Angeles, 1963.

8. B.C. Payne, D.C. Riedel, and T.B. Fitzpatrick, "The Character and Effectiveness of Hospital Use," in McNerney, et al., *Hospital and Medical Economics*, Hospital Research and Educational Trust, Chicago, 1962. See various other publications by these authors, particularly Payne, 1962 to 1968.

9. Yale University, BURP Progress Report, August 29, 1969, p. 1.1.

10. E.R. Weinerman, et al., "An Ambulatory Service Data System," Division of Health Care Statistics, U.S. Department of Health, Education, and Welfare, Arlington, Virginia, 22203, May 1969, p. 89.

Index

Abdellah, F. G. and Levine, E., 315
absenteeism, 250, 315
abstracting process, 372
accidental occurences, 265
accounting data, 282-284
address, of patient, 365
admissions: in output, 334; records in CUPISS-BURP, 374; scheduling rules, 160; use rate, 81
age: and adjusted demand rates, 95; distribution, 349; specific rates, 39
aggregation, problems of, 337
all-planning decisions, 209
alternatives, 236; and operating expenses, 210
ambiguity, 342
ambulatory care facility, 235
American College of Physicians, 337
American College of Surgeons, 337
American Hospital Association, 337; Chart of Accounts, 298
analysis: criteria-based, 377; patterns of, 209
analysis of variance: and demand rates, 96-99; programs, 40
analytic solutions: and demand distributions, 131-133
Apgar Score, 349
application range, 168
approximation: and total value analysis, 130, 131
assignment: matrix, 187; patterns, 207; problems, 186
assumption of linearity, 177
attitudinal states, 281
attributes measure, 255, 265
autocorrelation, 54
Autogroup, 377
automated cart delivery system, 209

Balintfly, J. C., 207; menu planning model, 202
bed allocation problem, 136-139
beneficiaries, 234
benefit evaluation, 232
benefit scales, 233
Bernoulli process, 58, 59, 270-273, 315
Bernoulli trials, 265
bias, 253
binomial distribution, 57
Birth Abstract, 345
birth rate, 79-81
Blue Cross Plan, 374
boundary conditions, 177

breadth, 381
Briggs, G. P., 164
Browning, F. G., 101, 103
budgets, 238; technique, 209
building construction, 168
BURP (Basic Utilization Review Program), 373, 376-381

capacity, 177
capital: benefit decisions, 238; costs, 213; investments, 210, 236; requirements, 214, 222
case-by-case analysis, 337
case tabulations, 346
CASH (Commission on Administrative Services in Hospitals), 304; in California, 207; nursing audit, 260; nursing survey, 323-328
cash benefits, 212
cash flow, 211-214; maximization, 225; stream, 232
cash scales, 316
census: input information, 206
Central Limit Theorem, 259, 304
changeover event, 169
Chart of Accounts, 298
coefficients, form of, 200
Comiskey, J. A., 364
commentary: room for in forms, 342
Commission on Hospital Care, 79
Commission on Professional and Hospital Activities (CPHA), 337
commitment index, 76-78
community planning committee, 240
comparability, 297
comparator process, 303
comparisons: of new program activities, 237
compiler systems, centralized, 370
complaint, rates of, 250
computer capability, 192
computerized simulation models, 150
confidence limits, of simulations, 152
Connecticut Blue Cross Association, 374
Connecticut Hospital Association, 374
Connecticut Medical Society, 374
Connecticut Regional Medical Program, 374
Connor, R. J., 103
constant staff requirements, 204
constraints: in Balintfly's model, 202; kinds of, 200; of PAS, 342
continuity, definition of, 258; of care, 264
continuous income stream formula, 214
continuous variables, 40

397

control, 4; components, 245; function and supervisors, 301; limits, 256, 320
control limit, 256, 320; calculation example, 265
control problems, 372
control supervisors, 247
control systems, 245, 279
controlled constant strength, 247
controller component, 246
controller considerations, 256
controller elements, 279
conventional control systems, 332
cost, 252; accounting studies, 196; average at present value, 231; -based reimbursement contracts, 225; -benefit analysis, 210, 225; control systems, 252; data collection, 98, 165, 192; estimates, 209; estimating assumptions 219; evaluation, 226; improvement component system, 332; and input devices, 342; intangibles, 117; of management, 220; matrix, 197; measurement, 212; minimization, 210; monetary, 280; overall, 196; of production, 211; renovation, 213; and size and complexity, 297; system development, 373; tradeoff, 175
CPM (Critical Path Method), 168
CPHA, processing of information, 345
criteria, patient classification, 105–107
CUPIS (Connecticut Utilization and Patient Information System), 373; CUPIS-BURP, 374
cybernetics, 245

data: census-based, 364; identifying in forms, 338; pooled, 365; and sensitivity analysis, 192
data banks, 372
data collection: and analysis, 301; and nursing quality, 314; problems of, 78–79; systems, 257
data input: CUPIS, 374
data processing: and CASH inspection samples, 319
data reduction, 346; mechanical problems, 303, 304
data storage: and CUPIS, 375
daily scheduling problem, 186
death rate, 81, 79–81
decision making, rational, 113
defer category, 240
definitions, standardized, 372
degenerate integer programming problem, 207
degenerate solution techniques, 202
Delphi Forecasting, 109–111
demand analysis, 17

demand: in Balintfy's model, 202; data, 334, 372; distribution of, 195; forecast, 219; functional, 4; generation, 13; projection, 22; rates, 93–96; specification of the, 192
dental clinic, 236
depreciation, 217
depth: of information system, 382
diagnosis, 341; and medical audit, 355
dietary quality scale, 308
difference distribution, 303
direct cost objective function, 196
direct labor cost measurement, 211
discharge, as basis for statistics, 364; case abstract, 374; categorie of, 361; in data, 334; probability of, 160
discontinuity, 258
discounting formula, 239
discrete variable, 258
distribution, of hospitals, 285
dollar volume, 377
Donabedian, A., 331
Dowling, W., 177
Drosness, D. L. and Lubin, S. W., 80, 81
dual, 184
dual formulation, 185
"dummy task," 170
Dunn, R. G., 163
Dunn's Admission Scheduling Model, 159

economics, of computer services, 370
editing routines, 345
efficiency: concept of, 280; control of scheduling and staffing, 302; of human resources, 281; measures of, 282
elements, number of, 200
empirical frequency distribution, 57
empirical inference, 55
employee: accident rates, 315; productivity, 282; satisfaction, 315
endogenous events, 163
epidemiologic detection, 304
equal likelihood service area, 65, 68–75
equipment, 280
equivalency, 210
error signal, 236, 254, 255
estimated life, 217, 231
evaluation procedures, 210
exception report, 245
exclusions, 298
exogenous events, 163
expansion of abstract forms, 342
expectations, 5
expenditures, alternative, 210, 233; time distribution, 227
explicit demand, 21
explicit primary control systems, 248, 279

explicit sensors, 250
exponential smoothing, 53, 301

facilities: 280; constraints, 179
facility size questions, 139–140
feedback cycle, 247
Feldstein, P. J., and German, K., 47
Fetter, R. B., 140
finance committees, 239; recommendation, 240
financial activities: CUPIS–BURP, 374
fixed costs, 114
forecast, 17, 30
forecasting assumptions, 219
forecasting short-term techniques, 50
format, PAS, 342
formatting: and HAS data, 299
forms, specialized, 252
frequency distribution, 35
frequency, of observation, 308
fringe benefits, 212
future demand, 209

Georgopoulos, B. S. and Mann, F. C., 315
geographic boundaries, 70; goal achievement, 167, 209, 250

HAS (Hospital Administrative Services), 207, 284
health care investments, 234
Henry Ford Hospitals, 163
histogram, 56
historic comparisons, 299
historic data, 55
home care, 235; demand for, 100
hospital output, 178; planning committee, 239; production problem, 177; technology matrix, 178; statewide use, 47–49
Hospital Utilization Research Project, 80, 81, 86
Housekeeping CASH checklist, 304
human resources, 250

identifiable costs, 211
idle capacity rates, 250
immediate finance category, 240
implementation, 209
incentive pay schemes, 283
income stream, 216
information: additional in abstract forms, 341; processing by CPHA, 345; uses of, 355
information system: for hospital management, 372, 373
in-hospital production, 211
impatient care: and PAS-MAP, 364
input data, 40, 334 input device: for PAS, 342

input-output coefficient, 178, 192, 200; in Wolfe's model, 203
inspection samples, 319
intangible factors, 224
integer programming, 201
interaction, 380
interest rate, 214, 227, 228; varying, 236
interhospital comparisons, 297
internal rate of return, 218, 223, 239
Internal Report, 285
International Classification of Diseases, 341
intuitive control systems, 247
inventory: control problems, 121-124; model, 214; reorder decision, 369; example of, 262
investigation: and forms, 341
investment decisions, 209, 223
isomers, 182
iterative loop, 11

job satisfaction, 250
Joint Commission on Accreditation of Hospitals, 249, 332
Joint Committee, of AHA, 67
judgment, 22
Johnson, E. A. and Vivaldo, L., 334

Kavet, J., 151
kidney dialysis unit, 236
Klicka, K. S. : quality of care, 331

lead time, 209
least cost alternative, 117
Lee, R. I. and Jones, L. W., 94
Leighton, E. and Headley, P., 376
Lembcke, P. A., 336, 337, 376
Lembcke, P. A. and Myers, R. S., 350
length of stay: in BURP, 377
Length of Stay Package, 349, 361
limitations: of PAS-MAP data, 364
linear approximation, 200
linear equations, 200
linear formats, 176
linearity assumption, 178, 179
linear programming: assumptions of, 201; limitations of, 200; models, 167
linear projection, 24
linear regressions, 26–28
linkage, 58
liquidity, 219, 224
logic: in multivariate analysis, 38
lost time, 169
lot testing, 249
lot samples, 304

MacEachern, M. T., 334, 337
McPherson Community Health Center, 107

make-or-buy decisions, 210
management of care data, 350
management: data, 21; decisions and model difficulties, 287; goal, 210; problems and variations, 257; style of, 281
Management Monitorying Systems Project, 300
manipulation: of information by PAS, 345
manpower, 280
Manpower Input Decision (MID), 301
manual data collection procedures, 90, 91
manual information-gathering systems, 334; limitations, 336
marginal costs, 118
marginal value analysis, 124, 185
mathematical programming models, 167
measurement, 22; difficulties, 41; problems of, 125, 126
Medical Audit Program, 342, 349
Medical Audit Report, 355
medical care process, 8
medical record information: and forms, 338
medical record librarian, 335
memory functions, 370
Michigan Blue Cross, 226
modelling, 113, 177
model precision, 192
monitor components, 246; considerations, 254; elements, 279; function, 3; systems, 316
Monte Carolo Simulation, 146
Morrill, R. and Earickson, R. L., 82-84
most likely: definition of as a category, 173
motivation, 287
multiple regression analysis: computer programs, 46; difficulties of, 44; equation, 41
Multivariate analysis, 37-41
Myers, R. S., 337, 350

National Center for Health Statistics, 47
near-term expenses, 238
need: contrasted with demand, 20, 21; measures of, 99
net cash inflow, 239
net internal rate of return, 224
net present value, 218
noncritical tasks, 173
nonemergency patients, 160
nonexistent services: demand for, 99-110
nonexplicit human systems, 248
nonlinear production relationships, 201
nonlinear programming, 179, 200
nonlinear projection, 24
nonlinear regression, 28-30
nonmonetary benefit projects, 226
nonmonetary considerations, 210, 239

nonnegative numbers, 182
nonnegativity constraints, 182
nonphysician-related information: and manual system, 335
nonprofit organizations, 226
nonquantitive systems, 279
nonrecurring decisions, 369
nonstationary: as a condition, 163
nonsurgical measurement: and forms, 341
normal distribution, 61-62
normal operating experience, 194
nursing care: 253; definition of, 313; estimate, 103; measures of, 314-317; nonclinical aspects, 317
nursing care task values, 205
nursing judgement, 207
nursing quality, 311; instrument, 323-328

objective function, 167, 175, 177; selection of, 195
omission: as a problem, 337
on-line computer use, 371
operating costs, 211-213
operating funds, 225
opportunity costs, 186
optimal mix, 203
optimistic: definition of as a category, 173
optimum patient mix, 177
Organization CUPIS, 373
output: 21; measures, 251; potential, 251; reports, 284; routine and special, 372
outcome: measures of data collecting, 334; in Sheps, 33; statistics and manual systems, 335
overflow, 158
overhead, 211

pacing estimations, 302
Parker, G. E., 337
Partially Computerized Procedural Outcome Measurement System, 337
participative management, 255
PAS (Professional Activity Study), 337; case abstract, 251; input form, 338; data 363; format, 342; input form, 338
PAS-MAP, 252; error signal generation, 346
patient: capacity for, 179; charts and CASH, 325; evaluation team, 104; welfare, 313, 323
pattern of use, 67
Payne, B. C.; Fitzpatrick, T. B. and Riedel, D. C., 377
payroll procedures, 301
patient care: determination, sample size, 107-111; plan, 318
Patient Census: evaluation, 104-107
Patient Condition Checklist, 104, 105

peak load condition, 281
performance, 3, 4, 210; expectation, 246
perinatal care: and input device, 342
PERT (Program Evaluation Review Technique), 168; cost functions, 175
pessimistic: definition of as a category, 174
physical resources, 280
planning, 4
planning region: definition of, 67
Poisson distribution, 59, 60, 136-139, 265, 315
Poland-Lembcke Procedures, 68-75
policy: questions, 382; selection concept, 113
population: definition of, 19; density and functions, 382; general and demand rates, 93, 94; special and demand rates, 94, 95
Population Studies Center, 85
preference matrix, 197
prenatal care, 253
present value calculation, 217; equation, 218
Preston, R. A., 103
primal: as a condition, 184
primary control systems, 245-248
primary diagnosis: and PAS, 346
primary responsibility center, 300
Principles of Accreditation, 333
procedural measures of quality, 333
procurement process, 250
professional activity measures, 251
professionalism, 283
Professional Performance Report, 334
profit, objective function, 195
Program in Hospital Administration, Yale, 374
programming models, 177
programming problems: elements analyzed, 177
progressive patient care hospital, 206
Progressive Patient Care Hospital, Estimating Bed Needs (PPC), 103-107
probabilistic prediction, 17
probability: estimates, 174; limits, 303; low individual, 265-269
problem formulation, 177; procedure, 206
production chores, 369
production coefficients, 177, 178
production possibility frontier, 181
project life: guidelines, 217

quality, 257; and CPHA, 338; demand for and background factors, 7; of performance, 372; problem areas, 332; variation, 364
quality control, 355; systems for, 250, 303; techniques, 346; statistics and interpretation of, 275; statistics and tests of, 272-274
quality scales: in CASH, 375
quantitative approach, 335
quantitative reference signal, 255
quantity of resources, 187
queuing theory, 136; models, 140-146

random access storage file, 365
random demand processes, 249
randomness, 55
ratio-correlated method, 86
realistic objective functions, selection of, 186
records, 250
recurring management decisions, 370
recurring operating expense, 209
recurring process decisions, 369
reference distribution, 298, 299
reference signal, 279
reference statistic, 258
regional comparisons, 356
Regional Medical Program, 365, 374
regression analysis, 240
reject: as a category, 240
relevance index, 75-78; service area, 65
reliability, 252; of subdivision, 192
reports, 346
reporting form, 305
resource allocation, 167, 282; difficulties, 120, 121; measures, 284; problems, 113; procedures, 118-121; and stochistic procedures, 135-140
resource control systems, 280
resources, 4; in Wolfe's model, 203; shortage, 20; supply processes, 249; utilization, 372
response time, 246
retrieval of data, 375
revisions, on abstract forms, 342
risk, 224
Rochester Regional Hospital Council, 337

Sales Management, 85
salvage value, 216
sample size, 308, 319
sampling procedures, 251
Sanders, H. D., 299
scheduling, 369; model, 196; policies and simulation, 153, 154
seasonal indices, 301
secondary service area, 74, 75
selection of sample and inspection, 320
sensitivity analysis, 192, 219, 230, 236, 253; calculation, 193; of simulations, 152
sensor component, 246; considerations, 250
sequential scheduling problems, 168

service: data, 350; quality of, 114–118
service area: definition sampling, 87–90; identification of, 70; population, 65; population calculation, 71–73; population forecast, 85–88
service bureau: concept of, 369
shadow prices, 177, 184, 201
Sheps, M. C., 333
simplex: method, 182; solution, 201
simulations, 136, 164; applications, 152, 153; and facility size problem, 146–153; output, 159; routines, 147–150, 194
skin condition: as indicator of nursing care, 314
slack resources, 182
slack variables, 182, 189, 190
Smalley, H. and Freeman, J., 212
Smith, R. L. and Horn, B. L., 277
software costs, 371
solution space, 177
source of payment, 349
Southwestern Michigan Hospital Council, 337
special training, costs of, 213
spoilage, 213
stability: of demand, 282; of reference population, 298
staffing: increment, 206; process, 282
standards, 254, 281
Stapleton, J. F., and Zwerneman, J. A., 363
stationary demand, 50
stationary Poisson process, 265–269
statistical analysis, 22
statistical deviation, meaning of, 274–276
statistical quality control, 256, 257
statistics, selected, 285
stochastic situation and total value analysis, 126–130
stochastic distributions, 177
stochastic fluctuation, 302
stochastic function, 187
stochastic variation, 209, 281
structural controls, 249
structural measures: of data collecting, 334; and manual systems, 334; of quality, 335
subjective judgement, 305
subjective nonquantitative policies, 208
subjective value system, 196
subprocess control systems, 250
subsampling, 308
subsidiary processes, 210
substitution, 233
subsystem information gathering, 332
sunk cost, 213
super controls, 245, 248, 303, 380; and statistics, 264; and systems, 279
supplies, 280
surgical simulation model, 150–152
surgical treatment: and forms, 341
survey: doctors' intentions, 101; of intentions, 100; personnel attitudes, 250
system: design, 249; hardware, 375

tableau, 189
tasks, in PERT, 168
technical manipulation, 204
technology matrix, 178
Thompson, J. D., 140
Thompson, J. D. and Fetter, R. B., 146
time lag: HAS data, 299
time series, 18–23
total present value, 215
total project time, 169
total service: and demand, 187
total systems, 279
total value analysis, 114–121, 167
transportation: model, 186; solution, 201
treatment: in data, 334
trial solutions, 189–193
trustee representation, 239
turnover, 315

unexpressed demand, 21
University of Iowa, 314
University of Michigan, Bureau of Hospital Administration, 300
urban setting: and service area, 82–85
urgent admissions, 163
use rate forecast, 85, 86
U. S. Public Health Service, 67, 103
utilization: measures of, 285; medical audit report, 355; variables, 378
Utilization Review Screening, 363, 374

validity, 252
variable budget, 300
variable cash flow, 215
variable cost basis, 212
variables measures, 255, 304, 377; analysis of, 258; calculation example, 260
variable staff approach, 205
variation, assumptions of, 37; cyclical, 52; in estimates, 173
variety index, 356
visual scanning, 345

waiting lists, 251
Warner, O. M., 207
weighting, 308; and CASH scale, 316
White, K. L. and Preston, R. A., 101
W. K. Kellogg Foundation, 337
Williams, J. E. and Donaldson, B., 302

Williamson, J. W., 110
work: measurement, 204; sampling, 302; standards, 282
workloads, 211
Wolfe's Nurse Staffing Model, 203
Wolfe, H., 207; task groups, 203

Yale University School of Medicine, 374
Young's Admission Scheduling Mode, 154, 155
Young, J., 158-164

Zimmer, J. G., 103

About the Author

John R. Griffith, Professor of Hospital Administration at The University of Michigan, has been Director of the Program and Bureau of Hospital Administration at that University since 1970. He received a Bachelor of Engineering Science degree from the Johns Hopkins University in 1955 with a major in Industrial Engineering and a Master of Business Administration in Hospital Administration from The University of Chicago in 1957. His career as a researcher, teacher, and practitioner has included special emphasis on the introduction of new methods and programs into hospitals as well as the applications of systems analysis to general hospital management problems.

His research has included studies in the implementation of home care and progressive patient care systems in community hospitals, the development of measures for forecasting need for hospital facilities, and most recently the development and installation of practical scheduling, planning, and control systems for community hospitals. His publications include *Progressive Patient Care, An Anthology*, and *The McPherson Experiment: Expanding Community Hospital Services*, both published by the Bureau of Hospital Administration at The University of Michigan. He was the founding editor of *Abstracts of Hospital Management Studies*, published by the Bureau, and has served on the editorial boards of *Medical Care, Inquiry*, and *Hospital Administration*. He is a Fellow of the American College of Hospital Administrators and the American Public Health Association and a member of the Health Applications Section of the Operations Research Society of America.